A "wake you up" manifesto and plant-based lifestyle plan to buck the system that keeps us fat, sick, and tired—from the Badass Vegan

As John Lewis, aka the Badass Vegan, says, when most people meet him, *vegan* isn't the first word that comes to mind. He's six-foot-six, African American, with the build of a guy who played Division I college basketball. Not bad for someone who hasn't had any animal protein in fifteen years.

Lewis became a plant-based eater when he saw how the conventional American diet was utterly failing his community. As he describes, heart disease, type 2 diabetes, high blood pressure, and chronic pain are killing Black people faster than any gun. The issue of food injustice is huge and complex, but as Lewis tells his strong community of followers, one solution is simple: *Wake up now* and do better in your own life. Want to give the middle finger to the processed-food and pharmaceutical industries that are keeping you fat, sick, and tired? *Go plant-based.*

Badass Vegan offers an irreverent, eye-opening four-part master plan to help readers shift their mindset and enjoy the massive health benefits and pure pleasures of a plant-based lifestyle. Lewis demystifies going vegan and makes it realistic—even if you're intimidated by a whole avocado (Lewis once was, too)—with rock-solid advice on stocking a pantry, getting your nutrients, building strength, shedding excess weight, and ultimately creating sustainable change for a lifetime of health. Complete with 85 recipes for delicious food that'll keep you motivated, from Jack U Up Street Tacos to Cucumber Watermelon Smoothies to Kimchi Nori Maki Rolls, *Badass Vegan* is a timely and profoundly needed manifesto for living a life with a lower risk of disease and making a positive impact on the world.

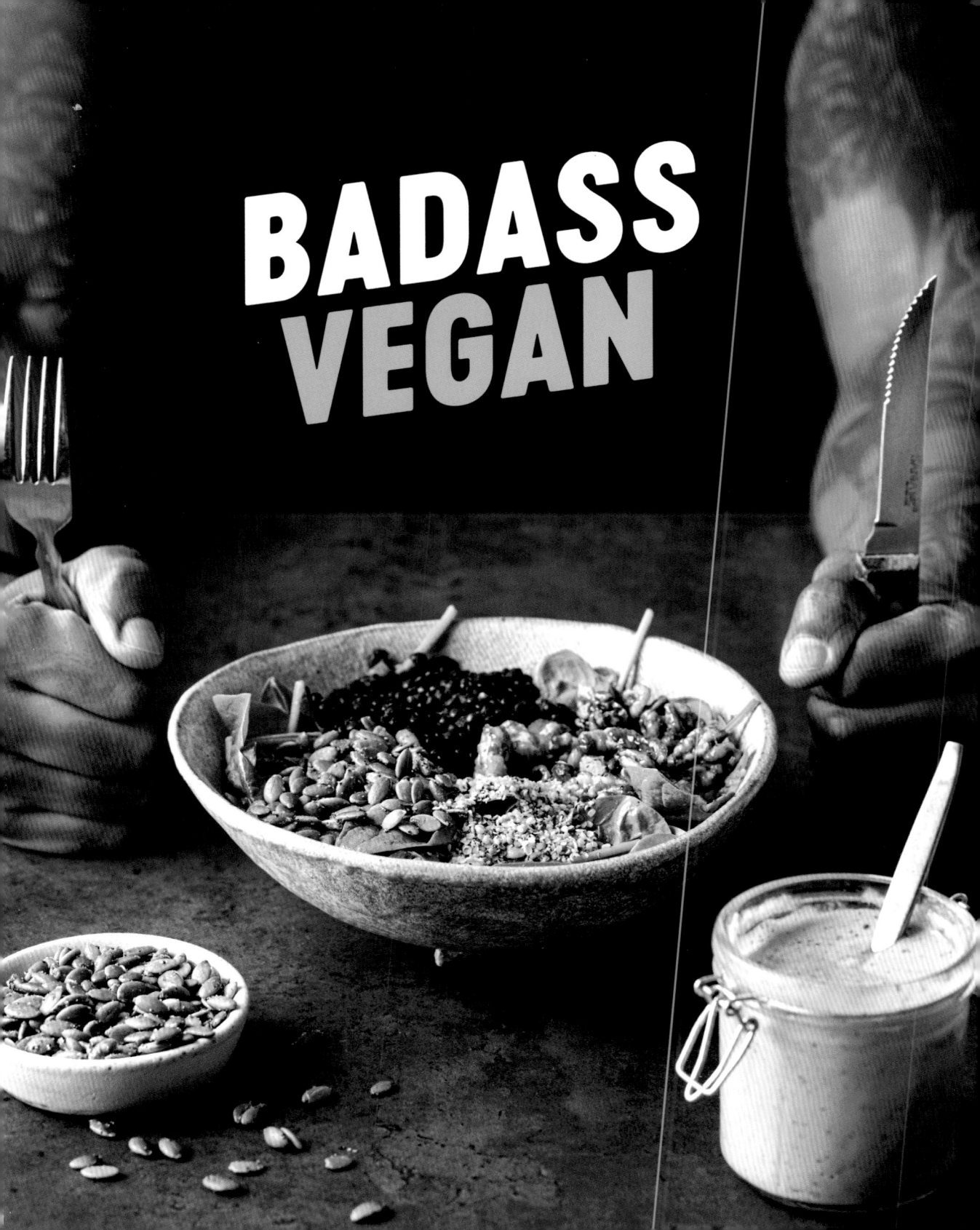

BADASS
VEGAN

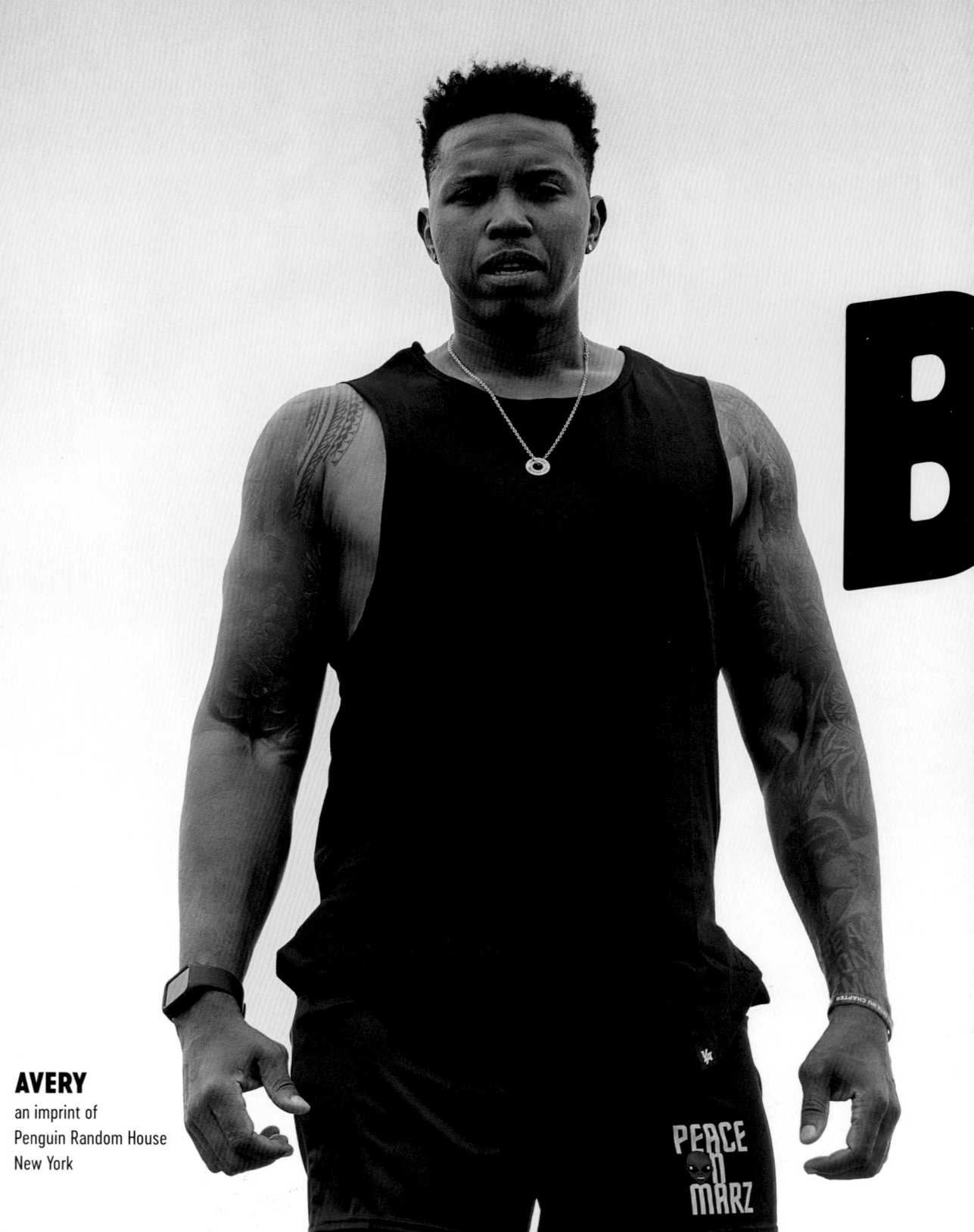

AVERY
an imprint of
Penguin Random House
New York

JOHN LEWIS

ADASS

VEGAN

FUEL YOUR BODY, PH*CK THE SYSTEM, AND **LIVE YOUR LIFE RIGHT**

CREATED WITH Rachel Holtzman

RECIPES IN COLLABORATION WITH Chef Tara Punzone • **FOOD PHOTOGRAPHY BY** Jackie Sobon

LIFESTYLE PHOTOGRAPHY BY Cassie Fuertez, Adam Codeus, and Davy Greenberg

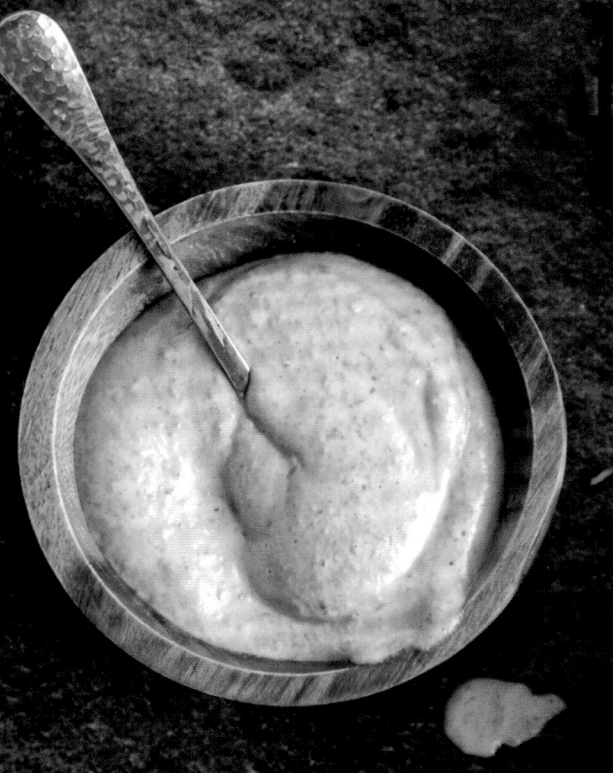

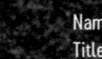

AVERY

an imprint of
Penguin Random House LLC
penguinrandomhouse.com

Photographs by Jackie Sobon, Cassie Fuertez,
Adam Codeus, and Davy Greenberg

Most Avery books are available at special
quantity discounts for bulk purchase for sales
promotions, premiums, fund-raising, and
educational needs. Special books or book
excerpts also can be created to fit specific
needs. For details, write SpecialMarkets@
penguinrandomhouse.com

Library of Congress Cataloging-in-Publication Data

Names: Lewis, John (Fitness expert), author.
Title: Badass vegan: fuel your body, ph*ck the
    system, and live your life right / John Lewis.
Description: New York: Avery, Penguin Random
    House, [2023] | Includes index.
Identifiers: LCCN 2022012159 (print) |
    LCCN 2022012160 (ebook) | ISBN 9780593420737
    (hardcover) | ISBN 9780593420744 (epub)
Subjects: LCSH: Vegetarian cooking. | Vegan cooking.
    | LCGFT: Cookbooks.
Classification: LCC TX837.L369 2022 (print) |
    LCC TX837 (ebook) | DDC 641.5/636—dc23/
    eng/20220714
LC record available at https://lccn.loc.gov/
    2022012159
LC ebook record available at https://lccn.loc.gov/
    2022012160

Printed in China
10 9 8 7 6 5 4 3 2 1

Book design by Ashley Tucker

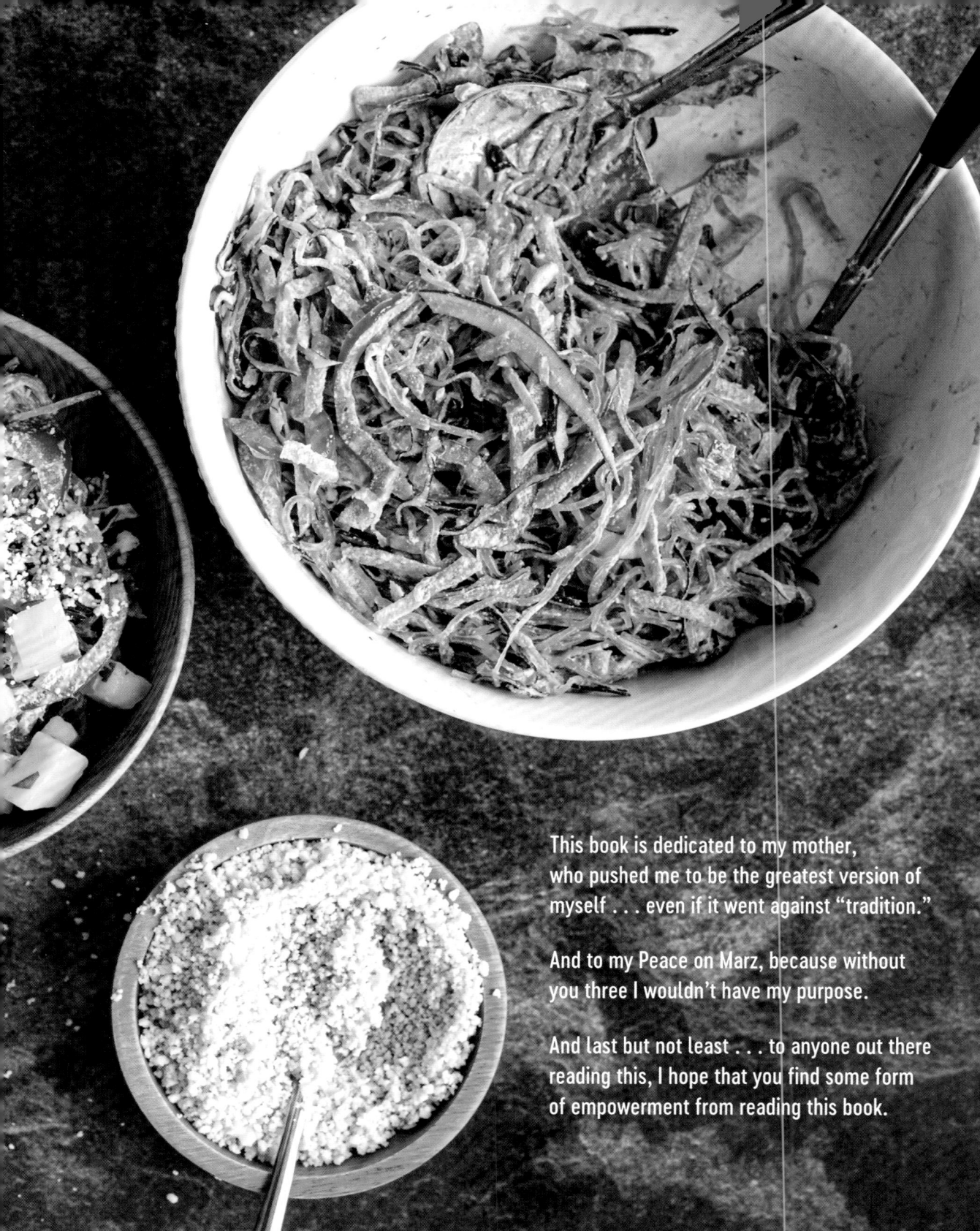

This book is dedicated to my mother,
who pushed me to be the greatest version of
myself . . . even if it went against "tradition."

And to my Peace on Marz, because without
you three I wouldn't have my purpose.

And last but not least . . . to anyone out there
reading this, I hope that you find some form
of empowerment from reading this book.

CONTENTS

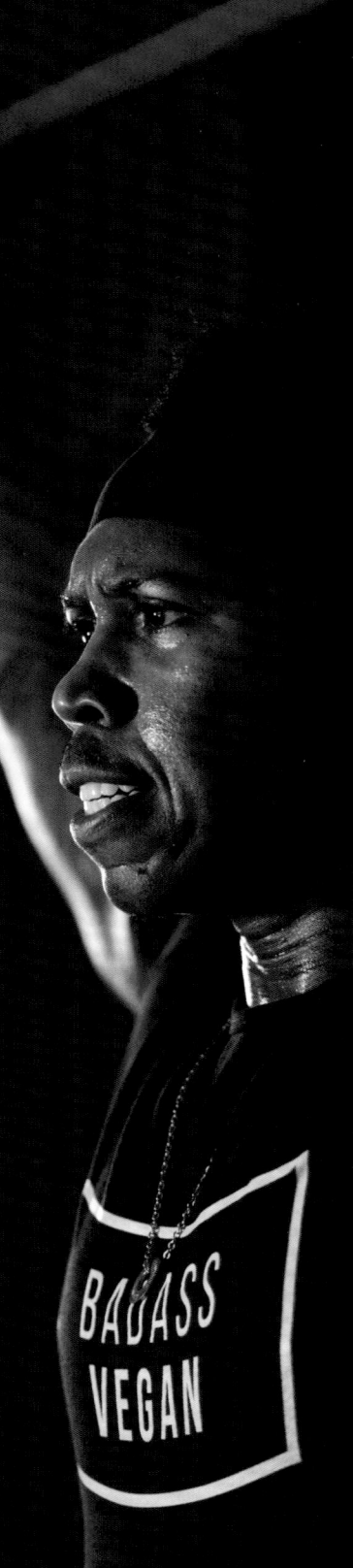

INTRODUCTION:
BECOMING A BADASS VEGAN

When most people meet me, *vegan* isn't the first word that comes to mind. I'm six-foot-six, African American, 240 pounds, and have the build of a guy who played Division I college basketball. Not too bad for a forty-four-year-old who hasn't had any animal protein in fifteen years.

People are also surprised that I'm . . . how should I put it . . . normal? Cool? But I'm just a guy living my life, *enjoying* my life; I just so happen to sometimes hang with other plant-based folks who just so happen to play for the NBA or make chart-topping hip-hop records, and we talk about how powerful eating plants can be on a physical, social, and environmental level. Again, not exactly what people picture when they think about a bunch of vegans. But I'm used to it—I've been surprising people since I gave up meat in grad school and started spreading the word about the benefits, busting stereotypes, and telling it like it is with a healthy side of sarcasm and language your mama probably wouldn't approve of. It's what has earned me the title "Badass Vegan."

What's driven me to get the word out to others is that I want to show people—the committed, the curious, the skeptical, all of them—-that I'm not part of some special class of people who were born with the superpower to have great stamina, endurance, strength, concentration, mood balance, clarity, and good-looking hair and skin. There's nothing exceptional in my

DNA. I was born to a drug-addicted mother and raised by my grandmother, who I now call Mom; I grew up overweight (I was pushing 315 pounds by the time I was thirteen); and I come from the hood, surrounded by the violence of Ferguson, Missouri. But when my IBS got so bad that I (and my grad school roommate) decided I had to do something about it, I followed the advice of a campus doctor who was clearly ahead of his time and initially gave up meat as part of a thirty-day experiment. By day fifteen, I was getting better, and I was sold. Shortly after that, my mother was diagnosed with colon cancer, and I asked the doctor how this could have happened. His answer? It was animal foods, not genetics. I realized that even though I wasn't eating meat per se, so long as I ate things like cheese, eggs, and butter, I was still eating the kinds of animal proteins that would set me up for chronic disease. I gave them all up that day, and I have never looked back. It has made my health better, my ball game better, my entire life better. And the food cravings? They weren't nearly as bad as all the folks saying I was gonna die if I gave up meat.

I am the ordinary guy here to tell you that **THE EXTRAORDINARY CAN BE DONE. YOU CAN CHANGE YOUR LIFE** and leave behind health ailments that bring you down every single day.

As I like to think of it: I am the ordinary guy here to tell you that the extraordinary can be done. You can change your life and leave behind heart disease, type 2 diabetes, high cholesterol, high blood pressure, digestive issues, joint pain, and all the other health ailments that bring you down every single day. You can have the energy and strength to do the things that you love, and the things that you never thought were possible. You can feel like you're riding an emotional high all day, every day. You can have the body, hair, and skin that you've always wanted. And while you're at it, you can give a big Fuck You to the system that keeps you fat, sick, and tired while draining your bank account and making this planet an increasingly dangerous place to live. If that's not badass, I don't know what is.

But nobody's gonna do it for you. Nobody's coming to do the work while you sit back and wait for your life to change. *You* have to make the decision; *you* have to put in the time. But what if you could also make that work easier? What if you could finally have the plan you've been waiting for? That's why I am writing *Badass Vegan*. This book is for anybody who wants to explore a plant-based lifestyle but doesn't want to lose their cool. You don't have to shop in fancy grocery stores. You don't have to spend a lot of money on food. You don't have to buy expensive appliances. You don't have to give up being an athlete. And you definitely, *definitely* don't have to give up good food. Though, you do have to admit that you may have been sleepin' on some of this shit. And that's okay—it's not like I've been a vegan my whole life either. Nobody's perfect.

I'm going to break down how exactly you can find the kind of success I have. (I'll give you a hint: Going plant-based is a lot like starting a new relationship—you gotta keep things exciting and a little sexy.) But first, let's make one thing clear: Being healthy is a *right*, not a hobby. And especially now, we have to fight for that right. Almost half of all Americans have some form of heart disease. Seventy percent are overweight, and by 2050, one in three of us will have diabetes. And in places like Ferguson and the many, many other Fergusons that exist around the country, it's even worse. Black women are 60 percent more likely to die of heart disease than white women. One out of every three Black Americans living with type 2 diabetes ends up needing an amputation. And when it comes to cancer, we have the highest death rate and lowest survival rate of any racial or ethnic group. We've all had that uncle/aunt/cousin/brother/sister who passed away in their forties, and it wasn't from a bullet or a car accident. People hate to admit it, but diet is killing Black people faster than any gun. We've got enough outside forces coming at us; let's not help 'em out.

Regardless of whether you're a person of color, take a step back and look at almost any hospital in the world. Want to know what they're not filled with? Vegans. No one's ODing on plants. Nah—these folks are living longer, reversing their heart disease and diabetes, lowering their cholesterol, avoiding Alzheimer's and dementia, getting less cancer, having fewer strokes, having less pain, and needing fewer surgeries, not to mention having more energy, losing unhealthy weight, gaining muscle, and yeah, having a better sex drive. I always say, "If it involves fresh juice, orgasms, and avocados, I'm probably down."

What about you? Thought so.

HOW TO USE THIS BOOK

I've organized *Badass Vegan* to make it easy and enjoyable for you to make the leap to a plant-based lifestyle. In fact, it looks a lot like my own transition: taking it thirty days at a time, giving myself permission to have fun with it, and not getting hung up on doing things "perfectly." I wasn't a health coach or wellness expert when I gave up meat, and I managed just fine. Though, granted, I did a ton of reading—consulting everything from *The China Study* to the World Health Organization to the CDC—to fill myself up with the knowledge that I needed. And let's just say I got through all the dense, boring research so you don't have to, and I've figured out all kinds of tips and hacks along the way. I always like to say to people: I'm not a scientist; I'm a *realist*. I'm all about what's going to work in real life. So I'm gonna break all this down for you in a way where you're like, *Damn, that makes sense*. Because if it makes sense, you're gonna do it. Here's how it will look:

Step 1: Wake the Fuck Up—Day 1

Before you change a single meal, I want you to first change your *mind*. Clearly you're already at least a little intrigued by what this plant-based thing is all about or you wouldn't have opened this book and made it this far. But now is when I want you to take that curiosity and turn it into burning passion. I can make going plant-based as easy and as fun as it can possibly be, but it's the drive that you bring that's going to create lifelong change. So at this point, I don't care how many veggies you may or may not have in your fridge or what you had for lunch. All I care about right now is that you start to dig deep into what's calling your name and motivating you to make this change. Is it your health? The planet? The animals? The fucked-up system that is purposely keeping you fat and sick so that other people can make money off you? Not sure yet? All good—this section is where I'll spell it all out and give you the dirty little secrets that you were never supposed to find out. By the time you finish reading, you'll be begging me for the broccoli.

Step 2: Getting It On—the First Thirty Days

I said it before: In the beginning, you're gonna want to treat going plant-based like you would a new relationship. Think about it, when you first connect with someone you like, you're getting it on everywhere, all the time. In the library, in the car, daytime, nighttime—you don't care. You're getting to know each other and reaping the benefits. The same goes for your food during these first thirty days. This transitional phase is all about having a good time—all the time—experimenting, figuring out what you like, with no restrictions (except keeping it vegan). I'm not saying get filthy with it, but in addition to trying all the fruits and vegetables, you're also free to have the vegan nachos, vegan burgers, and vegan wings. Or try some of my recipes here, like Jack U Up Street Tacos (page 255), Badass Sweet Potato Soup (page 193), or Pika-Chew Smoothie (page 174). Don't like something? Cool, scratch it off your list. Oh, and no calorie counting, portioning, or worrying about macros (especially if you have no idea what those are yet). But that doesn't mean you aren't going to see results—because you most definitely are, while also discovering that there's a lot more to vegan life than wheatgrass shots and salads with no dressing.

Step 3: Getting into It—the Next Three Months

I like to tell people that they can do anything on a plant-based diet that they could do on a conventional one (except a conventional diet doesn't cure heart disease and reverse diabetes). By that I mean that you can lose, gain, or maintain. Want to slim down? You can do that with plants. Want to gain muscle and bulk up? Same thing. Want to keep things as they are in the weight department once you're starting to feel good? Again, the plants have your back. These next three months are dedicated to adjusting your meal-time approach to meet your goals, one month at a time. You can still eat the foods you've figured out that you love, but now you'll be working them into an even bigger formula.

Step 4: Making It Last

There certainly are a lot of people out there talking about how to become vegan. But where a lot of these "experts" miss the boat is with getting people to *stay* vegan. They aren't talking about what to do when you go to your cousin's cookout and people are eating things like steaks or ribs—the foods you've loved your whole life—or you see a fast-food commercial for something that triggers a craving. Figuring out your why is one very powerful way to do that, and you're already ahead of the game from your first thirty days of becoming a badass vegan. After all, it's a lot harder to take a bite of those ribs when you remember that you'd be letting down yourself, your family, your planet, your community, and the pig, who doesn't have a say in the matter. Pretty heavy shit, but real. The other part of staying vegan is knowing how to surround yourself with good food. By that I mean food for real people with real lives and responsibilities and maybe not the most time in the world. But food that also tastes so damn good.

/////

I wrote this book because I want you to see what you can achieve when you stop telling yourself the same story. I want you to experience the incredible health and success that I've created for myself, and for my followers and readers, and more importantly, to avoid the same mistakes that I initially made. I'm not some kind of wellness guru, and I'm not flawless, but I have a lot of real-life experience, and I'm a good listener. And talker. That's what has set me up to be the best person to open this door for you, show you the way inside, and keep you moving toward all the things you want out of this evolution.

I used to be all up in people's faces about being vegan, and if you weren't, you could go to hell. That's how strongly I felt about it. But then a friend pointed out, *Yeah, that's not working.* I thought I was helping to heal people by being so hard core. But he was right—if people weren't listening, how could I help them? So I started *listening* to the people instead. I started going to where the people are, in their real lives with their real problems and their real obstacles. I realized how hypocritical I had been, putting things out there like it's all or nothing. I used to be a butcher; I've sold drugs; I've done it all. So how could I be judging other people? I'm not here to guilt or shame you into joining me in some mystical vegan world. I'm here at your doorstep, asking how I can help you where you are today. Together, we're going to leave behind past mistakes. We're going to be okay with the fact that maybe we fucked up a little bit before and that's what's gotten us into our current situation. But now look at what we're about to do. You ready for it?

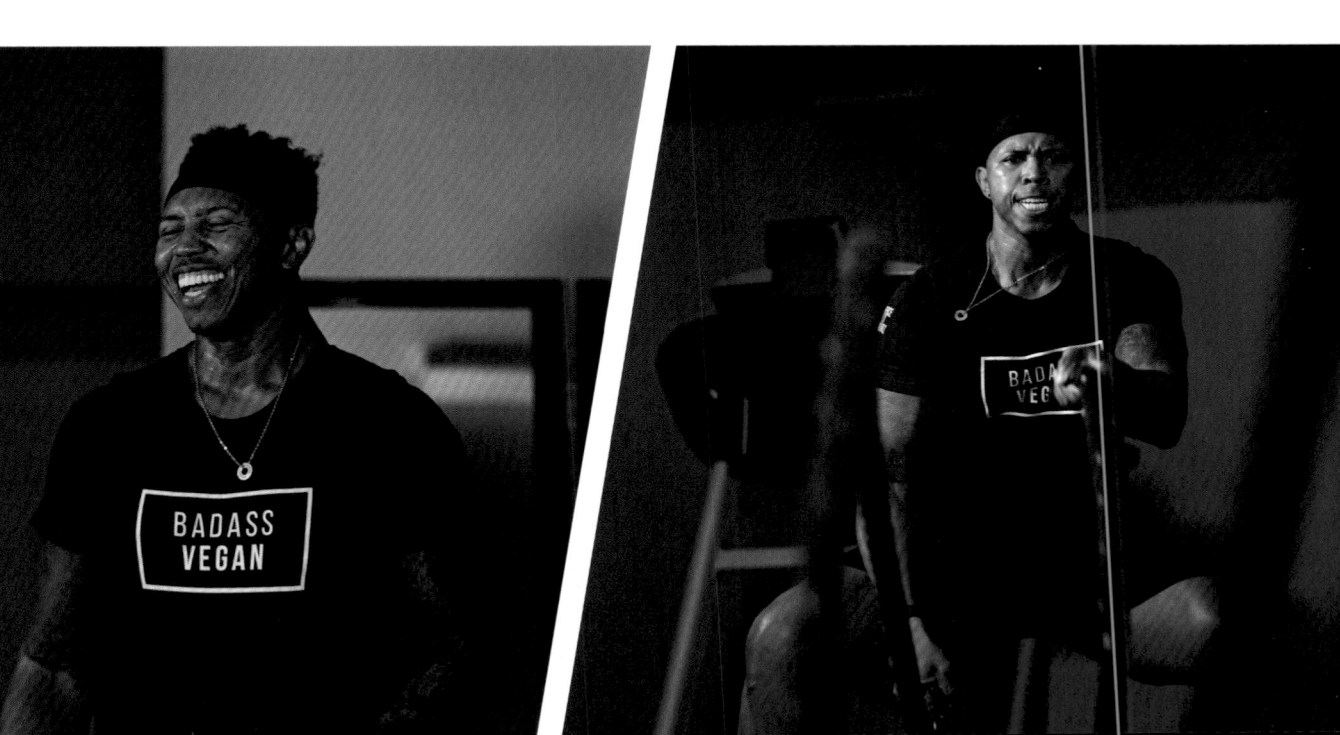

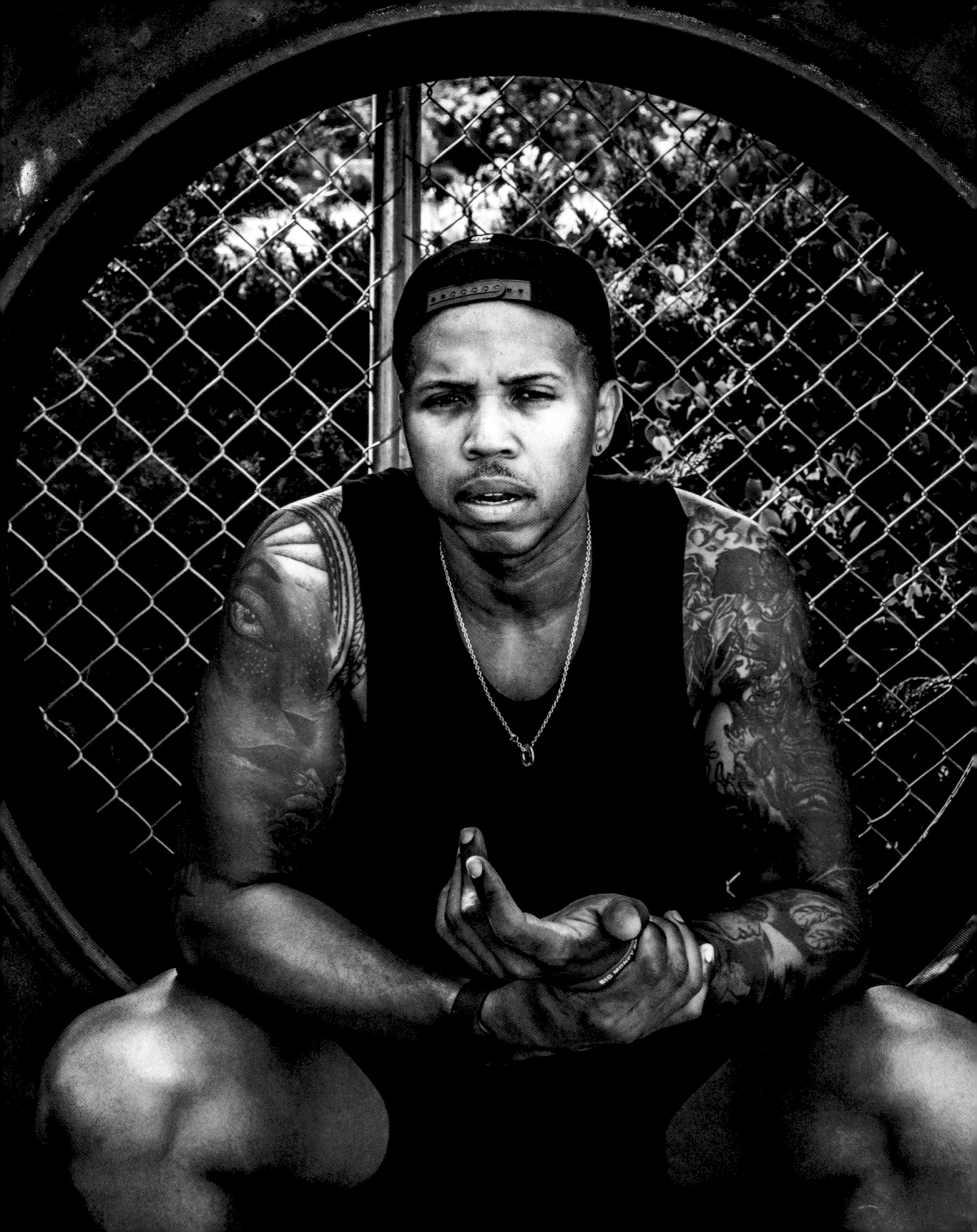

FROM THE BUTCHER TO THE VEGAN

Once I got to high school and began playing basketball with the hope of making it to the NBA (spoiler alert: it didn't happen for me), the 315 pounds I'd been carrying around started turning into muscle. I continued playing basketball through college, and by the time I got to grad school, you could say that I was a pretty solid athlete. But my body was telling another story. In Saint Louis, there wasn't a lot of food to choose from. There was fast food and fast food. My typical day of eating was usually something chicken and something fried. My mom had a Sam's Club card, and our deep freezer would be stocked with huge packages of processed food and the pantry with sugary cereals. So when I moved to Fort Lauderdale for school, there was a culture shock. Suddenly I was trying tons of different foods—Asian, Haitian, Jamaican, Dominican, Cuban. And my stomach was like, *Okay, time out. We can't handle this.* I had digestive issues so bad that my roommate made me go see the doctor on campus. I told him about my "complications," which he diagnosed as IBS. He also asked if I ate a lot of meat. I was like, "No, of course not." But luckily he could see through what I perceived to be not a lot of meat (I was definitely eating meat at every meal), and suggested that I try giving it up for thirty days to see how it felt. I said, "Do you see how big I am? I need my meat!" And I left it at that.

That was early October 2004. But on October 31, my good friend and frat brother from Saint Louis passed away from sickle cell anemia. And out of respect for him and the pain he went through, and out of respect for me and my body, I made a vow then and there to take better care of myself. That meant going vegetarian for thirty days. Before that point, I'd never gone a single day without eating meat. I had worked at a butcher shop in high school, for God's sake. It was a meat market outside Ferguson called Frost Meat, where I'd gotten a job because my best friend at the time, Craig (who, it turns out, is now a vegan too), knew I needed one. I'd been working at Big Al's burgers in the mall (the same Big Al's from the show *Happy Days*), but he convinced me to come prepare meat to order as a butcher: dismembering chickens, preparing ten pounds of pig snout, and everything in between, including mixing the expired ground meat with the fresh to help it get that bright red color again. (That's right; we did that shit, and it is common practice in pretty much all stores nationwide.) I guess it shouldn't come as a surprise that I gave up meat so easily . . .

But back to that moment in the doctor's office. I thought I needed meat to be healthy and strong. And there were rarely vegetables on my plate, or if there were, they were cooked in butter. It was the classic down-south mentality—we think it's made with love, but really, it's just a lot of butter or a ham hock. My buddies also thought I was nuts. These were big, athletic guys and they were coming at me with all the classic myths: *We're put on this earth to eat meat! You're gonna die! There's no way you'll stick with it.* But I was already all in at that point. And you know what? I didn't die. In fact, after just fifteen days, I felt like a million bucks. My training wasn't affected, it didn't change my size or my ability on the court, and the cravings were less of a problem than all the annoying-ass people saying I have to eat meat or I'm going to die.

What worked for me was twofold: I just felt good. Plus, I lost the rest of the extra nonmuscle bulk I was carrying around and put on even more muscle. I figured if I could feel this amazing after fifteen days, then I wanted to see what fifteen more could do. And fifteen more after that. Also, I was real about it. I didn't just go straight to eating only berries and carrot sticks. I was still eating french fries and finding salads on the menu when I went out to eat. But what really rocked me was the real food I discovered. Before I moved to Florida, I'd never had a fresh plantain or a mango. I'd had mango soda, but no real mango whatsoever. But once I had that fresh-ass fruit, I didn't need the soda anymore. It was like an awakening—I could feel healthy and not eat a boring diet.

That said, the real flashbulb didn't go off until two years later, when my mom was diagnosed with colon cancer. I was so confused about how this could happen to her, and when I asked the doctor, do you know what he said? *Too much animal food.* I asked him whether it could have just been hereditary. *No, it's a lifestyle disease,* he said. Up until then, even though I wasn't eating meat, I was still eating things like cheese, milk, and eggs. But after going through this health scare with my mom—and thinking about all the other family members of mine who'd had heart attacks and strokes and who'd had legs amputated from diabetes complications—it prompted me to do more research about the effect these foods also have on your health. Sure enough, I saw that *all* animal foods were at the root of chronic ailments like hypertension, type 2 diabetes, heart disease, and cancer. Now, I'm a big believer in learning from my mistakes. But I'm an even bigger believer in learning from other people's mistakes. If something's not working, you gotta change it up. And it was clear in the findings of these studies: Animal foods were causing diseases, so why the hell would I continue putting them into my body?

I'm not one of those people who needs a month to prepare to do something. No—that day, there and then, I was done with all animal foods. I wasn't looking to start a movement or a company based on these ideas; I was just thinking selfishly about my health and how I didn't want to spend one more day setting myself up for potentially dangerous outcomes. This is one of the reasons why when people ask me, "How do I start?," I say, "Just do it." If someone told you that something was going to make your life better, why would you wait to make your life better? If your doctor told you that you could increase your quality of life, you wouldn't say, "Maybe I'll just start next year," would you? Or say that you'll go vegan and still eat meat sometimes? That's like getting an oil change but putting the old oil back in! For me, it's always been about getting positive about change and getting in control of your own destiny. (Coincidentally, "Creating My Own Destiny" was the first tattoo I ever got.)

Once I made these changes, I felt the difference immediately. I really did feel *that* good. My overall health improved: My pounding headaches stopped completely, and my IBS was gone. I was sleeping better at night. I lost excess body fat and put on *twenty-two pounds* of pure muscle. I didn't feel weighed down and sluggish after I ate. I felt more alive and ready to take on the world. I'll never forget, there was this one time when I was playing basketball and went up for a dunk, and—I'm not kidding—I felt this bolt of energy that traveled up from my big toe, to my arm, to the ball, to the basket. I just went, *Holy shit.* But I couldn't tell anybody on the court because they'd be like, *Dude, you're crazy.* Can you imagine? *Guys, now that I'm a vegan I can feel the energy traveling through my body.* Forget it! But when I called my one friend who was a vegan, she was just like, "I told you."

The more time I spent on my own personal journey, the more I learned about the other aspects of a vegan lifestyle as well—especially the environmental, compassionate, and social justice elements. I grew up seeing the effects of food on my community, how it ravaged our health and left us prisoners of a broken health-care system. I realized that I had been ignorant of the feelings of animals that are a lot smarter and emotionally evolved than I ever knew them to be. And I saw how our current food system is literally poisoning our planet and making us all sick. But you just gotta have that bacon, right?

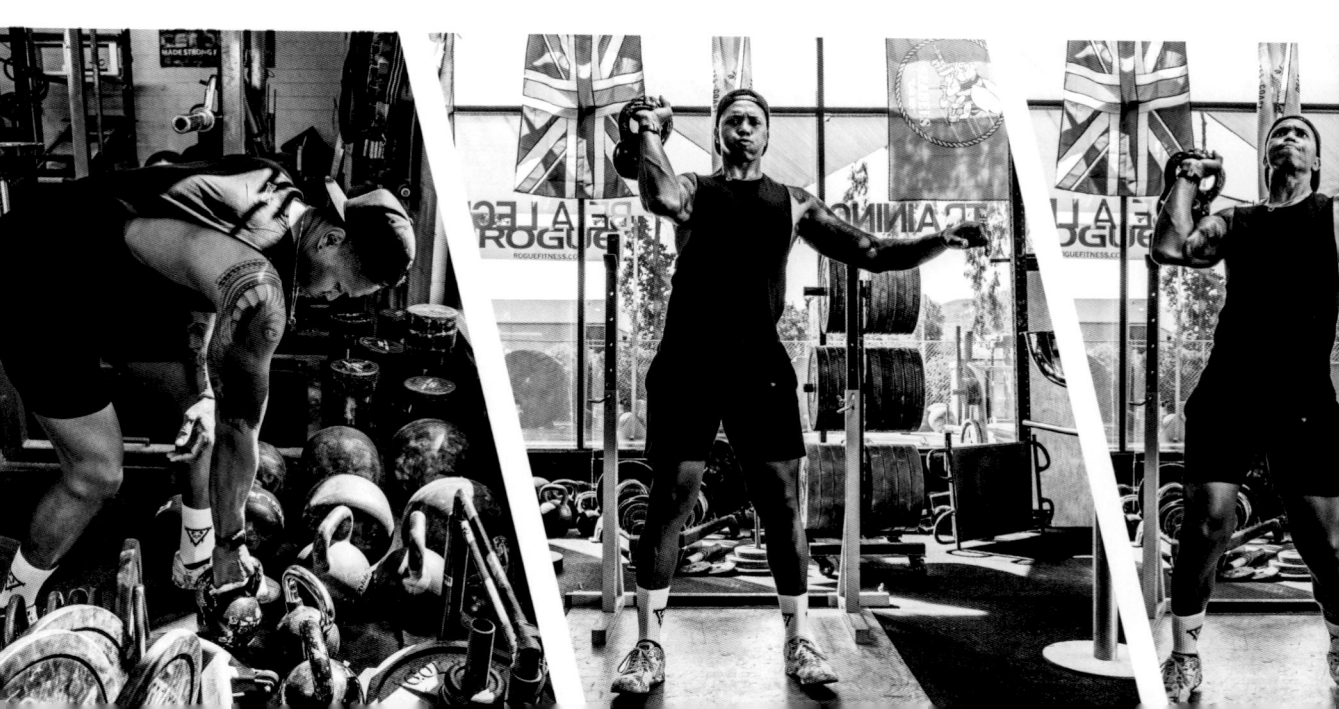

Giving up animal foods became bigger than just me getting healthy. That's when Badass Vegan started to take root—so I could bring in people from all these different paths and give them an online platform where they could relax and not worry about meat being thrown in their face. It began in 2010 with my website and a Facebook group. And eventually, like me, people started realizing that the movement was more than just what brought them there in the first place, whether it was feeling better after giving up animal foods, which they did in the name of saving the planet, or saving the planet in the name of extending compassion and kindness toward animals. The same goes for this book: No matter what path you're on or what matters to you most, the fact remains that when you choose a lifestyle made up of plants and not animals, you're going to be making a much bigger, much more positive impact on this world.

If I Can Do It, You Can Do It

Believe me, I understand that it can be scary to break away from the tradition or norm when it comes to food. But I can also tell you that as an obese kid coming out of Ferguson, Missouri, whose family owns some of the most popular barbecue restaurants in the South, as someone who used to be a

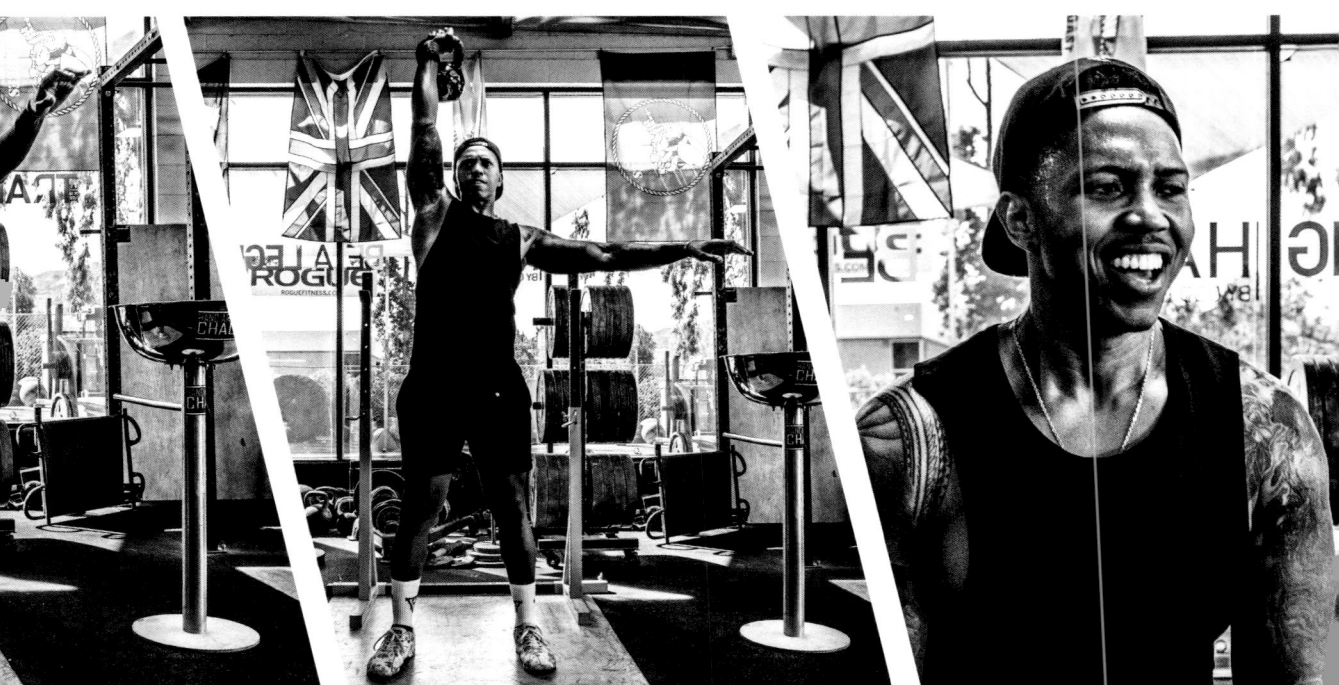

butcher and who was born to a mother addicted to crack cocaine . . . it's not the hardest thing I've done in my life. Those are just a fraction of the challenges I've faced, and changing my diet doesn't rank up there as one of them. I'm not saying that for some kind of bragging rights; I'm telling you so you can understand that I'm not special in any way. I don't have DNA that makes it easier for my body to be vegan. In fact, it's sort of the opposite—if you believe the blood-type diet, which recommends mostly animal foods for a type O negative guy like me, I should have been dead fifteen years ago. If I can do it, so can you.

Maybe you're reading my story and thinking it's bullshit, that there's no way that something as simple as changing my diet could make such a big impact on my health and my life. Well, let me tell you something—the one thing I hear from friends, family, clients, connections on social media, and people I meet while touring is: "I wish I had done this sooner." That's because they're losing weight, putting on muscle, dropping medications they no longer need, dropping diagnoses for chronic conditions they thought they'd have to live with forever, thinking more clearly, and finding more energy and intention.

By comparing going plant-based to life in the hood, I'm not trying to scare you into thinking that what you're about to do is super hard core. While this might feel like a challenge, it might just be one of the easiest things you've ever done in your life. *Especially* if you've faced hardships and survived tests. This, my friend, is not one of those hardships. When you're used to struggling, it's easy to focus on your health and get yourself feeling better because there's nowhere to go but up. Plus, I'm going to make it even easier for you. We're going to get you eating delicious, satisfying, nutritious food that won't have you thinking twice about what you're leaving off your plate. I'm going to make things so simple that you'll be telling everyone how much fun you've been having. And all you have to do? Keep reading.

IT'S NOT OUR DNA, IT'S OUR DIET

For many of you reading this, you've grown up being taught that things like heart disease, hypertension, type 2 diabetes, asthma, and various forms of cancer are your destiny. We're told that they're a "Black thing"—an unavoidable tax that we pay just because we're Black. No, no—it's because you're Black *and you're feeding the disease* with things like animal and processed foods. Yeah, you might be more predisposed to these conditions, but it's not 100 percent fact. Actually, by changing your diet, there's a significant chance that you won't develop any of them. If I told you that there's a 70 percent chance that you'd win a million dollars by following these guidelines, you'd jump on board, right? **THE ONLY WAY TO END GENERATIONAL TRAUMA IS FOR ONE GENERATION TO SAY, "ENOUGH."** Just because your mom/uncle/cousin had diabetes/heart disease/cancer doesn't mean that it's your life sentence.

These diseases aren't always hereditary; the lifestyles that *cause* the diseases, however, are. You can either pass down habits and choices that help the next generation, or ones that hurt them. Personally, I hope you'll make the choice to take another look at our traditions and second-guess whether they're doing us any favors. Too many times we **MISTAKE TRADITION AND WHAT IS "NORMAL" FOR WHAT IS RIGHT**, whether it's the idea that we humans were put on Earth to eat animals or that having turkey on Thanksgiving is the correct thing to do. Just because things have been done a certain way for generations doesn't mean that they're correct. In fact, that's pretty much the definition of insanity—doing something over and over expecting different results. As in, eating the same foods over and over again and expecting them to nourish us or make our lives better, but instead we watch our friends and family buried way too young. Don't think that just because you don't follow your loved ones into the grave that you don't love or respect them. Instead, let's figure out how you can honor your ancestors and loved ones with **BETTER HABITS** and **BETTER CHOICES** that work with your DNA, not against it. Let's pray over tables of food that will heal us, not kill us—you can't pray away poison. It's time to say, "Enough."

PHUCK THE SYSTEM

BREAKING FREE
FROM THE SAD DIET

BEFORE WE EVEN GET INTO WHAT TO EAT on a plant-based diet, we gotta get down to *why* you want to do it in the first place. Is it for your health? (And hell yeah, looking good is included in that!) The good of the planet? To protect the animals? To break free of an oppressive, damaging, and inherently racist system? These are all equally valid "tracks," and **I'LL WALK YOU THROUGH EACH OF THEM** so you can figure out which one(s) speak most to you. Your why can be different from my why, your sister's why, your best friend's why, your neighbor's why. In fact, the more individualized it is to you and your beliefs and experience, the stronger it will be. At the end of the day, that's what will create the most significant, most lasting change, no matter how many tasty smoothie recipes I throw at you. Even if you think you have an idea of why you're ready to stop eating animal foods, don't skip this section. **I GUARANTEE YOU THAT THESE NEXT FEW CHAPTERS WILL OPEN YOUR EYES** even more to the pretty fucked-up damage that these foods are doing to our health, our planet, our fellow creatures, and our quality of life. Take it from me: I was already all in on going plant-based, but after researching the detrimental effects of animal food for my documentary, *They're Trying to Kill Us,* my resolve went to a whole new level. I'm willing to bet that after the first person comes at you wanting to know why you don't eat animals and you hit them with just a fraction of this knowledge that I'm about to give you, you'll never feel self-conscious or anxious about what other people think. In fact, you'll probably find a lot more people who are willing to see the world the way that you do. As far as I'm concerned, there are just two kinds of people: vegans and those folks who haven't been educated yet.

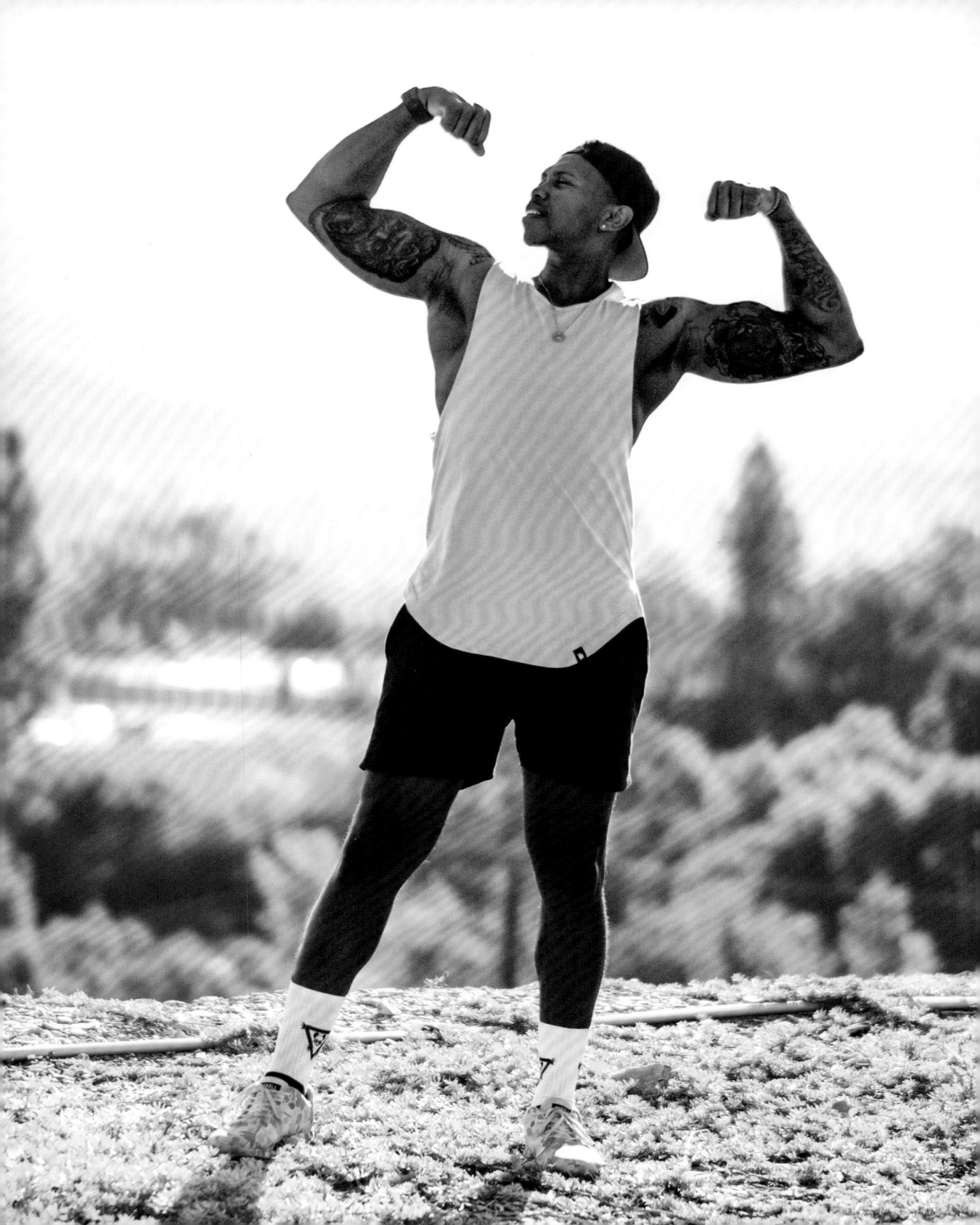

CHAPTER 1

PICK YOUR LANE
Figuring Out Your Why

When people tell me that they're interested in going plant-based, the first question I always ask them is "Why?" I'm not trying to give them a hard time; I'm trying to help them get some clarity so that they have something powerful to reach for when they feel challenged. Going vegan without a why is like hopping in the car for a road trip without any map or plan. Not knowing the final destination of the trip or how to get there, you'd be zigzagging all over the place and maybe even arriving at the wrong destination. Your why is your reason for getting in that car, what keeps you going in the right direction, and what will help you keep going when you do stall out or accidentally take a wrong turn. It's what's going to motivate you and keep you focused. Your why is what you're going to reach for when you're at that barbecue, when you have that urge for foods you used to depend on to make you feel good, when everyone's talking shit about how eating that *one piece* of pizza isn't going to kill you. Your why will be a beacon of light if things ever get a little dark, because, let's be honest, it will happen. If that sounds like bullshit to you, just think about it: Have you ever been in a situation where things aren't going your way and that little voice starts creeping into your mind, that voice going, *What makes you think that you can do this?* It happens to the best of us. But when you know that why, and you have that purpose, then you're a lot less likely to get deterred from your goal.

For me, my why was looking around at the diseases that were plaguing my family and my community and not wanting to be a part of that. When my mother was diagnosed with colon cancer and the doctor told me that it wasn't caused by something hereditary, I decided to be the one to break from the generational trauma at the root of so many chronic ailments. I didn't want to keep loving food that wasn't loving me back, especially because I was overweight and in pain—pain that I didn't realize I was in until I stopped eating animal foods. Now that I'm a dad, my kids have become part of my why. It adds even more fuel to this journey because I know that they're watching me and how I live and enjoy life—and I want to instill in them the same values, and for them to have the same remarkable quality of life. Over time, my why also evolved to include the deadly impact that the meat and dairy industries have on poor communities and people of color, and how the waste pollutes the soil, the water, and the air for anyone living in the vicinity (usually poor people of color). And as I've spent more time visiting animal sanctuaries around the country, I've also come to include in my why that these creatures have valuable lives and are just as entitled to peace as I am.

Your why should be personal. And it doesn't have to be what you think people will want to hear it is. Some vegans go plant-based out of their love for animals. You, on the other hand, might not care that much about what

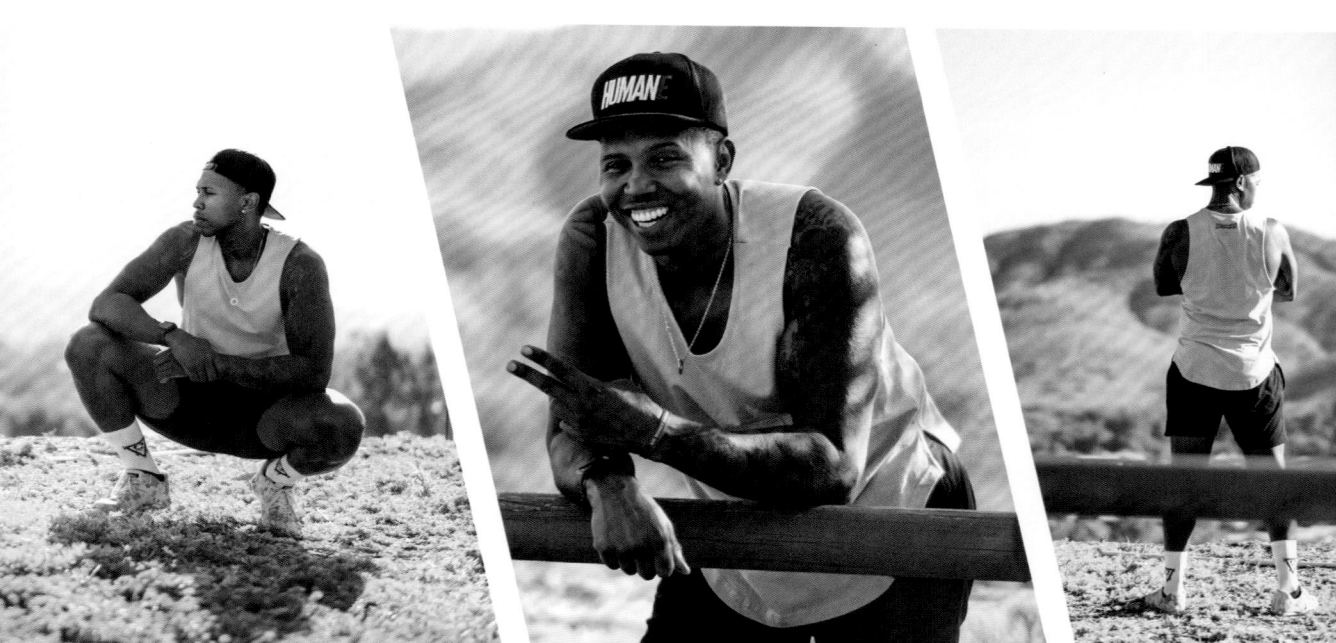

happens to a cow when it's living on an industrial feedlot, but you do know that every dollar you spend on a burger ends up in the paycheck of the folks keeping you, your family, and your community down and out. In these next few chapters, I'm going to lay out all the data-supported reasons you can arm yourself with, whether it's:

○ Preventing or reversing a chronic disease

○ Looking good and feeling better

○ Being more compassionate toward animals

○ Saving our planet

○ Not wanting to keep throwing cash at a broken system that keeps you fat, sick, and tired on purpose

Think of this book as a very large highway—there may be a lot of different lanes, but we're all going to the same place. Pick which lane or lanes feel right to you. If you're here for the health stuff, stick to the health stuff. You don't care about the (poor, defenseless, adorable) animals? Skip that stuff, Choose Your Own Adventure–style. Then, once you find the why or whys that speak most to you, revisit those sections of the book from time to time. Hey, it wouldn't be so ridiculous if you read it every night before bed. Do it until you feel it in your bones that you're ready to do this thing.

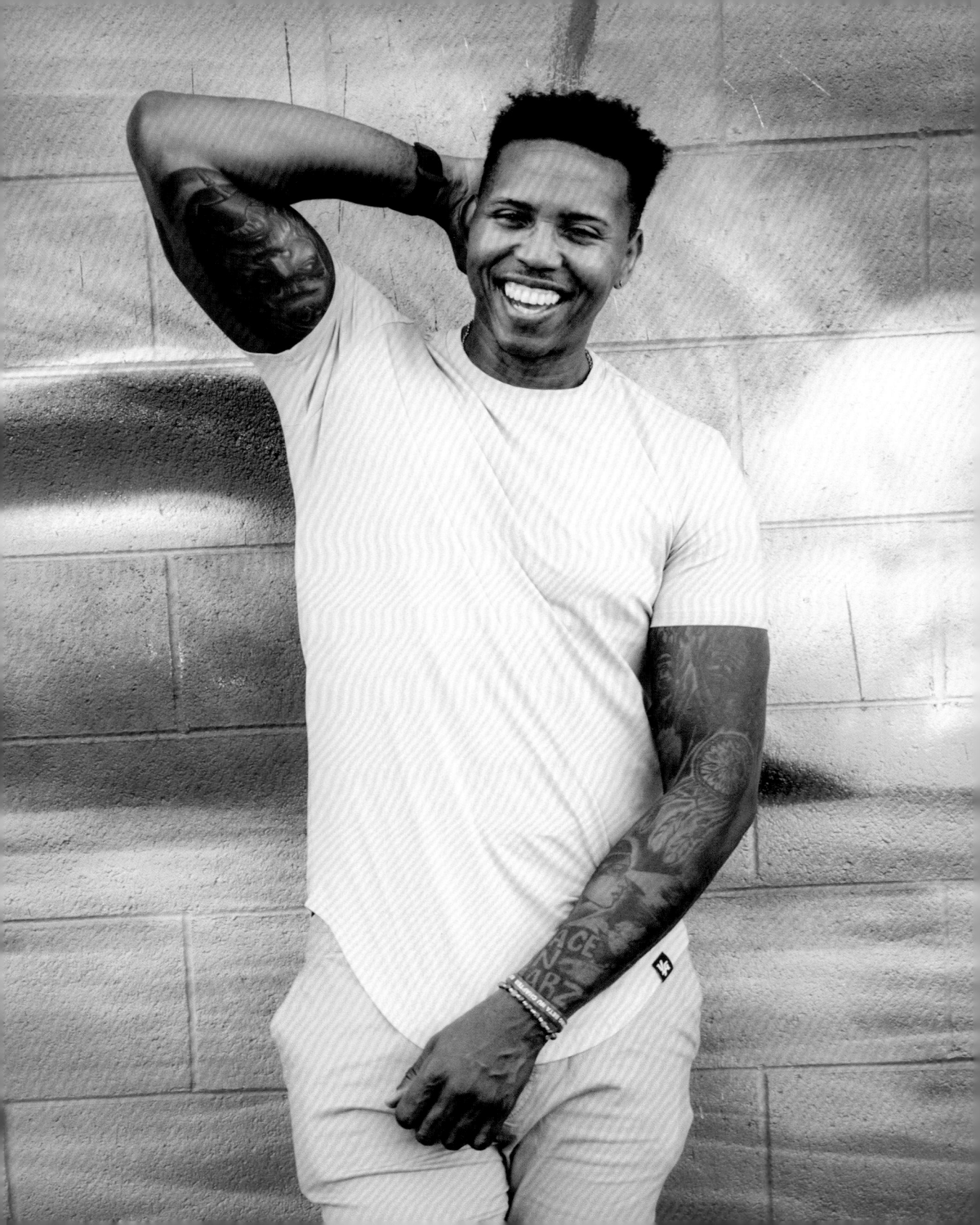

CHAPTER 2

HEALTHY IS THE NEW GANGSTER

One of the most powerful advantages of adopting a plant-based diet is that it completely—and I do mean completely—transforms your health. I used to give a talk called "Vegans Aren't Filling Up Hospitals" because it's true: No one's rushed to the hospital for having a salad that day. There's no "Oh man, what happened?!" "His heart just couldn't take all those leafy greens." No doctor's going to tell you to eat only meat and no plants. They'd be trying to kill you if they did (though, that does happen in this country—but more on that in chapter 5). The key to unlocking truly great health, the kind that's free of chronic disease, aches, pains, excess weight, bad skin, brain fog, emotional turbulence, and hormonal imbalance, is eating plants. I think that's pretty gangster when you compare it to the alternative—a life full of sickness and pain all because you wouldn't cut out the addictions that have been passed down to us, generation after generation (which we'll also get into in chapter 5).

Health definitely doesn't have to be your primary reason for going vegan, but it's a pretty damn compelling one. I mean, if you're gonna go after it in the name of the planet, the animals, or social change, don't you want to stick around long enough to make a difference? And I'm not saying that to be melodramatic; eating an animal-filled diet is one of the best ways to roll the dice on cutting your life short, especially if you're a person of color. Again, we'll be getting into that whole nasty ball of wax where health intersects with race, government, and economics. For now, let's focus on what animal foods are and aren't doing for your body.

Animal Foods: The Silent Assassin

If you thought something like gun violence or a car accident was more likely to take you out than any kind of illness, think again. The *number one* cause of death in America right now is heart disease. Any guesses as to what one of the most common causes of heart disease is? Yep, diet. Heart disease is directly linked to a diet high in animal protein, including meat, milk, and eggs. These foods contain large amounts of dietary cholesterol and saturated fat, which create plaque buildup in your arteries, which then restricts blood flow to your vital organs. That right there is a recipe for congestive heart failure, a heart attack, or a stroke. Or if that doesn't get you right away, it's also the primary underlying cause of erectile dysfunction. (Which for some dudes might be worse than a death sentence.)

Researchers at Harvard found that people who eat red meat three times a week were 10 percent more likely to die an early death, while over in Finland they found that during a twenty-year period, men who ate more animal protein in their diet had a greater risk of early death than men who ate more plant-based protein sources. That makes sense when you consider that *50 percent of all deaths* can be linked to diseases such as heart disease, stroke, cancer, diabetes, chronic kidney disease, nonalcoholic fatty liver disease (NAFLD), and autoimmune and neurodegenerative conditions, such as Alzheimer's—all of which have one thing in common: They're linked to diets containing animal foods.

Did you know that today half the American population is either diabetic or prediabetic? Complications from diabetes lead to things like cardiovascular disease, nerve damage, kidney damage, Alzheimer's disease, hearing and vision impairment, and the loss of limbs. Despite the fact that doctors want you to believe that diabetes is caused by a metformin deficiency, we now know that a diet high in saturated fat is what contributes to insulin resistance, the underlying cause of diabetes. Well, the top two sources of saturated fat are meat and dairy. Eating just one serving of processed meat

ANIMAL FACE KILLAHS

It makes sense that animal foods are one of the most vicious killers in this country when you consider that a diet rich in them is directly linked to:

- Obesity
- Type 2 diabetes
- Hypertension
- High cholesterol
- Organ failure
- Cancer
- Dementia and Alzheimer's
- Neurological disease
- Rheumatoid arthritis

Then there's all the other stuff that won't necessarily kill you but will make your life a whole lot less great:

- Low sperm count
- Erectile dysfunction
- Infertility
- Hormonal imbalance
- Polycystic ovarian syndrome, endometriosis, and painful periods
- Mood turbulence and disorders
- Brain fog
- Eczema, psoriasis, and acne
- Hair loss
- Weight gain
- Low energy
- Muscle aches and joint pain
- Inflammatory bowel diseases such as Crohn's disease and ulcerative colitis

a day increases your risk of developing type 2 diabetes by 51 percent. No other food comes even close to that.

And then there's the big C. The World Health Organization itself has acknowledged that meat (especially beef, pork, lamb) and processed meats (hot dogs, lunch meats) have been linked to the development of certain cancers—specifically colorectal, pancreatic, and prostate. What's even crazier is that this link between meat and cancer is just as strong as the one between smoking and developing lung cancer, to the point where processed meat is now classified as a Group 1 carcinogen. And researchers have also found that drinking dairy milk is associated with a greater risk—up to 80 percent—of breast cancer in women, and that the milk protein casein can stimulate the production and spread of prostate cancer cells. For men with prostate cancer, eating chicken increased the risk of their disease progressing by 400 percent.

Last, but certainly not least, is stress. People who eat meat have higher levels of the stress hormone cortisol in their blood. While cortisol can be beneficial in small doses, it will ravage your body if left unchecked. And one study found that eating meat increases stress hormones *higher than if you lost a spouse*. Consistently having high cortisol levels is a strong predictor of cardiovascular death, as well as a contributor to a depressed immune system, anxiety, depression, digestive issues, and memory impairment. It also messes with your sleep, which is probably the most important thing for your health. Without good rest, you have a dramatically higher risk of developing high blood pressure, diabetes, heart attack, and heart failure or stroke, in addition to obesity, depression, impaired immunity, and lower sex drive.

There's a reason why Dr. Neal Barnard, on behalf of the American Society for Nutrition, advised that both adults and children should avoid consuming animal products if they want to live a longer, healthier life. I mean, as if things like pandemics, gun violence, and natural disasters weren't bad enough—do we really need to add food-related disease to the mix?

Don't Feed the Animals (to Your Body)

One reason why animal foods suck so bad for your health (to be scientific about it) is because they cause *inflammation*. Inflammation is one of those terms that gets thrown around a lot when it comes to your body, so let's break it down.

Basically, inflammation is a tool that your body uses as part of its immune system. In fact, it's technically supposed to help keep you healthy. When your immune system senses outside "invaders" like bacteria or viruses or a splinter in your foot, it unleashes a vicious counterresponse—it's called "fighting off a cold" for a reason! Immune cells are sent to attack what's perceived to be foreign bodies, blowing up anything it doesn't like the look of. Your affected tissues dilate, sending more blood to the area (which is why inflamed areas get red and hot), and immune system hormones purposely irritate the surrounding nerves so that your brain receives a pain signal, which keeps you from using the part of you that's under repair.

While this process is helpful when it comes to keeping the body healthy in the long run, it can take a toll on your body in the short run. Which is why it's meant to be called upon only every once in a while. Just think about how drained and run-down you feel after being sick or getting injured. So you can imagine what would happen if your immune system repeatedly gets "alerts" that it's being attacked and your body is consistently in a state of inflammation. You'd not only have a situation where your body is constantly being bombarded by an aggravated immune system but also be draining your body's energy and resources. That kind of chronic inflammation is when you start running into some real health issues.

You see, your immune system doesn't just get amped when it detects viruses or bacteria, it can also get triggered by *the food you eat*. And I bet you can guess by now which foods consistently cause an inflammatory response? That's right: animal foods like meat, dairy, and eggs. It's no wonder that chronic inflammation is the most significant cause of death in the world today.

Another reason why animal foods don't do right by us is because they're high in sulfur amino acids. A 2020 study published in *The Lancet* found that eating too many foods high in this amino acid—especially eggs, fish, red meat, and chicken—can lead to a higher risk of heart disease, stroke, diabetes, and nonalcoholic fatty liver disease. When the researchers were asked what could reduce these risks, want to know what they said? That's right, a plant-based diet.

DAIRY'S GUILTY TOO

Thanks to very clever marketing by the dairy industry, we've come to believe that milk does a body good. What's more powerful than seeing some of the biggest figures in sports and pop culture with a milk mustache telling us that drinking milk will give us stronger bones? But just like the meat industry and fast-food industry, dairy has a stake in getting you to drink the stuff at any cost.

Historically, dairy isn't native to the United States. It was brought here by the Europeans, who introduced a style of cooking that depended heavily on things like cream and butter—which is not how Indigenous people were eating. By contrast, their food included no dairy. That's most likely because dairy isn't native to the human body. **IT'S THE PERFECTLY DESIGNED FOOD . . . FOR A BABY COW**. And if you aren't a baby cow, then it's not perfectly designed for you. Sure, dairy products are made up of a collection of edible compounds that people can ingest, but **IT'S NO MORE OF A FOOD GROUP FOR US THAN TOBACCO**. You don't need it, and not only that, it's not good for you. A diet that includes dairy is linked to heart disease, stroke, a variety of cancers, and autoimmune disease, as well as a lot of gastrointestinal issues like gas, bloating, and IBS. All the way back in the 1960s, researchers were thinking about lactose intolerance as though it were a disease. They tested a large group of prisoners and found that Native Americans, Black Americans, and Asian Americans have a very high rate of lactose intolerance—which is common in most places in the world. Seventy-five to 80 percent of African Americans are lactose intolerant. That number is closer to 90 percent in Asians and 95 percent in Native Americans. But here we are, still talking about it like it's a small problem. If you're eating something you can't digest, then it's not going to be good for you.

DAIRY HAS ALSO NEVER BEEN SHOWN TO BENEFIT BONE HEALTH. The Nurses' Health Study, which is among the largest investigations into the risk factors for major chronic diseases in women, found that the participants who ingested the most dairy were at the highest risk of hip fracture. Dairy is also the number one source of saturated fat in the American diet, which is a strong risk factor for heart disease. It's also high in estrogen that your body doesn't make, or exogenous estrogen, which attaches to hormone receptors in the body—in the breasts, prostate, ovaries, and uterus—and makes them grow. And finally, dairy is associated with aggravating many inflammatory and allergic conditions, including high blood pressure, diabetes, digestive issues, asthma, eczema, psoriasis, and some cancers.

That's what makes it particularly insidious that government agencies promote and push dairy. There's economic incentive to make kids drink it in schools, people drink it in hospitals, and prisoners drink it in jail. It's also the **CRUELEST INDUSTRY** on the planet, which we'll get into in chapter 4. The bottom line: You don't need dairy in your diet from a nutritional perspective. All nutrients you'd hope to gain from eating it you can get from other sources, namely plants—and with none of the other bullshit.

Plants Do a Body Good

I want you to do something for me: If you've been diagnosed with a chronic disease, if you struggle with an ongoing ailment, even if you just don't feel great, I want you to for one minute let go of any diagnoses or labels you've been given for your health. Instead, think of that diagnosis or label as a *symptom*. When your blood pressure is high, it's not a disease; it's a symptom. Same thing with diabetes, or joint pain, or even weight gain. It's your body saying something's not right here. It's time to do better by that body.

What I'm going to say to you next might sound shocking, and maybe even a little over-the-top, but here it goes: A plant-based diet can prevent or reverse almost every single ailment listed on page 33. I repeat, a plant-based diet will make you look better, feel better, and straight up save your life. Thanks to little to no saturated fat and tons of fiber, vitamins, antioxidants, and other nutrients (all things we'll talk more about in part II), plants are truly nature's miracles when it comes to your health. They're the most cost-effective, low-risk medication you can take to live longer and better.

A plant-based diet can **PREVENT OR REVERSE ALMOST EVERY SINGLE AILMENT** listed on page 33.

Remember when I told you that animal foods were so bad for you because of how they fuck with your circulation and blood pressure and ultimately cause problems for your heart, among other systems in your body? Studies show that a plant-based diet will reduce your blood pressure, which reduces your risk for all those associated conditions. An article published in *JAMA Internal Medicine* looked at the results of thirty-nine studies and concluded that people who gave up meat had lower blood pressure on average than those who didn't. A 2019 study published in the *Journal of the American Heart Association* found that eating a plant-based diet may reduce the risk of developing cardiovascular disease by 16 percent and dying of heart disease by about 31 percent. Another study in the *Journal of the Amer-*

ican Heart Association found that a plant-based diet lowers the risk of death by cardiovascular disease by 19 percent and all causes of mortality by 25 percent.

You can't have this conversation without talking about diabetes, one of the best examples of a condition that has negatively affected so many families, and yet everyone assumes that it's something you can't avoid. Dr. Neal Barnard and his colleagues conducted multiple peer-reviewed and replicated studies (meaning, legit and trustworthy) showing that when people suffering from type 2 diabetes remove animal products from their diet and replace them with whole foods and vegetables, they're able to reverse the disease, become more insulin sensitive, and in many cases, get off insulin altogether. Plants reduce the risk of developing type 2 diabetes by 34 percent, lower your LDL cholesterol levels, and slow the progression of rheumatoid arthritis. Think about that the next time you're with a friend or family member who is suffering from any one of these conditions, or maybe even all three. It doesn't have to be that way. The same thing goes for certain cancers. Plants can slow the growth of some cancers and increase the chances of breast cancer survival.

That's because plants heal us at the place where health really begins. A 2019 review published in *Frontiers in Nutrition* found that diet has the most influence over the makeup of our gut microbiomes and that plant-based diets encourage greater microbial diversity—the key to a healthy gut. A healthy gut contributes to things such as a strong immune system, a healthier heart and brain, improved mood, better sleep, better digestion, and prevention of some cancers, autoimmune diseases, obesity, and type 2 diabetes.

And you can't forget about your brain—because your body doesn't just stop at the neck. Some research has shown that a plant-based diet may slow the progression of Alzheimer's and reduces the risk of cognitive impairment and dementia. Researchers have also found that nonmeat eaters report significantly less negative emotion than omnivores—and not just because they're not sick all the time; but because they experience less neuroinflammation and because plants can boost the happy hormone, serotonin. So that's at least one thing to be happy about . . . not to mention the fact that a cool, clear head is one that can plan better, be better, and succeed better.

Oh, and did I mention the fact that plants make you sexy as hell? Plants make you superfine not only on the inside but on the outside too. Plants help with weight control, treat cellulite, clear up acne, and can slow the physical effects of aging.

It's no wonder that vegans report higher sex drives—which is also thanks to more of that clean, healthy blood pumping to all the right parts. And vegans are also more, shall we say, up for anything. When you take high cholesterol, obesity, diabetes, prostate cancer, inflammation, and hormonal imbalance out of the picture—as a plant-based diet does—then you no longer have the physical underlying causes of impotence.

Do You Even Lift, Bro?

A lot of people are under the (incorrect) impression that a plant-based diet is for skinny folks who have no desire to put on real muscle or excel athletically. But what research shows, what tons of professional athletes have proven, and what I've experienced myself is that a plant-based diet is one of the greatest performance-enhancing drugs there is. Plants increase circulation, oxygenate the blood, calm inflammation, nourish your muscles and organs, and keep your brain sharp—all of which adds up to gains in the gym and on the field, court, mat, what have you.

Thanks to emerging research, we now know for a fact that:

○ Plant-based proteins can build muscle and strength just as well as animal proteins.

○ A vegan diet will not negatively affect endurance or muscle strength. Actually, these qualities might be better in vegans than they are in omnivores.

I can tell you firsthand that once I went plant-based, I didn't shrivel up—the opposite is true. I'm not playing college ball anymore, but I've been doing CrossFit, playing recreational basketball and football, and lifting weights, and let me tell you, I feel just as strong as when I was a twenty-year-old kid (just maybe not as fast). Or don't take it from me, take it from the number of professional elite athletes who manage to win championships and world titles fueled only by plants. Jim Morris, my mentor who passed away, was probably the strongest person at Gold's Gym in Venice Beach—even including folks half his age—and he had been a vegan for almost twenty years. Then you got Tyrann Mathieu, a Heisman Trophy finalist who played for the Kansas City Chiefs and has been nicknamed "the honey badger" for his ruthless no-fucks-given playing style; twenty-three-time Grand Slam singles winner and tennis legend Serena Williams; Colin Kaepernick, the NFL player whose veganism is as much about his activism as it is about his fuel; Torre Washington, a top professional bodybuilder; Cam Awesome, a US title- and Golden Gloves–winning boxer; Olympic skier Seba Johnson; pro surfer and Olympic hopeful Tia Blanco; world champion race car driver Lewis Hamilton; Rich Roll, who is synonymous with endurance athletes and ultramarathoning; Toni Deion Pressley, a defender for the Orlando Pride of the National Women's Soccer League; and vegan bodybuilder Jehina Malik.

And you definitely can't talk about vegan athletes without mentioning Chris Paul, the Western Conference finals champion who is considered one of the highest-level point guards in the NBA. When I interviewed him for my documentary, he said that he almost didn't want to tell people that he went plant-based because he felt like he'd found some kind of cheat code. It was an advantage that he had and his competitors didn't, and he didn't want anyone stealing his edge. But now you know. And if anyone comes at you saying that plant-based athletes are inferior in any way, just show 'em this list (and tell them to STFU).

To view the references cited in this chapter, please visit badassvegan.com/citations.

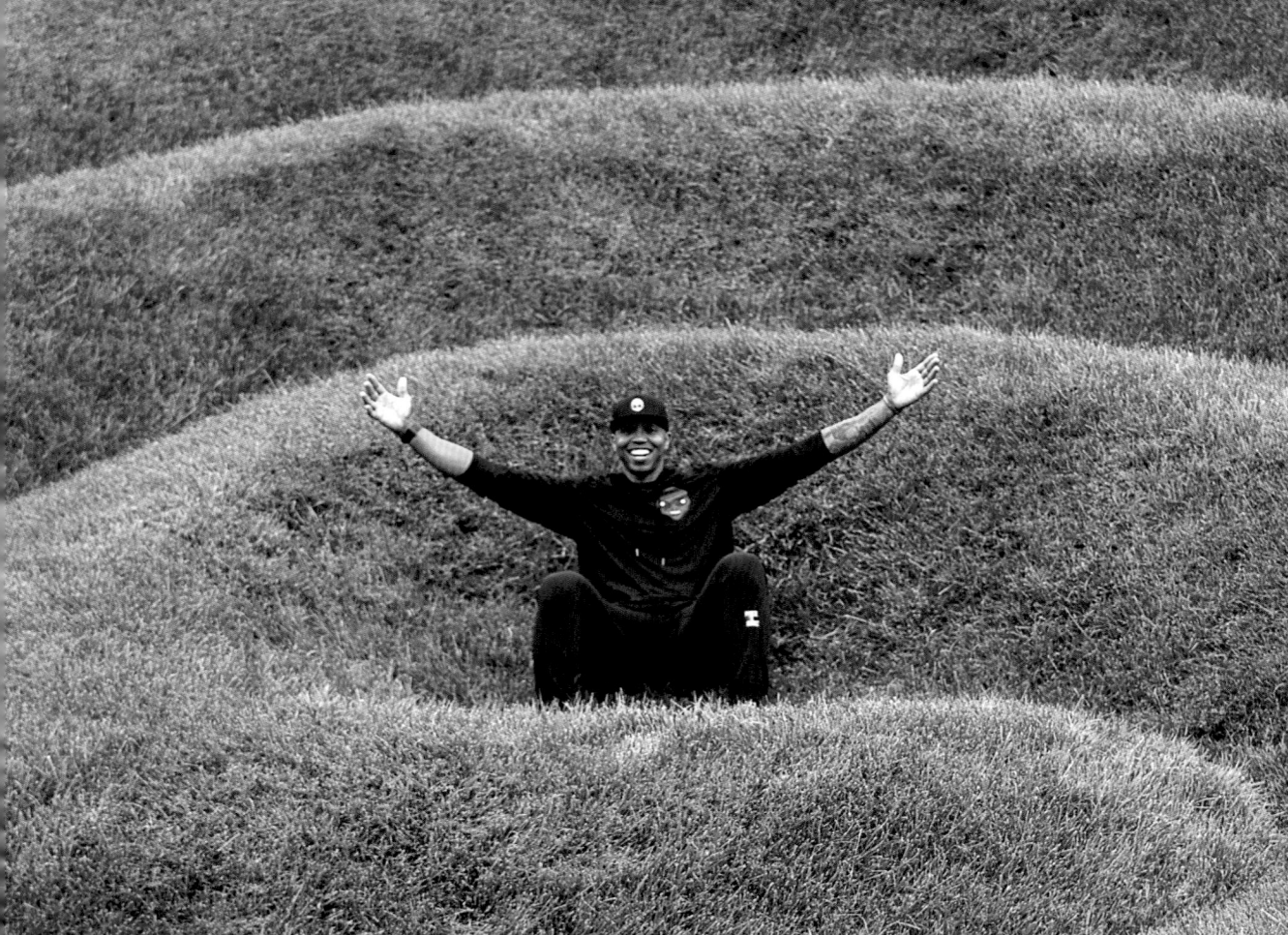

CHAPTER 3

PROTECT YOUR HOME

When we were filming *They're Trying to Kill Us*, my codirector Keegan Kuhn and I wanted to show all the ways the meat industry can affect our lives, especially those in poor communities. There were some things that seemed obvious—in certain communities, only fast food is available, and this cheap food is made with cheap, processed ingredients that are actively making people sick. But what we weren't expecting was how animal farming can affect us even when we aren't eating meat.

We went on a tour of a hog farm in Lillington, North Carolina. As part of showing off his enormous operation—the farmer thought we were there to learn how a hog farm worked—he pointed out one of the enormous lagoons on his property. He told us that the lagoon collects six million gallons of hog waste each year. And there are *three* of them on that farm—enough feces and urine to fill fifteen thousand Olympic swimming pools, the waste equivalent of sixty million people. After all, you raise a lot of pigs, you get a lot of shit—and it's not like there's a big market for pig shit. He explained that they would take that wastewater and hose it over crops, something called a "spray-field system." In addition to that being one of the foulest things I've ever heard, it's also incredibly damaging and potentially dangerous.

You see, it's not as though their fields go on for miles and miles.

Communities border these fields, and as you may have guessed, the people who live there are people of color. And we all know that if it's raining or the wind blows, that shit water is going to run into the soil, into the water, and into the air. Johns Hopkins actually stepped in and did a test in which they swabbed the walls of some of the homes near the hog farm, as well as kitchen surfaces, appliances, and toys. They all came back with fecal matter. Those lagoons aren't just poisoning the ground and the water, they are poisoning the people, too, whether they are breathing that tainted air in, inadvertently getting it into their mouths, or eating the fish who are eating the hog waste. And what's really fucked up? There are more hogs in the state of North Carolina than there are people. Imagine this on the scale of our entire country, let alone our entire planet. We now know that factory-farmed animals in the United States produce forty-four times more waste than humans—virtually none of which is treated.

///

I like to joke with people and say that to be a vegan, you have to be a little bit of a conspiracy theorist—you have to be skeptical of everything and pretty much assume the worst in people when it comes to what the government, Big Pharma, and Big Business are trying to sell you. But in the case of how eating animals negatively affects the environment, you don't need to just believe the conspiracies; you can look at the actual data:

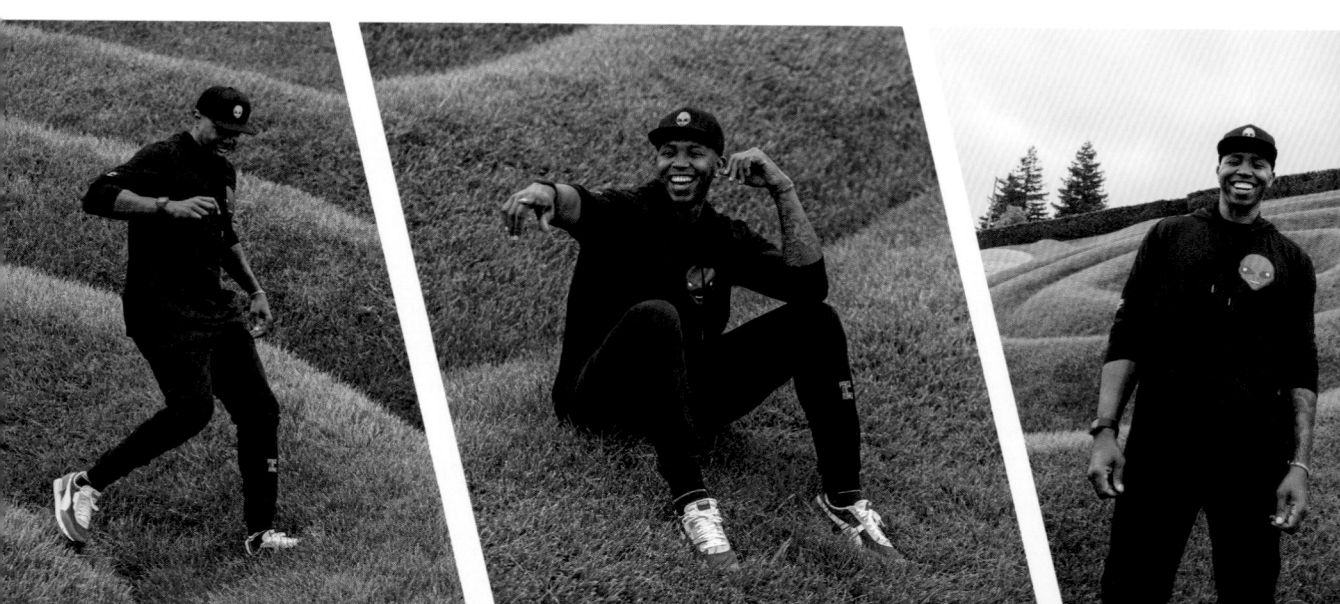

Meat causes climate change.

The industrial meat industry's carbon emissions are roughly the equivalent of all the driving and flying of every car, truck, and plane in the world. This is mainly because farming livestock—and the animals themselves—sends up a ton of carbon dioxide into the atmosphere, plus the fossil fuels burned and emitted just to transport the meat. And then there's the billions of tons of CO_2 that are released into the atmosphere when forests are clear-cut to make room for more farmland. It's expected that by 2030, the industrial meat farming sector will have used up half (49 percent) of the total quantity of greenhouse gases that *all humans worldwide* can emit if we have a chance of hitting the goals outlined by the Paris Agreement.

Meat sucks (up the water).

It takes an overwhelming amount of water to raise livestock—for example, 1,910 gallons per pound of beef to raise a cow from birth to burger, largely because of the feed that it needs. Not to mention the fact that toxic runoff from factory livestock farms seeps into our water table and pollutes all our water sources.

Meat causes deforestation and forest fires.

Right now, the lungs of the planet—the Amazon rain forest—are being clear-cut to make room for raising even more livestock. This isn't just to service the good people of Brazil. No, this is for meat that's distributed globally, including to fast-food chains like Burger King, McDonald's, and KFC. Heard of 'em? (JBS, the largest company in the industrial meat sector, is also estimated to produce around half the annual carbon emissions of fossil fuel heavyweights such as ExxonMobil, Shell, and BP.) In fact, industrial meat is the single biggest cause of deforestation. This is a problem because clearing forests, in Brazil and elsewhere, releases global warming–causing CO_2 into the atmosphere. It also depletes trees, which naturally offset CO_2 emissions. And in some cases, this clear-cutting is done with deliberate slashing and burning, which is a leading cause of forest fires, including the tragic Amazon fire in 2019.

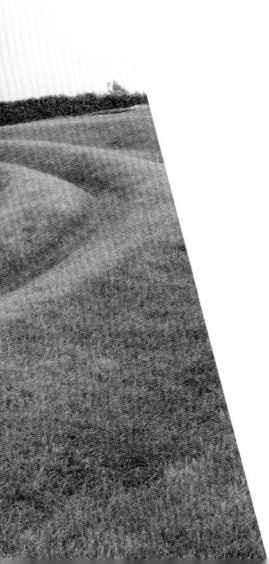

Deforestation is also a major public health issue, which leads me to my next truth bomb:

Meat is increasing the risk of future pandemics.

When natural habitats of wild animals are destroyed (such as through deforestation), it forces those creatures to live closer to one another, as well as to humans. When that happens, there's a greater chance of deadly viruses passing not only between various animal species but also between animals and humans—and it's estimated that three-quarters of new diseases affecting humans come from animals. Factory farms also increase the risk of disease spread between animals and humans because the cramped conditions for the animals are ripe for rapid transmission and these animals tend to have weakened immune systems and are therefore more likely to get sick.

On the other hand, a new report from *The Lancet* found that not eating animals can reduce these effects—surprise! Right now, food production accounts for 30 percent of all greenhouse gas emissions, with animal products making up the vast majority of that. The researchers found that vegan and vegetarian diets were associated with the greatest reduction in greenhouse gas emissions. If everyone cut their animal consumption even by half, our food production would require 37 percent less water overall. Considering that agriculture accounts for about 70 percent of freshwater use, that's a big deal. And if Americans ate more vegetables and less meat, our agriculture would require 42 percent less land, leaving more for the trees and animals.

To view the references cited in this chapter, please visit badassvegan.com/citations.

CHAPTER 4

WE ARE ALL ANIMALS

I was once asked during an interview on CNN: "What if you were on death row (for something you didn't do)—you mean to tell me that you wouldn't ask for a tender, juicy steak?"

My answer: "Why would I want another being to die just because I'm going to die?" The interviewer looked at me, shook his head in agreement, and said, "That actually makes sense."

That's just it: We are all animals. It's not just meat at the end of that fork.

But people try to justify eating animals any way they can. The first thing they say is that we've been doing it for a long time. You know what else we've been doing for a long time? Enslaving people and putting them at a systemic disadvantage. Remember when doctors used to prescribe cigarettes to patients? Or when we just threw trash out the window before we knew littering was bad? Precedent doesn't always make it right.

I say it's 2023, and it's time to call bullshit on killing another sentient being for pleasure. If you wouldn't go hunting and hang your trophy's head on the wall (also fucked up and egotistical), why would you kill another creature for your dinner? The idea that we have a right as humans to eat other animals is a top-of-the-food-chain lie that people have been telling themselves for way too long in order to go with the status quo.

Once someone asked me what the difference between eating plants and animals is in terms of ethical considerations. I told the guy that it's simple: "If it has parents, I don't eat it." He responded by saying, "Well, the tree is technically a fruit's parent." "Okay," I responded, "but I can eat a fruit and plant the seed and get another tree. I can't eat you and put your heart back into your mother and get another you." As you can probably imagine, he didn't have a response to that.

///

Animals are living creatures, just like us. They have thoughts, feelings, and family, and want to enjoy their lives. An animal's life is as important and irreplaceable to them as ours is to us. But as children we are conditioned to view cows, pigs, chickens, sheep, and fish as inferior beings whose reason for existence is to provide us with meat, milk, eggs, and clothing. This way of seeing other species is known as speciesism. It's time for us to change the way we see the other animals with whom we share the planet. We need to stop thinking of them as just resources, and to start viewing them for who they are: individual sentient beings whose lives deserve to be respected and valued.

Scientists who have studied the topic agree that all vertebrate animals—mammals, birds, reptiles, amphibians, and fish—are, to varying degrees,

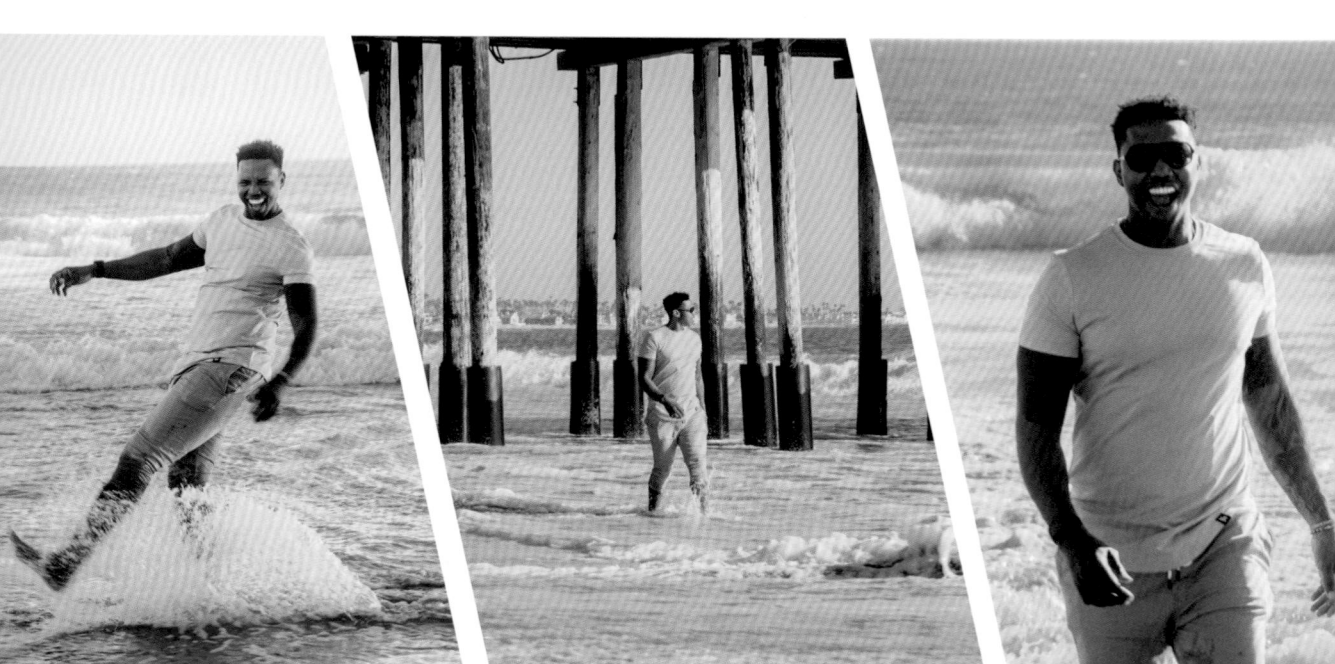

sentient. Many of the animals that we eat are highly intelligent creatures capable of feeling fear and empathy. In a range of studies, rats, pigs, goats, and even honeybees have all been shown to have what's called the pessimism/optimism response (what scientists call "cognitive bias") to uncertain outcomes. That means that these animals have the ability to reflect on their experiences and use them to figure out how to feel about what happens next—not just experience the fleeting emotions of a given moment.

Until recently, most people were unaware that pigs are as smart as dogs. They use tools, understand symbolic language, can be house-trained, wag their tails when happy, control their environment, and are empathetic. Researchers have found that domestic pigs can quickly learn how mirrors work and will use their understanding of reflected images to examine their surroundings and find food—a sign of advanced intelligence shared by dolphins and apes. Other researchers have found that pigs are very good at remembering where food stores are cached and how big each stash is relative to the rest; that they learn to follow other pigs who show signs of knowing where food is; and that they will try to deceive other pigs into not following them once they know the location of the secret stash. Pigs are among the quickest of animals to learn a new routine and can be taught to make word-like sounds on command, herd sheep, close and open cages, and play video games with joysticks. They are also slow to forget—they remember their experiences, good and bad, and modify their behavior accordingly. According to a new paper published recently in the peer-reviewed scientific journal the *International Journal of Comparative Psychology*, pigs perform as well as or better than dogs on some tests of behavioral and cognitive sophistication, and they aren't too far capability-wise from chimpanzees, our closest human relatives, in addition to other primates. And recently, an international team of biologists at the University of Illinois Urbana-Champaign released the first draft sequence of a pig genome, which they concluded is similar to the human genome.

Cows are also more like us than we may realize. They have a unique bonded relationship with their calves—researchers have observed that when listening to recordings of their mothers' vocalizations, calves responded more quickly to the sound, were more likely to walk toward the loudspeaker emitting the noise, and were more likely to call back in response to their own mothers than to calls from other females. And even less intelligent animals like chickens, rats, and mice demonstrate empathy.

You also can't leave fish out of this conversation. Studies indicate that the cognitive abilities of fish often match or exceed other vertebrates, and fish experience pain in a manner similar to the rest of the vertebrates. Fish have been observed to show fear, excitement, anger, pleasure, and anxiety, and their brains produce the same compounds that accompany emotions in mammals. It takes forty-eight hours for fish hormones to return to normal after they've been handled roughly, such as when they are caught by anglers and put into small buckets. In a study led by Robert Elwood at Queen's University Belfast, it was proven that unless a prawn who has had their antenna pinched received a follow-up application of a local anesthetic, they spent more time grooming and rubbing their antenna than unharmed prawns. And just as touch is therapeutic for humans, so, too, with fish. In a study from the University of Lisbon, captive surgeonfish had lower levels of stress hormones when they could sidle up to a mechanical wand that delivered gentle strokes.

///

Now that you realize how these creatures are so much more than the meals they make, consider this: Over fifty-six billion farmed animals are killed every year by humans. (You can go to animalclock.org to see the exact number that have been killed this year to the second.) That doesn't even include fish and other sea creatures whose deaths are so great in number that they're only measured in tons. But what might be even more tragic is how these animals are treated while they're still alive. A majority of them are held in concentrated animal feeding operations (CAFOs), industrial-size livestock operations that house anywhere from hundreds to millions of animals. Pigs, cows, and chickens are often confined for at least forty-five days out of the year in an area without vegetation, either in open feedlots or in windowless buildings confined to boxes or stalls. They're subjected to being separated from their offspring at birth, having tags torn out of their ears, and being left inside without adequate ventilation when it's sweltering outside. Herding dogs that bite monitor the animals, and it isn't uncommon for them to receive an overdose of growth drugs because workers mix it into their feed incorrectly.

In order to get chickens eating and growing, industrial farms restrict their sleep by keeping lights on almost all the time. As they grow, meat chickens become even more crowded together, making sleep even more difficult. And as chickens die, their bodies are sometimes left among the living, making the conditions even more stressful and unhygienic. As for the roughly 330 million egg-laying hens in the US, they're mostly raised in long, windowless sheds containing rows of stacked "battery cages" barely bigger than an 8½ × 11-inch sheet of paper. Living in such unnatural conditions leads to abnormal pecking behavior and cannibalism. Instead of fixing the housing issue, farmers will burn or cut off a portion of the hens' sensitive beaks. Because they're so crowded in there, it's impossible to monitor whether any of the hens are sick, injured, or dead. Since there's no market for male chickens in the egg-laying industry, male chicks are killed at the hatchery. And hens whose egg production drops due to age are also of no value, so they're sent to slaughter—but oftentimes not before proper nutrition is withheld in order to shock the bird's body into a final laying cycle.

Of the 120 million pigs slaughtered for food each year, the vast majority are raised in barren crates or pens without fresh air or sunlight. They live on hard, slatted floors that don't accommodate their natural urge to root. These barren surroundings can cause frustration, which leads to abnormal behavior like tail-biting. Again, instead of fixing the accommodations, the industry has adopted the common practice of cutting off a portion of pigs' tails or their teeth, without painkillers. Most female breeding pigs in the US are confined to a gestation crate barely bigger than their bodies, without enough room to turn around. They're artificially inseminated on a constant cycle, being removed from their stall only to birth their babies, then being sent right back to be inseminated once again until they're sent for slaughter.

Cattle raised for beef are the only farm animals still raised largely outdoors. But they spend the last few months of their lives in feedlots with hundreds of thousands of other cows. Without the pasture their bodies are designed to eat and with a new corn- and soy-based diet meant to rapidly increase their weight, many of these animals suffer from digestive distress and ulcers, in addition to heat stress and respiratory issues from the suboptimal conditions.

In addition to being severely inhumane, CAFOs are also breeding grounds for disease. Animal factories are incentivized to raise as many animals as possible, as quickly as possible, while keeping costs as low as possible, in order to make the most profit. That adds up to overcrowded conditions, poor sanitation, forced rapid weight gain, and compromised animal immune systems—which is a recipe for the spread of disease. In addition to making animals live knee-deep in their own waste, often among the carcasses of their dead friends, industrial farms also rely on the rampant use of animal drugs and feed additives to produce rapid weight gain. This further stresses the animals' bodies and immune systems. That would explain why approximately 80 percent of all medically important antibiotics in the United States are sold for use in animals—a number that is steadily increasing. And that comes at a cost: The overuse of animal drugs has resulted in the spread of drug-resistant bacteria and even more contaminated toxic runoff that infiltrates our water table and harms environmental and human health.

These wretched living conditions also have the epidemiological community concerned. CAFOs are a breeding ground for new strains of diseases, one of which could be the next pandemic. Scientists estimate that more than six out of every ten known infectious diseases can be spread from animals to people, and three out of every four new or emerging infectious diseases in people come from animals. In fact, more than 150 known enteric pathogens may be present in the untreated wastes, with one new enteric pathogen being discovered every year over the past decade. Such pathogens pose a particularly heightened risk to people of color—African Americans were more than three and a half times more likely to die from COVID-19 than white Americans, and the Indigenous communities were hit just as hard. Over half the COVID-related deaths in New Mexico were Native people.

///

If compassion toward animals isn't your thing, consider no longer supporting industrial meat farming operations because of the horrible effects they have on people. Consider that:

○ Workers at slaughterhouses and factory farms are typically immigrants who don't have a legal permit to work and so are very vulnerable. They're paid low wages and are very exposed—they can't speak up against the terrible working conditions and poor treatment. In some slaughterhouses they have to wear diapers because they can't take breaks. They also are more likely to have psychological problems owing to the gruesome nature of their work, and are more likely to be infected with respiratory and immune-compromising illnesses that can then be spread to their entire community.

○ Some meat processing facilities use prisoners as labor. People serving time for nonviolent crimes can be forced to violently kill, dismember, and butcher hundreds of animals every day. African Americans are disproportionately wrongly convicted, charged, and sentenced versus white counterparts for the same crimes. As a result, prisons are filled with people of color who are being forced to work for the system that put them there. It's nothing short of modern-day slavery.

///

Don't you wish there was a way to put an end to all this nastiness? There is a very simple way you can do it: by adopting a vegan lifestyle. By no longer eating animal products, you can personally save up to ninety-five animals a year, and thousands during your lifetime. Plus, where you spend your money is the biggest statement you can make, sending meat producers and legislators the message that their product is undesirable in a language they can understand. Choosing a healthy, varied vegan lifestyle means respecting the lives of animals and refusing to take part in their exploitation. If you have been thinking about it, go for it. You have nothing to lose and everything to gain.

To view the references cited in this chapter, please visit badassvegan.com/citations.

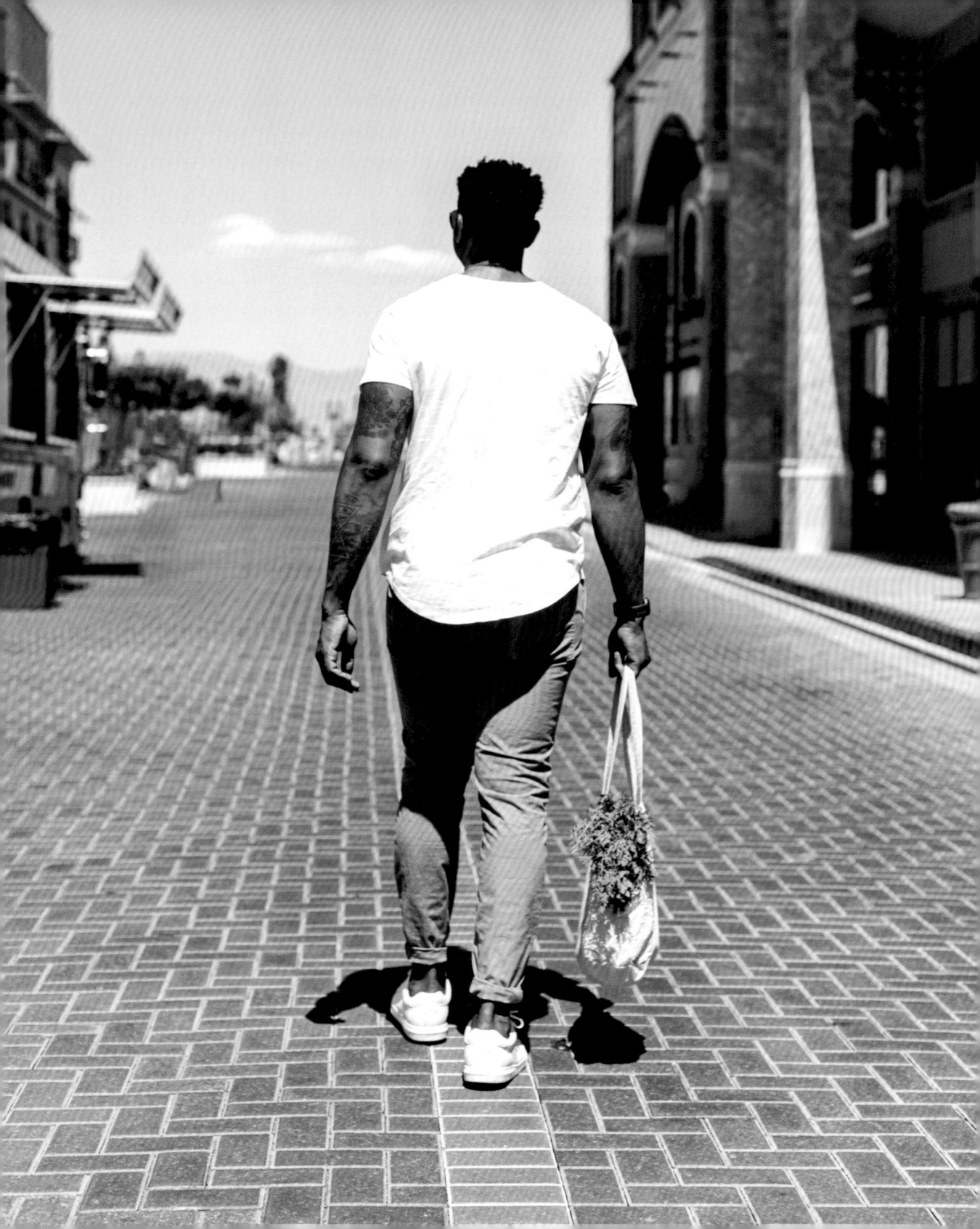

CHAPTER 5

THEY'RE TRYING TO KILL US

Even though I list this as a single lane for choosing to go plant-based, it's actually a combo platter of all the other big whys. It's where health, environmental, financial, compassionate, and social issues meet at one big, complicated, super-messed-up intersection. Because where all these angles meet is where it's clear to see that they're put together by design. And the design is to keep us fat, sick, and tired—especially if you're a Black American, a Native American, or another person of color. But even if you're not, that doesn't mean that these reasons shouldn't motivate you to take another look at how simply by choosing to eat a different way, we can put an end to harmful, even deadly, systems. The game can't stay rigged if everyone learns how to play.

Are You Hungry for Justice?

It's not a coincidence that this is also the name of the documentary I made with Keegan Kuhn, which took a closer look at the relationship between structural racism and chronic disease. The truth is, people—mostly Black and brown people—are dying at higher rates than any other population from preventable disease. At the height of the crack epidemic, there were close to fourteen thousand crack and cocaine overdose-related deaths in the US every year. That's not even *one-fortieth* of the deaths from heart disease in the Black community. Heart disease also kills way more people than inner city violence, or even police brutality. Poor diet is killing more brothers than pistols, and it's not an accident. What we're looking at here is *diet* brutality.

Many of the chronic diseases that used to be associated with older people, such as hypertension, high cholesterol, cardiac disease, and diabetes, are now manifesting in millennials. And the more the numbers go up of how many people are affected, the more it's clear that a disproportionate number of Black Americans are among them:

○ Almost half of all African Americans have cardiovascular disease, and close to one in five have diabetes. Black Americans are 30 percent more likely to die from heart disease than white Americans, 40 percent more likely to die from stroke, twice as likely to die from diabetes, and twice as likely to die of stomach cancer.

○ African American men are also 60 percent more likely to end up with prostate cancer than white men, and when they do, they're more likely to develop a more aggressive and deadly form of the disease and are twice as likely to die from it.

○ A 2017 study in *JAMA* showed that a poor diet high in sodium, sugar-sweetened beverages, and meat is responsible for half the deaths from stroke, diabetes, and heart disease. What also emerged from the study is that among Blacks and Latinos, the preventable deaths due to those ailments were even higher as it relates to poor diet.

○ African Americans are twice as likely to end up blind or visually impaired as a result of complications from diabetes, 2.3 times more likely to lose a lower limb, and 3.5 times more likely to end up on dialysis than whites.

○ Johns Hopkins compared two communities in Baltimore, one affluent and white and the other poor and Black. There was a *twenty-year life expectancy difference.*

Why are Black folks dying from these diseases at such high rates? Do they have a genetic susceptibility to certain diseases? No. What these causes of death all have in common is that diet is driving the disease and preying on our vulnerabilities.

Most of the heart disease, cancer, diabetes, stroke, high blood pressure, IBS, and autoimmune problems like lupus and rheumatoid arthritis are direct outgrowths of the way that people eat. Nearly half of all deaths from heart disease, stroke, and diabetes are directly attributable to a poor diet—not genes, not family history, not a sedentary lifestyle, and not smoking.

We know that there's a diet that can prevent or reverse heart disease, diabetes, and some cancers; save millions of lives every year; and make life better for millions more. So, shouldn't that be the default diet? It's obviously not. And there are a few powerful reasons why.

The first reason is generational trauma.

Black people are trying to preserve some of their culture by eating soul food. But soul food is from slavery. Enslaved people were forced to eat their captors' scraps. While the masters ate "high on the hog," enslaved people got the pig skin, pig's feet, intestines, bones, snout, and lard, plus chicken necks, feet, and gizzards. These foods, along with the few vegetables that they could cultivate in their gardens, became the foundation of soul food. And today, if you show up to just about any cookout or holiday meal, you still see the vestiges of slavery on our plates—the fried chicken, the chitlins, the greens boiled with ham bones. These foods are woven into our traditions—we even named it soul food because it became a way of showing love to our families when there wasn't a whole lot of happiness to go around. We took our great-grandmother and -grandfather's scraps and made them a delicacy; we pray over this food. And yet it's the very reason why we'll always have a relative who has died of heart disease or that uncle with the amputated leg who never leaves his room. Not to mention negative effects on our own health. If you eat how your mama ate, then you're gonna have the same diseases that your mama had.

By contrast, let's look at the traditional diet in West Africa, where the slave trade originated. They had agrarian communities and diets built

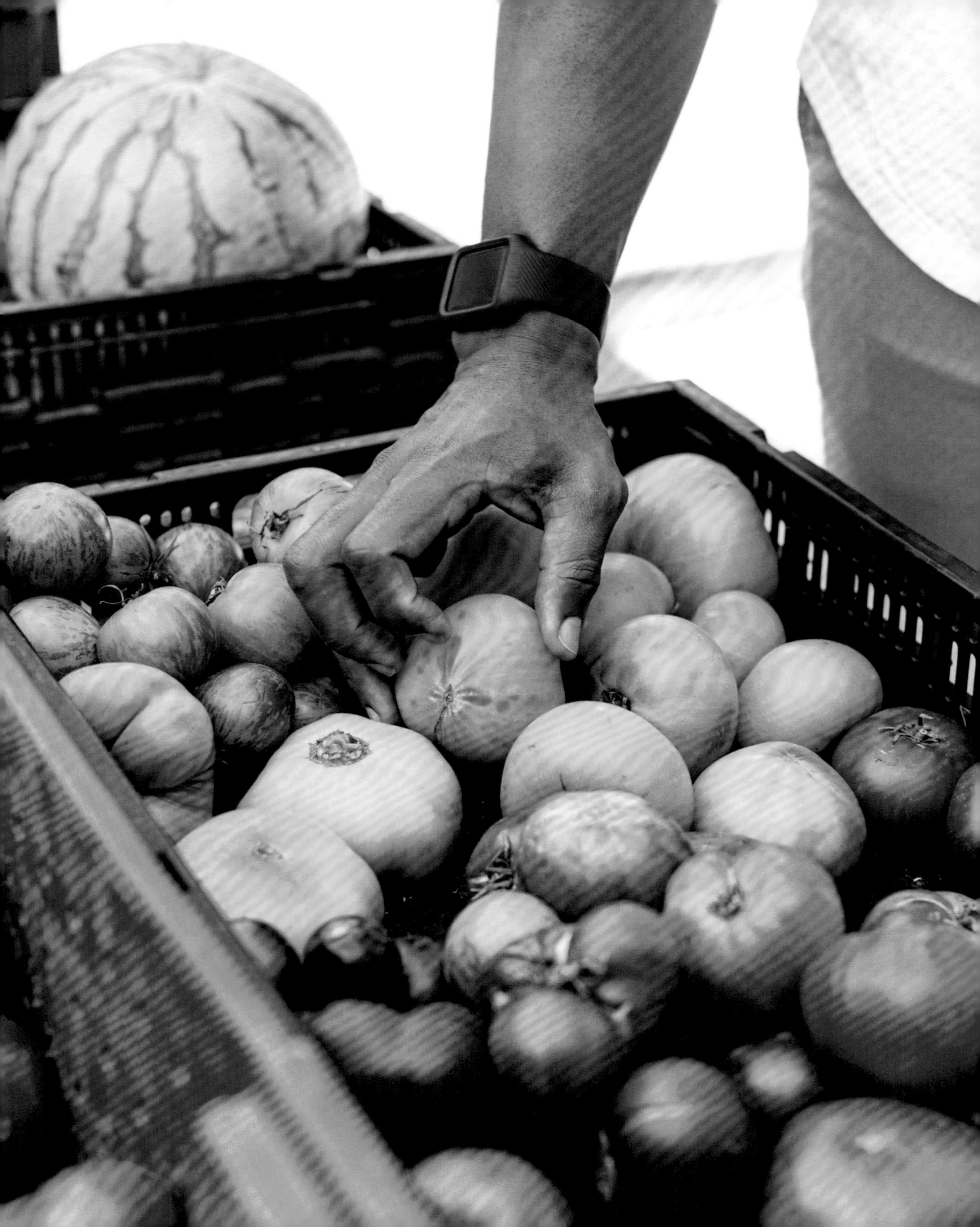

around whole foods, whole grains, no dairy, and very little animal food. If they did eat meat, it wasn't all the time, every day, all day long. A study conducted by the University of Pittsburgh showed that when Black Americans adopted a more traditional African diet, which was high in fiber, fruits, and vegetables, low in fat, and with little to no meat, after only two weeks they started to produce more anticancer molecules that are proven to protect against colon cancer in particular. In the same study, when Black Africans switched from their traditional foods to an American diet, their bodies created cancerous microbiota. We've also seen that African Americans suffer more than double the rates of hypertension than in West Africa. And as the Western diet starts to pervade Africa, hypertension goes with it. It's clear: Our higher rate of disease isn't due to genetic factors that we brought over from Africa. It's the food.

Our higher rate of disease isn't due to genetic factors that we brought over from Africa. IT'S THE FOOD.

The second reason why it's beneficial for folks of color to continue eating food that kills them shouldn't really come as a surprise. It's power.

One of the primary means that the government has used to control minority populations is to place them in positions of food insecurity. Because if you can control a person's access to food, you can control the person. What did our government do when it wanted to control the Native Americans? Run the First Nations off their fertile land. They deliberately burned and destroyed the crops. Then they deliberately moved them onto land that was infertile, arid, and impossible to cultivate. They starved them out and made them dependent on the government for their food. In turn, they were provided with white rice, white flour, canned meat, sugar, and alcohol—all things we know are associated with chronic disease. Generations later, almost 245 years later to be exact, that food is still at the center of the table, wiping out more and more Native people with preventable lifestyle diseases. Tell me that's not part of the plan to annihilate Native Americans.

If you can control a person's access to food, you can CONTROL THE PERSON.

The same thing happened to African Americans. They were dragged out of West Africa, locked into slave labor camps—or plantations—and fed the garbage that has now become part of our damaging food traditions. And we're still being told what to eat, this time in the form of food deserts. Food deserts describe areas that lack access to fresh food. Want to see an example? Drive through any poor, predominantly Black neighborhood. Do you see Whole Foods, Trader Joe's, and Aldi competing for customers? Or do you see McDonald's, Burger King, and Taco Bell? When adjusted for income, Black and brown communities have less access to food than their poor white counterparts. And in affluent white communities, that problem is nonexistent.

When adjusted for income, Black and brown communities have **LESS ACCESS** to food than their poor white counterparts. And in affluent white communities, that problem is nonexistent.

And while food deserts in urban African American communities are terrible, they pale in comparison to what Indigenous people face. The Navajo Nation, an area the size of West Virginia, has only ten official grocery stores for the entire population. The rest are convenience stores that carry only packaged junk food. It shouldn't surprise you then that the three top killers of the Navajo people are diet related. The latest statistics show that 30 to 35 percent of the population has type 2 diabetes, including young people and children.

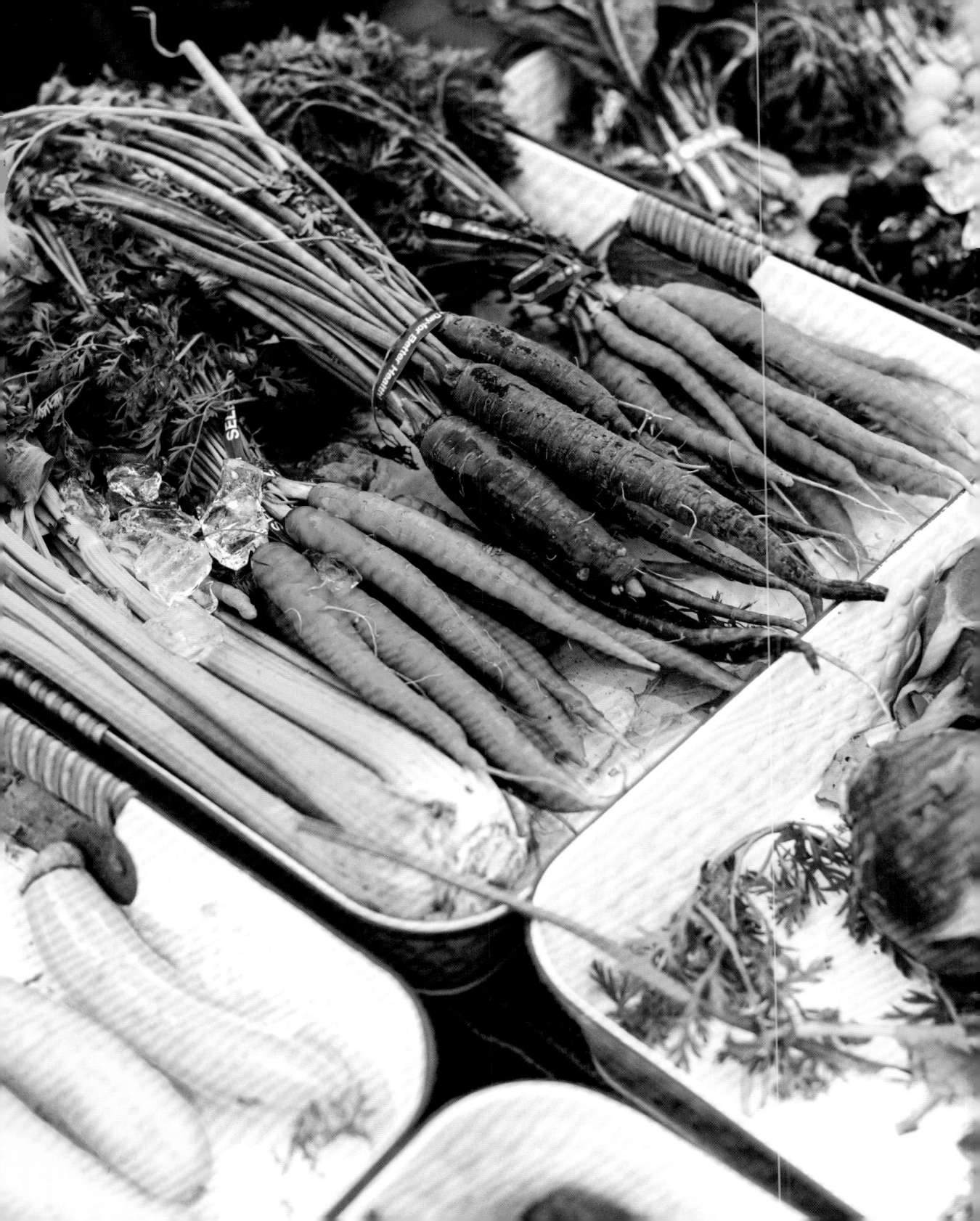

Isn't that just because these people are poor, so they need cheap food?

Okay, I see where you're coming from—after all, if you live in poverty, you have to make your money stretch, and that Dollar Menu is definitely one way to do it. But why is fast food so cheap?

Is there really no money in these neighborhoods, where fast-food restaurants and liquor stores are actually thriving?

Let's follow the money. To say that there's no economic activity in these poor neighborhoods is an excuse that's clouding the real argument. All those fast-food places and liquor stores *are* making money. So, if the reason for not giving these communities access to fresh food isn't the cash, there must be something else: what's being allowed into the neighborhood. City councils and planning commissioners will often permit more liquor stores in communities of color than they do in white communities. And not only are there fewer grocery stores, but some chains actively prevent other grocery stores from opening after they've left, including clauses in their leases that a similar business can't operate in that space for ten to twenty years. They do this in order to protect themselves from a potential competitor moving in and driving business away from their new location, even if it's no longer in that same neighborhood. What they're not concerned about is that they're robbing that community of food. Then there are other systemic limitations to getting fresh food, such as the bag limit that many cities have on public transportation. In these places, a bus or a train is the only way many people can get to the store, but if they can bring only two bags back, that affects what they're going to buy and whether it's worth it to go in the first place.

The money also leads to the issue of why fast food is cheap. That's not an accident; hamburgers aren't magically inexpensive. No, the price of fast food stays low because of federal subsidies—the government essentially pays to keep the meat and dairy industries in business; keeping feed for cows, pigs, and chickens cheap and profit margins wide. These industries receive *$38 billion* a year to prop them up and keep unhealthy food costing less. *That's more than the entire spending for all Section 8 housing vouchers.* That's the real welfare issue. The truth is, the industrial animal farms couldn't survive without taxpayer subsidies because of how unsustainable their business practices are. They use huge amounts of electricity and fuel, not to mention millions of gallons of water to attempt to hose things down. If you took government welfare away from the meat and dairy industries, a four-dollar Big Mac would cost eleven dollars.

If the reason for not giving these communities access to fresh food isn't the CASH, there must be something else: what's being allowed into the neighborhood.

Why is the government doling out cash to an industry that we all know is at the root of epidemic chronic disease and the climate crisis?

Because food corporations are paying for the reelection of Congress members through their lobbyists, members of Congress are in turn pushing through the legislation. Over the last thirty years, the meat, dairy, and egg industries have given over $134 million to United States Congress members. It's a pay-for-play system that becomes shockingly apparent when you consider that the United States Department of Agriculture (USDA) and the Department of Health and Human Services (HHS) are responsible for creating the dietary guidelines for Americans. These guidelines, formerly known as the food pyramid, dictate all federal food policies. And the committee responsible for creating these guidelines is made up of people who have received money from companies and entities such as the National Dairy Council, the North American Meat Institute, the Sugar Association, Dannon, McDonald's, Coca-Cola, General Mills, Kellogg's, Kraft, and Anheuser-Busch. So the people responsible for telling us what and how much to eat are being paid off by the meat industry, dairy industry, fast-food industry, and sugar industry. Sure, the people in our government may not have been the ones to put this plan in motion . . . but have they done anything to stop and eradicate it?

Over the last thirty years, the meat, dairy, and egg industries have given over **$134 MILLION** to United States Congress members.

Who suffers the most from the rigged system?

Any guesses? That's right, poor people of color. Just look at food assistance programs. SNAP, formerly called food stamps, is the main food welfare program in the United States. It provides food assistance to about 10 percent of the population. Well, these participants are more likely to be obese, or suffer or die from almost every single diet-related disease. That's because every year $80 billion in government money is being used to buy animal products under the guise of helping poor people. That way, the meat and dairy industries can overproduce cheap commodity foods and dump them into poor communities. And lobbyists from companies like Kraft and Coca-Cola are fighting for guidelines that dictate where SNAP dollars can be spent—primarily on junk food. When health advocates urged the government to include more fruits and vegetables in the WIC package—another major assistance program for women, infants, and children—the meat and dairy industries lobbied against it, denying low-income women and their children access to healthier foods. These folks get richer while the people get sicker. And the government, who has all the power in these matters, does nothing about it. When a government agency knows a product is bad for a group of people and pushes it on them anyway, that is systemic racism.

When a government agency knows a product is bad for a group of people and pushes it on them anyway, that is **SYSTEMIC RACISM.**

The meat and dairy industries are perpetrators of systemic environmental racism too.

Communities of color not only have toxic food dumped onto them but also literal toxins. African Americans are three times more likely to die from pollution than white people and experience 63 percent more pollution than they create themselves. A prime example of what's generating that pollution is factory farms, where most animals in the US are raised. In chapter 3 we talked about how these enormous operations produce literal tons of waste, which are sprayed over fields and enter the water, air, and homes of surrounding people—usually people of color. That's because CAFOs, concentrated animal feeding operations, are strategically located in or near communities of color. In the example of the hog farms of North Carolina, you're more than twice as likely to live near one if you're Black or brown. If you're an Indigenous person, you're three times as likely. It's no mistake they're there. It's not happenstance. It's the avenue of least resistance. There's the least amount of political and economic power to fight them off. The state could stop permitting CAFOs to be built in these communities, but they won't. There's a lot of pork money up in that legislature.

Big Pharma's in on it too.

This one's especially personal for me. My uncle died of heart disease, and it shook our family to the core. The fact that so much pain for us was caused by a treatable condition made it hurt that much more. I wondered why we aren't hearing more doctors talk about that—the fact that we can prevent and reverse diseases that are tearing families, entire communities apart. We hear them talk about the basic physiology of the disease and about the medication. But not nutrition, the single biggest cause of the disease and also the *treatment*. It's just not part of the paradigm of Western medicine. Our doctors get their information through their continuing medication education, which is funded in part by the pharmaceutical industry (studies have shown that it's not uncommon for a portion of a medical school's budget to come from the drug industry). That's pretty messed up when you think about the fact that the only way this industry makes money is if sick people stay sick.

There's no money in things that keep people well. Most medications in the drugstore or pharmacy aren't designed to cure your disease; they're designed to manage it. If taking a pill actually solved our problems, we'd be the longest-living population because we objectively consume more medications in this country than in any other country in the world. Seriously—Americans take over half the world's pharmaceutical drugs, and we're only 5 percent of the world's population. (We also pay more for these meds. We're charged, on average, 300 percent more than the world average for medications, making our health-care system the most expensive in the world.) Sure, modern medicine is a great tool, but there also has to be a plan to get off those medications at some point. Instead, the pharmaceutical industry is printing money at your expense, and everybody's getting paid, except you.

Most medications in the drugstore or pharmacy aren't designed to CURE your disease; they're designed to MANAGE it.

Now, I am not saying that medication is never needed, but let's be honest—if 10 percent of individuals taking prescription drugs were able to get off them because of a change of lifestyle, the pharmaceutical industry would tank. Don't think so? Consider this: According to market research, the worldwide pharmaceutical market was worth nearly $1.3 trillion in 2019. Ten percent of $1.3 trillion is $130 billion. Now does that seem like such a small dent? Hopefully now it's clearer than ever: Pharma doesn't want a healthy world; there is too much money to be made in keeping people sick. In fact, in general, hospitals, doctors, pharmaceutical companies, and even the government (the pharmaceutical industry spends more on lobbying the government than any other industry) are all making billions keeping us hooked on medication. Just like the fast-food and junk food industries are making billions keeping us addicted to their product. If it seems like they're working together, that's because they are.

Jeff Kindler, former CEO of Pfizer, the largest pharmaceutical company in the world, was also the executive vice president of McDonald's. Three more of McDonald's executive board members also have ties to Big Pharma: Miles White (Abbott), Lloyd Dean (Upjohn Company), and Robert Eckert (Amgen). Coca-Cola's VP of Strategic Securities Kelly Johnstone comes from the FDA. PepsiCo board member Daniel Vasella was chairman of the pharmaceutical company Novartis. Cargill Protein, one of the largest meat companies, counts among its board members Bernard Poussot, the former president of pharma company Wyeth; Richard Anderson of Medtronic, the world's largest medical device company, which generates most of its profits from the US health-care system; and Stephen Hemsley, the former CEO of UnitedHealth Group, an insurance provider and the fifth largest corporation in this country.

That's just a small sample. Companies providing life and health insurance own over $1.9 billion worth of stock in fast-food industries, investing in the very food that's making people sick, then charging higher premiums to individuals who end up with heart disease, diabetes, and cancer from these same foods. This isn't just greedy corporations, though. The previous head of the US Department of Health and Human Services (the people who make the dietary recommendations for all Americans), Alex Azar, was a senior executive for pharmaceutical giant Eli Lilly, and the current US secretary of agriculture, Tom Vilsack, was a lobbyist for the dairy industry.

Companies providing life and health insurance own over $1.9 BILLION worth of stock in fast-food industries, investing in the very food that's making people sick.

It's like they're TRYING TO KILL US.

If this isn't a giant conspiracy to make people sick—because of power, money, or both—why on earth would fast-food, junk food, and meat companies want pharmaceutical board members when these industries have apparently nothing in common? You put poor food in the communities; you put disease in the communities. It's like they want to make us sick. It's like they're trying to kill us.

Systemic changes need to happen, but we can't wait on the government. WE CAN START TODAY, with our food.

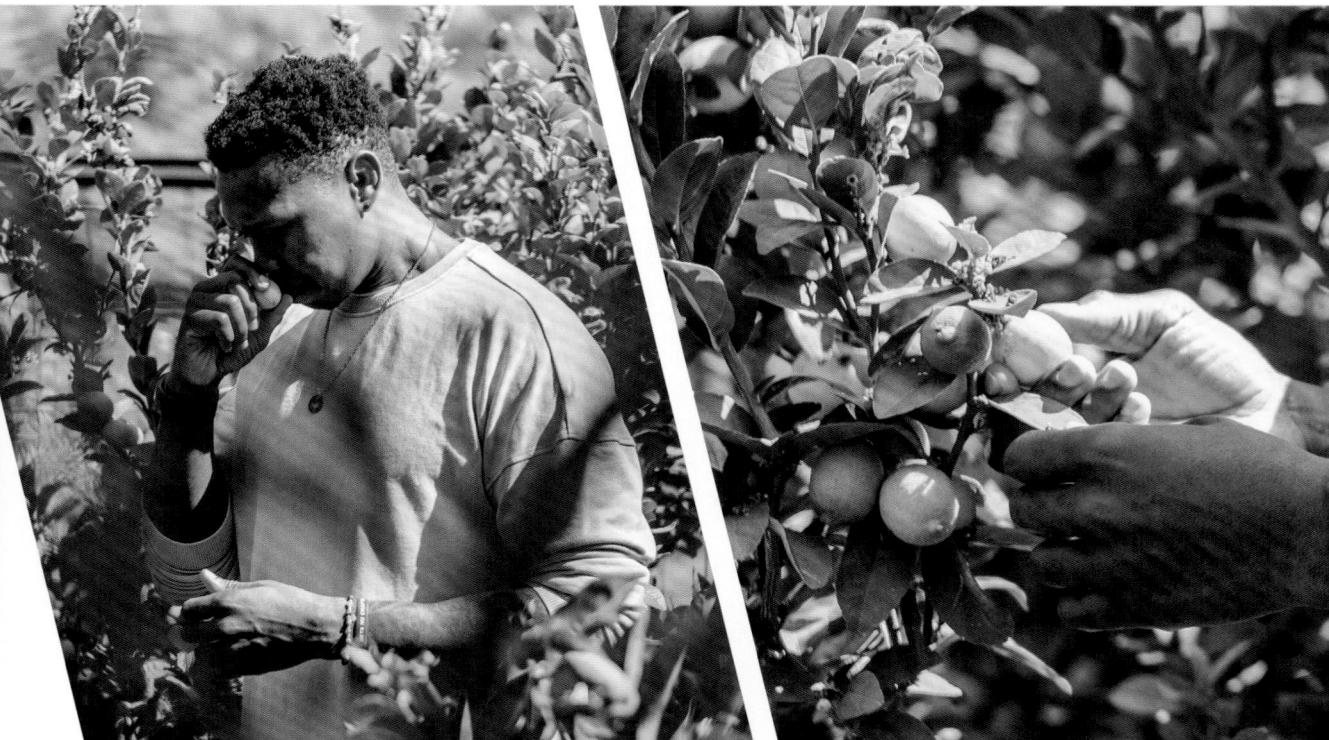

Like Maya Angelou said, "Do the best you can until you know better. Then when you know better, do better."

You can fight systemic racism by saying, "I don't want any of your chicken, your beef, your cheese. No thanks." When I did that in my own life, I didn't just find a new vitality that I hadn't experienced since I was a kid, or put on muscle in the gym in a whole new way, or feel younger now than I did at twenty-three; I also couldn't help but imagine what the world would be like if we all ate a different way. If we reclaimed our health and our communities. This system doesn't just affect Black people. We can all take this power back from these industries. The billions that we spend on health care could go back into our neighborhoods and families and build generational wealth. Half the world's grain, which is now fed to livestock, could be fed to the eight hundred million starving and malnourished people around the planet. We could reverse climate change by getting rid of animal agriculture entirely and allowing the forests to grow back. We could prevent new pandemics from emerging from the factory farms. We could stop industries from polluting our air, water, and food. We could literally save our planet and ourselves. I know it may seem hard, but I can tell you that as a Black man in America, going vegan doesn't even come close to the hardest things I've ever done. I know that systemic changes need to happen in our policies and laws, but we can't wait on the government. We can start today, with our food.

To view the references cited in this chapter, please visit badassvegan.com/citations.

LOVE THE FOOD THAT LOVES YOU BACK

THE FIRST THIRTY DAYS

Remember when I said that we're going to treat your plant-based adventure like a new relationship? Well, **THIS IS WHERE THINGS GET FUN.** It's where you and your food are having those long, deep conversations about the future without worrying whether any of it will come true—when every date uncovers something new and titillating and every interaction is a little flirty and a little dirty. This is the time when you just can't keep your hands off each other. We're talking full-on exploration of your wishes and fantasies, anytime, anywhere. With your food. We're talking about food here.

These first thirty days are all about that **FRESH EXCITEMENT** and no-guilt, no-shame, no-pressure experimentation. I want you to eat whatever speaks to you, so long as it doesn't include animal foods. You want to eat three meals of guacamole and chips? Go for it. Vegan doughnuts? You got it. Prepared foods, frozen foods, even fast foods? Good deal—so long as you leave out anything that once went moo, oink, cluck, and whatever sound fish make. Just don't go thinking that you can get where you want to go with eating *fewer* animal foods or still eating them every once in a while. I know some people say, "Everything in moderation," but you know who also says that? Crackheads.

I know what you're thinking right now: *Whatever I want? What's that?* That's what I hear all the time when I first tell people that eating plant-based can really be as simple as eating whatever plants sound good. It's almost like people are asking me, "What *do* I want? What sounds good to *me*?" Well, friend, I can't tell you that. But what I *can* do is introduce you to all the options you have and give you some guidance for how to put them together as simple meals and snacks. **BUT AS FAR AS WHAT YOU WILL ACTUALLY EAT, THAT'S WHEN YOU DO YOU.**

We'll get into things like micro- and macronutrients in the next section, but for now, just relax into the basics. This is the time for you to get to know your food, especially how delicious and satisfying it can be—while also ruling out because you'll be eating only plants doesn't mean you need to love all of them. Not into asparagus? No problem; there's like twenty thousand other vegetables for you to choose from. Harder-to-digest foods like beans also aren't for everyone, especially if your digestive tract is still healing after years of being beat up by Cheetos and Coca-Cola. Again, **YOU'RE NOT GONNA GO HUNGRY.** Check out how many varieties of fruits and vegetables there are besides apple slices and mashed potatoes. Learn about all the different grains and legumes and finally figure out how to pronounce "quinoa" (no spoilers). Figure out what the deal is with soy and why it's not always bad for you.

I'll give you some quick-hit "recipes" to get you started in chapter 10, but chapters 8 and 9 are your menu for exploration—consider them your formal introduction to all the plants you might come across in your grocery store. Mix and match from all the different categories: fruits and veggies, grains, alternative proteins, and good fats. **CHALLENGE YOURSELF** to reach beyond your comfort zone and try some new things. Dress that shit up—some plain rice and beans or roasted vegetables go a long way with sauces and condiments. That's why Mother Nature gave us hummus and hot sauce! No one's ever died from a plant experiment gone wrong. No one's ever been rushed to the hospital because they put salad dressing on their grain bowl, or cauliflower in their smoothie. And mess around with not just tastes but textures too. You might figure out that you enjoy a meal more if it has something crunchy, or that you like your smoothies more if they're extra-thick and creamy (the trick is to load 'em up with frozen bananas—try two instead of just one). Again, do whatever YOU want. This shouldn't feel like boot camp; there should be light *in* the tunnel, not just at the end of it.

That's also why I included tons of recipes at the end of this book to get you through breakfast, lunch, and dinner, plus dressings and sauces, sweets (yes, sweets), and a bunch of smoothies thrown in because they're basically a vegan rite of essed by a monk, no ingredients that are eighty bucks an unce. We're talking straightforward *and* crave-worthy. But hey'll also be delicious because I'm all about flavor. You ould tell me that something's going to help me live for an xtra hundred years, but if it tastes like shit, I'm not ating it. Sorry. I'm guessing you feel the same way too. hat's why I think food needs to be a party in your mouth. t's gotta be *mouthgasmic*. If it's not, why would you eat it?

bove all, I want you to be in the mindset that this journey ou're about to go on is going to **CHANGE YOUR LIFE.** And nstead of focusing on what you will miss out on, try ocusing on what you'll gain. Of course, you gotta understand hat any beneficial change can be uncomfortable at first, but he more you practice, the more reps you get in, the better ou'll get. A lot of times people ask me what it's like to go egan or what they can expect. I like to tell them that it's ike trying to explain losing your virginity. We all have ifferent experiences: some good, some bad. But it gets etter the more you do it. If you stick to a plant-based diet or the next thirty days, I guarantee that you're going to ee results. You're going to **LOOK BETTER, FEEL BETTER, BE BETTER.** You're also going to see what you have the power to o when you put your mind to something. Believe in this shit, ecause it works. And believe in yourself because you're onna make it happen.

f You Want to Make a Change, You Have to Shake Sh*t Up

f there's a goal that you're not reaching and you've been oing the same damn thing day after day, the message is lear: It's not working for you! If you want to make a hange, you have to shake shit up. I want you to get honest vith yourself about what your goals are and what you've been oing to reach them all this time. How's that been working or you? A lot of times what happens is that we do the same hing over and over again expecting to get exponential esults. But my guess is that if you're reading this book

then your previous habits have left something on
So even though leaving behind the food that's beer
plate for most of your life can be difficult becaus
there for you when you've felt excited, or sad, or
it reminds you of special memories, consider this
official step toward something new. And not just th
something that'll work.

Don't worry; **WE'RE GOING TO DO IT TOGETHER.** So of
starting something new, we fill our heads with junk
if I mess up? What if I have to start over? But do
kinds of thoughts actually get us anywhere or prot
anything? They don't. So instead, I want you to ca
yourself when you find those same types of thoughts
in, and I want you to replace them with something
Here's what's going to happen when I stick to my g
it in your mind, commit to it. Understand that you
this power inside of you; you just needed someone
your shoulder, wake you up, and make you realize *O*
been sleepin' on this shit. There are no losses he
lessons. If you slip up and eat cheese at 11:59, j
sure you're right back on the path at 12:00.

I get that you might be trying to break habits tha
had for twenty, thirty, even fifty years. I get tha

MAKING YOUR DOCTOR YOUR TEAMM/

If you're currently taking medication for t
high blood pressure, high cholesterol, thyr
issues, or diabetes, I recommend working wi
medical practitioner to adjust your dosage,
will soon require less medication. I also s
encourage you to find a plant-based practiti
because they will understand exactly how yo
food as medicine.

be trying to break generational trauma that's been going on for decades. But you can do it and you will do it because you can believe in yourself. And also because you have to realize that no one else is going to do it for you, and that there's no magic potion or miracle pill. That's why you're doing this right here, right now. This journey is going to make you reflect on things from your past and focus on things for your future—and that can feel big. But remember you are powerful. You're so powerful that you made it this far in life and that you've gotten to this point right here: understanding that it's time for a change. **IT'S TIME TO SHAKE SHIT UP.**

IF YOU'RE ALREADY A VEGAN

Maybe you've **ALREADY COMMITTED** to a plant-based diet, but you're reading this book to learn more about how you can make your diet work for you and your goals, or you want to **SHAKE THINGS UP** and **GET MORE EXCITED** about what you're eating. In your case, these thirty days should be about having fun too. I'm not saying you should go out and stuff yourself with processed food if that's not something you're already doing, but do get adventurous and see what happens. Maybe try out a new recipe from this book, or **CHALLENGE YOURSELF** to incorporate a new grain, bean, vegetable, or fruit you hadn't messed around with before. You might be surprised what you learn about yourself or what foods and flavors you discover. You could also just skip to the next section, but I think you might want to stick around because I'm about to drop some serious knowledge.

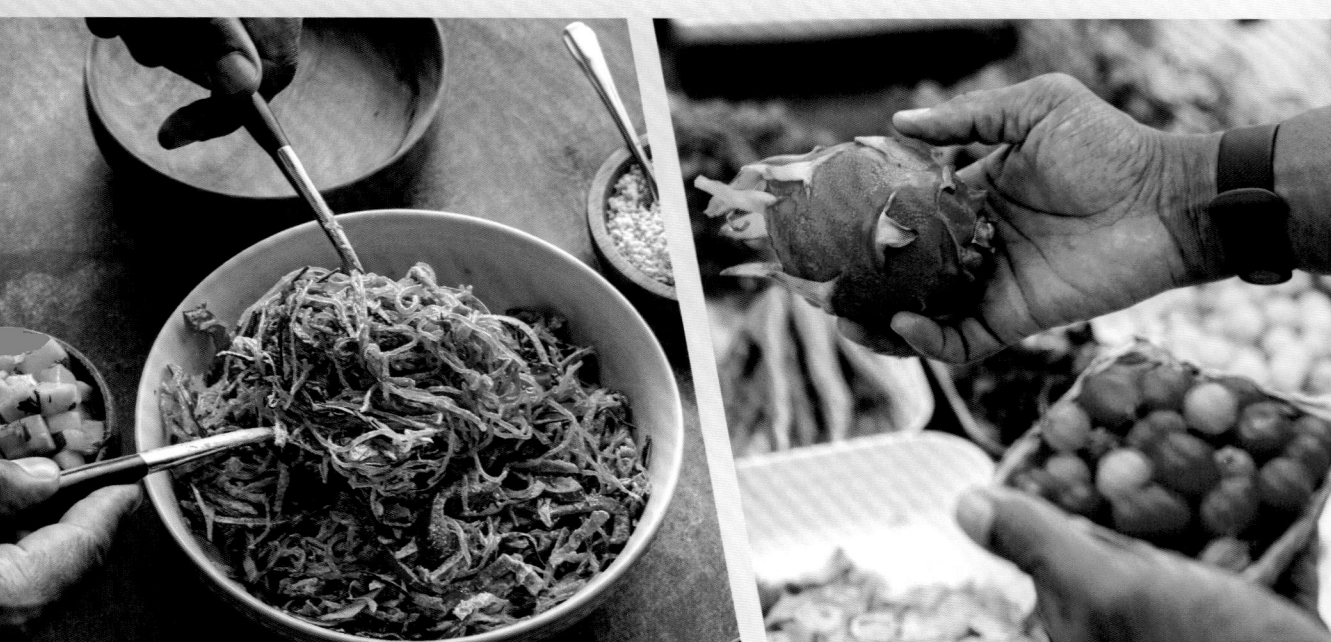

CHAPTER 6

PLAN YOUR ATTACK

It's one thing to get pumped up about going vegan and diving into things headfirst because of that excitement. That's fine and well; we want you getting right into that deep end. But once you're there, you're gonna need a flotation device. Even if you're someone who's been committed to living a healthy lifestyle but just hasn't been plant-based. Even if you're really, really committed to seeing changes in your life. Because that dinner out at your favorite restaurant is coming. That family gathering is coming. That road trip past all the billboards for your favorite foods is coming. *Life* is coming. And again, no matter how set on staying the course you might be, these challenges can be trying for even the most experienced vegan. That's why I want you to get prepared. Going vegan isn't some kind of life sentence; it's a downright pleasure if you let it be. But it's more difficult to unlock that pleasure if you're not giving yourself the tools you need to succeed.

If you've ever gone on a diet or started a new lifestyle program, you've probably read a similar section about how you need to get set up if you want to get the best, most sustainable results. It's no different with going plant-based. We're gonna have fun here, but we're gonna be serious about it. And that means:

○ Getting rid of all the animal products in your kitchen and your stash drawer at work

- Getting comfortable planning and prepping for your meals

- Investing in your cooking equipment (not a ton, but enough so you can do what you need to do)

- Finding some support

- Figuring out what you're going to do when it's time to eat outside of your house

As I said, I'm here to make sure that you and your food have the most delicious, exciting, mouthgasmic relationship possible. But in order to get you there, I've gotta be a little bit of a hard-ass too. Trust me, the more work you do now to lay a strong foundation, the easier it'll be when it comes time to make the transition.

Prep Your Kitchen

Before you do anything, take a look through your fridge, freezer, pantry, and cabinets to get rid of the obvious stuff—meat, dairy, eggs, seafood. You don't have to throw everything away—give it to a neighbor, or donate it to someone who needs it, if you can. Just because it's animal food doesn't mean it should go to waste. But no matter what, don't hang on to it. You don't want to tempt yourself into thinking that that one little frozen beef burrito or that one little pint of dairy ice cream doesn't really count, or that it sounds really, really good when it's late and you've been out and you deserve it. Don't even have it there talking to you.

Next, scan the labels of just about everything to make sure there aren't any animal products lurking. On the next page are some examples of what you might find.

Saving Money: Shopping Tips and Avoiding Food Waste

This may not be exactly what people associate first off with going vegan. All those fresh vegetables and fruits and fancy grains must get expensive, right? Hell no. If you buy smart (buy in bulk, buy on sale, buy in season), your

INGREDIENT	WHAT IT IS	WHERE YOU FIND IT
Albumin	The protein component of egg whites	Processed foods
Anchovies	Small, silver-colored fish	Worcestershire sauce, Caesar salad dressing
Animal shortening	Butter, suet, lard	Packaged cookies and crackers, refried beans, flour tortillas, ready-made piecrusts
Carmine (carmine cochineal or carminic acid)	Red coloring made from a ground-up insect	Bottled juices, colored pasta, some candies, frozen pops
Casein (caseinate)	A milk protein	Some soy cheeses
Gelatin	Protein from bones, cartilage, tendons, and skin of animals	Marshmallows, frosted cereals, gelatin-containing desserts, some candies
Glucose (dextrose)	Animal tissues and fluids (some glucose can come from fruits)	Baked goods, soft drinks, candies, frosting
Glycerides (mono-, di-, and triglycerides)	Glycerol from animal fats or plants	Processed foods
Isinglass	Gelatin from the air bladder of sturgeon and other freshwater fish	Alcoholic beverages, some jellied desserts
Lactose (saccharum lactin, D-lactose)	Milk sugar	As a culture medium for souring milk and in processed foods
Lactylic stearate	Salt of stearic acid (see stearic acid)	As a conditioner in bread dough
Lard	Fat from the abdomens of pigs	Baked goods, refried beans, some potato chips
Lecithin	Phospholipids from animal tissues, plants, and egg yolks	Baked goods, refried beans
Lutein	Deep yellow coloring from marigolds or egg yolks	Breakfast cereals, candies, chocolate, baked goods, vegetable oil sprays
Oleic acid (oleinic acid)	Animal tallow	Commercial food coloring
Stearic acid (octadecanoic acid)	Tallow, other animal fats and oils	Vegetable fats and oils, candies, beverages, condiments
Suet	Hard white fat around kidneys and loins of animals	Vanilla flavoring, baked goods, beverages, candies
Vitamin A (A_1, retinol)	Vitamin obtained from vegetables, egg yolks, or fish liver oils	Pastries
Vitamin B_{12}	Vitamin produced by microorganisms and found in all animal products; synthetic form (cyanocobalamin or cobalamin on labels) is vegan	Vitamin supplements, fortification of foods
Vitamin D_3 (cholecalciferol)	Comes from fish liver oils or lanolin	Supplements, fortified foods
Whey	Watery liquid that separates from the solids in cheese making	Supplements, fortified foods

home-cooked meals will ultimately cost you less because you'll be cooking more and going out less. Especially when you factor in the money you'd be shelling out down the road on things like doctor's visits, lifelong medications, and eventual surgeries. Chris Rock put it best: "Ain't no money in the cure; the money is in the medicine. That's how you get paid, on the comeback. That's all the government is, a bunch of motherfucking drug dealers on the comeback." You can pay the farmer now or the doctor later. Just sayin'.

Time Is Money: Planning and Prepping

Again, people hear the word *vegan* and think, *All that rabbit food must take a long time to prepare.* I mean, look at a head of broccoli or a whole squash—those things can be fucking terrifying. But as you get more familiar with using whole ingredients, you'll realize that while, yes, it's a little more work than throwing a potpie in the microwave, you don't have to quit your job just so you have time to feed yourself.

The first way you can set yourself up for success is by planning ahead. You don't need to know what you're gonna eat every minute of every day because that would be unrealistic and, let's face it, a total buzzkill. But you can have an idea of foods you like to eat that you want to have on hand, and maybe an idea of what meals you can make from those foods. Or the ingredients from a few of the recipes later in this book. In the beginning you're going to want to cook a new recipe every day. But slow up, Gordon Ramsay. Be realistic about how much time you actually have to make food or want to be making food. I've thrown away a lot of food in my day because of overenthusiastic meal planning. Don't count out easy meals like a bowl of grains with some kind of veg and some beans or tofu and maybe a dressing. Those are mostly things you don't need to buy fresh every week and can fill in the holes when you're not in a position to make a recipe from scratch.

In terms of food prep, I'm not gonna lie to you—having a fridge full of food that's ready to eat is the easiest way to make good decisions come mealtime. But I'm also a real person; I know that going to the grocery store is hard enough without having to come home and prep a week's worth of food. Hard pass on that (unless you have the time and it sounds like fun). I say be reasonable about it—if you're making a pot of rice, cook double and save the rest in the fridge. If you're chopping up a head of broccoli or an onion and only need half, save the rest in the fridge. Getting the idea?

One of the easiest ways you can plan ahead is to store your smoothie ingredients in individual jars or freezer bags. Throw in your cup of fruit, handful of greens, and whatever else you want in there—except the liquid—and stash it until you're ready to dump it into the blender with some nut milk.

Gear Up

You don't need fancy equipment to cook, but you do need some basics. Your goods don't have to be expensive, and you don't have to buy them all at once. I highly recommend checking out discount stores, where you can find good brands for a lot less money. This is especially helpful for bigger-ticket items like pots, pans, and appliances. And those of you who don't have a kitchen—I see you too. These things have got you covered:

A GOOD KNIFE: One goes a long way.

RUBBER SPATULA: Key for everything, whether it's getting smoothies out of the blender, cooking in a skillet, or mixing things in a bowl.

PIZZA SLICER: It just helps. I cut my kids' sandwiches with one—I don't know why nobody thought of that. No need to be worried about a big-ass knife cutting off your fingers. Just one slice and that's a wrap.

KITCHEN SET: Forks, spoons, knives, plates, bowls. It doesn't have to be fancy and you don't need enough to entertain a crowd. Ideally nothing disposable because nature's not down with that anymore.

MIXING BOWLS: One or two big ones. Bonus if you can find one with a fitted lid, which is great for mixing up salads.

MEASURING CUPS AND SPOONS: For obvious reasons. Though, I love using a shot glass for measuring because it's 2 tablespoons. And 2 tablespoons happens to be the ideal amount of dressing for a salad or maple syrup for a smoothie or oats.

PANS: At least one big skillet, a set of 'em if you can swing it.

POTS: A medium-size pot (6 quarts) that's big enough for grains and making pasta will get you pretty far, but I'd also throw in a smaller 4-quart pot for good measure.

BLENDER: I personally have a high-speed blender because I use it constantly for making things like smoothies and dressings.

RICE COOKER: This has saved me time and again because I can't cook rice to save my life.

AIR FRYER: These aren't just great for making things crispy without a lot of oil; they're also helpful if you need to heat/reheat something and don't have a microwave or oven.

TOASTER OVEN: This is another easy way to heat/reheat things if you don't have access to a full-size oven.

REFRIGERATION: Even a small refrigerator to store what you're eating for the week will help.

STORAGE CONTAINERS: You'll want a few different sizes or larger 4- or 5-quart ones with partitions that you can store leftovers or prepped food in. If you're short on space, I'm a big fan of silicone reusable zip-top bags, which store the same amount of food, but you don't have to worry about transferring it to a smaller container after a couple of days. So you can pack a whole lot more into your fridge or freezer. As an added bonus, find containers that are oven-safe so you can put your food right in there.

Squad Up

Making changes, especially ones that'll hopefully last your whole life, can take some hard work. And it gets even harder if you're the only one in your family making this commitment. (Though, give it a month or two before everyone starts eyeing your results and your tasty food.) It's easier to make a transition when you're in good company. Find a friend or a sibling/cousin/parent/aunt/uncle/child who might be interested in coming along for the ride even part of the time, or join a local vegan group for support. You could also check out any number of awesome organizations who are doing great work in the social justice, environmental, and all-around world-changing spaces, such as Food Not Bombs, Support + Feed, SÜPRMARKT, and Gangster Vegan. Getting involved in their efforts, or even just following their social media, is a powerful way to remind yourself that you're not in this thing alone, and that there are a lot of other people out there working their asses off in the name of positive change.

Know How to Eat in a Restaurant

Just because you're leaving meat and dairy off your plate doesn't mean that you can no longer be social or eat in restaurants. Even in spots like Applebee's or TGI Fridays you can find menu items that either are entirely vegan or can be made vegan by taking out a couple of ingredients. Nowadays you can also ask your server for their recommendations on how to make something plant-based. Twenty years ago they might have been like, *Wha??* But it's becoming more and more common for people with all kinds of dietary considerations to be eating out. Paleo, keto, gluten-free, dairy-free, nut-free—just to a name a few. What's a couple more special requests from you? So long as you're not a jerk about it, no one's gonna roll their eyes at the vegan. Another great option is to let the chef know that they have full license to do their thing with whatever plants they have back there in the kitchen. They usually love that—they get to cook whatever they want and just create. And if you're in a fast-food restaurant, I get it. It's not my top choice for you, but I understand that life happens. If all else fails, remember that french fries are technically vegan.

Put Yo Money Where Yo Mouth Is

One of the most common obstacles that people face when transitioning to a plant-based diet is sourcing good, fresh food. I get it—it's tough when all that's around is a corner store or bodega, or a grocery store that's a bus ride away. I want to include this section for three really important reasons:

1. You have to remember that hard does not mean impossible.

2. I'm not saying it'll be easy, but there will always be a healthier option available. It may not be the best possible choice, but it's the *better* one. Think a bean burrito from Taco Bell versus the Crunchwrap Supreme. Or even a protein bar from the bodega versus the bag of chips.

3. Last, and most importantly, the better choices that you make today pave the way for even better choices tomorrow. Think of your money as a vote—food companies keep track of those votes. Lupe Fiasco had a great line: "Complain about the liquor store, but what you drinking liquor for?" If you spend money at the fast-food restaurant instead of at the grocery store, then you're putting your money in the fast-food bank account. Believe me, if a grocery store chain notices that more people in your community are putting money in their bank account and want a certain kind of product, they're going to sell it there. In fact, they might try to make it as convenient as possible to get that particular product, maybe even opening up other stores that are closer and more convenient to you. Not because they necessarily care about your well-being but because they want your money. But hey, that's a win-win. The same goes for fast-food restaurants—KFC will never be vegan. Carl's Jr. will never be vegan. But they're seeing that there's money to be made with at least some vegan offerings. If more of us demand more than junk, we're going to get more of the kinds of food we want.

To view the references cited in this chapter, please visit badassvegan.com/citations.

CHAPTER 7

MEET YOUR FOOD

So we've got a plan: Eat more plants. Oh, but what's that you say? You've never eaten a plant before? Trust me when I tell you that, if that's really where you're coming from, you're not the only one. I've known people who have gone their entire lives without eating a whole fruit or vegetable except for what comes on top of their Whopper or under their General Tso's chicken. I remember being at a family reunion in Arkansas when my cousin, who's always nitpicking my food, pointed at my plate and said, "Ew, what's that?" I said, "You mean asparagus?" Seeing the expression on her face, even I couldn't give her a hard time about it—which is saying something. Because I've been there.

It took me a while to get to a place where I didn't think something looked nasty if I didn't know what it was, or where I wasn't totally confused by what many fruits and vegetables were. I'll never forget the time after I'd just moved to Miami and my roommate bought some plantains. I was like, "Dude, why you buying these funky bananas?" He told me they were plantains, but I continued to argue with him—to my mind, anyone with a brain could see that they were the saddest, mushiest, brownest bananas. In reality, they were rich, creamy, and just begging to be sliced, baked, fried, or mashed. I used to even give avocados the side-eye until I figured out how delicious they were. Oh man, and jackfruit? I thought it was an alien life form until someone told me that that's where the flavor for Juicy Fruit gum came from—remember that stuff?

For a lot of folks, that's how navigating the fresh produce aisle can feel, especially when everything's in its whole form. There's level one of celery, carrots, kale, collards, romaine, apples, pears, sweet potatoes, regular-old potatoes—nothing too crazy there. But then you get into level two with radishes, fennel, arugula, dragon fruit, and Japanese sweet potatoes. And forget grains, beans, and protein alternatives—keen-a-what? Freaky who? Gar-bozos? Satan? What do you do with quinoa, freekeh, garbanzo beans, and seitan? Suddenly this whole plant thing feels pretty complicated in terms of how to buy, eat, and prepare these foods, let alone identify them.

That's why I'm dedicating these next few sections to all the plants you might come across in your grocery store, so you can get more comfortable with buying and eating them. I'll walk you through what they taste like, why they're good for you, and in some cases, how to cook them. (For even more on that tip you can check out the recipes in part IV.) What I hope you'll come to realize is that this is an incredible abundance of food. So if you're ever feeling like this process is only about giving up food, I want you to revisit this section. I mean, you eat the same six animals all the time—pork, beef, chicken, lamb, turkey, fish. But when it comes to plants, look at the variety you've got! The boring is in the meat.

Carbohydrates Are Not Your Enemy

You'll notice that you'll be eating a lot more carbohydrates than before—and that's okay. In fact, that's *good*. As we'll talk about more during the next thirty days, carbohydrate-rich foods like fruits, vegetables, grains, and legumes are where you should be getting a majority of your calories because they're the body's perfect fuel source.

A lot of you will be coming to this diet with a diabetes diagnosis, either type 1, 2, or 1.5; prediabetes; or gestational diabetes. Or maybe you've just spent most of your life hearing people tell you how carbohydrates make you fat. But if all these fruits, vegetables, grains, and legumes are rich in carbohydrates, how are you supposed to eat? We'll get into this in much more detail in part III, but for now I want you to take a deep breath and forget

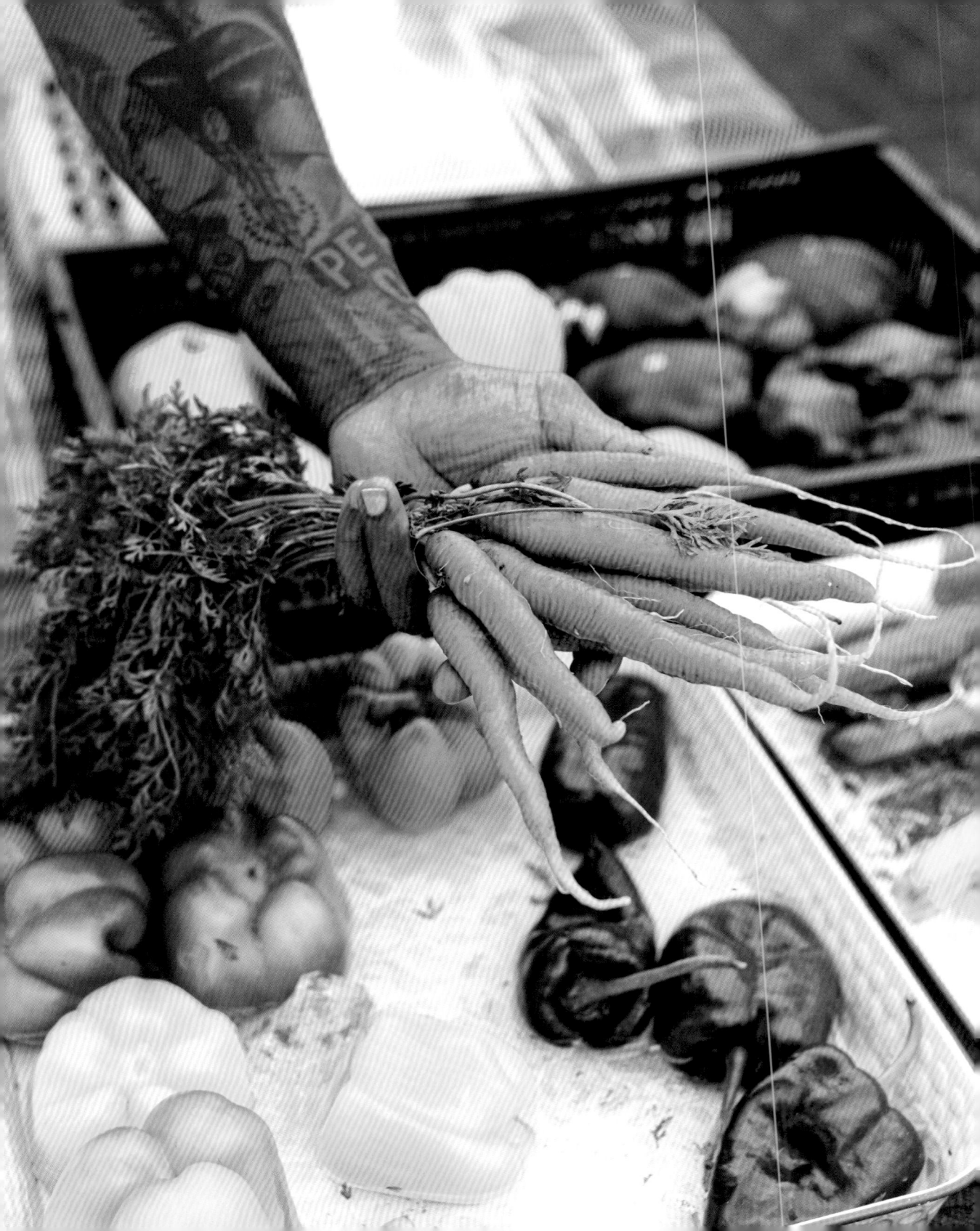

everything you think you know about food science and nutrition. The fact is, whole food, plant-based carbohydrates are healthy and will not lead to high blood sugar. Even fruit. Yes, you read that right. *Fruits and vegetables are not the root cause of your diabetes.* The sugar in these foods is wrapped up in fiber and contains the vitamins and nutrients your body needs to function optimally. It's not stripped down to a highly addictive white powder, and I'm not talking about cocaine—although it's just a few molecules off. (Yes, cocaine is derived from a plant, just like sugar is.) And speaking of fiber, you'll be getting a nice, high dose of the stuff now that you're committing to a diet of whole-plant foods, especially fruits, vegetables, and grains. Fiber not only helps regulate the way your body uses sugar and keeps blood sugar in check, but is also like those big spinning scrub brushes at the car wash. Fiber is too difficult to digest, so it scours its way through your intestines on its way out, taking harmful bacteria and other buildup with it. Let's just say you're not going to need Metamucil anymore.

And for those of you who may have heard that eating a ketogenic diet or low-carb diet is the key to losing weight and getting healthy, let's just put that to the side, shall we? In my own experience, I can tell you that when I tried doing keto, I just didn't feel as great. All that fat and protein made me

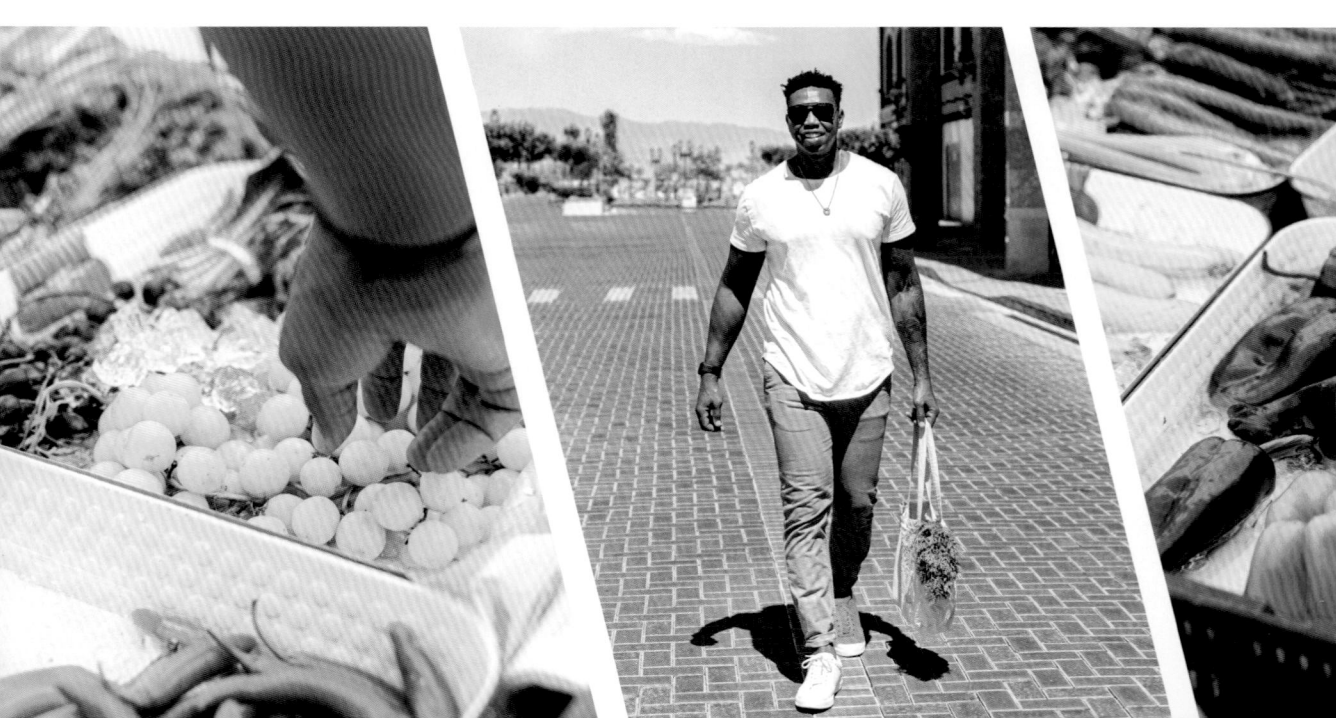

feel a little sludgy (yes, that is a word). When I'm eating mostly carbs, on the other hand, I see a difference in my performance for the better. We're talking running half marathons, playing at all-day basketball tournaments, weightlifting, and just generally being constantly on the go.

Depriving your body of carbohydrates does trigger ketosis and make your body dip into its fat stores for energy, but that's not healthy in the long term. Your brain needs the glucose from carbohydrates for fuel. And keeping your body in a constant state of ketosis can have a negative effect on your health, even leading to chronic disease. I can tell you right now that eating a diet rich in carbohydrates is not going to do that—and it's still going to help you reach your goals. Plus, you can reach ketosis through intermittent fasting without having to give up carbohydrates.

We'll eventually kick it up a notch with more information, structure, and guidelines for what you eat in a day. And yes, we'll talk a lot more about how you can use your daily food intake to build muscle or lose weight. But for now your objective shouldn't necessarily be going after the harder abs or bigger biceps; it's to get healthy—and to make that transition in a way that feels good. So for now, just get out there and enjoy your food, including all those carbohydrates.

Be the Fat Friend

This might come as a shock after years of believing that fat is the devil, but fat is a necessary part of your diet. You need to eat fat just to stay alive. It protects your organs, helps your body absorb nutrients, supports your metabolism, boosts immunity, regulates hormone production, decreases depression, prevents osteoporosis, produces important hormones, and supports cell growth. It's also required for giving your body energy. So let's just all agree that we're going to keep fat in our diets.

As we'll get into in more detail in chapter 11, we don't need a whole lot of dietary fat (we want our energy to come from carbohydrates instead), and not all fat is the same. But for our purposes during these first thirty days, all you need to keep in mind is that the fat on your plate should play a supporting role and that it should come from whole, plant-based sources. For example, a spoonful of nut butter in your oats, a few slices of avocado

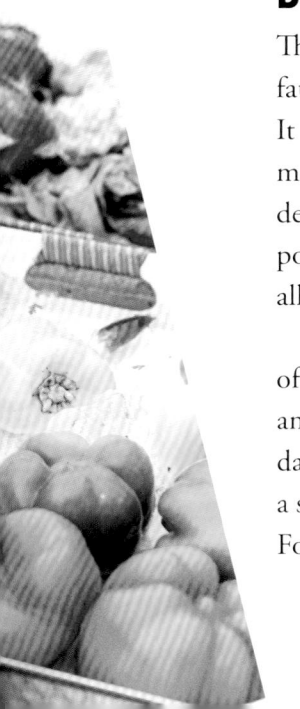

on top of your black bean soup, a sauce or dressing over sauteed greens, or some creamy tahini mixed into your grain bowl. Fat isn't the main attraction, but it makes everything a whole lot better.

Going Organic

As you're stocking up your kitchen with your new plant foods, one of the decisions you'll be making is whether to buy organic. This label gets a bad rap because it seems like another excuse to make food more expensive than it needs to be. But what's reflected in the price tag is quality and, in some cases, better health. Would you rather eat an apple that's been grown in soil that's depleted of any nutrients so that the trees need to be sprayed with man-made chemicals to keep insects and disease away? Or would you rather eat an apple grown from the most nutrient-dense soil possible so that it naturally grows to be strong enough to defend itself against attackers—strength that it passes on to you? Oh, and would it help to know that those man-made chemicals, known as Roundup, have been suspected to cause cancer? Just ask Edwin Hardeman, who was awarded $75 million in punitive damages because he developed non-Hodgkin's lymphoma after repeated exposure to Roundup. Now which apple are you going for?

If you're buying organic produce from a grocery store, at the very least you're getting plants that are raised without pesticides. It also means that you're getting plants that are not genetically modified organisms, or GMOs. GMOs are plants whose genetic material has been manipulated in a laboratory. Scientists mess around with crossing plant, animal, bacteria, and even virus genes in combinations that don't occur in nature. The result is a plant that can withstand the application of even *more* pesticides—meaning, they're sprayed even more liberally and frequently—and in some cases, produce their own insecticides. That's right, a plant that kills insects when they eat it. You can only wonder what that does to humans—especially because there have been no credible independent long-term studies about the safety of GMOs. I'm not saying that GMOs are killing us, but I don't have great evidence that they're *not* killing us either. I can't tell you that it's wiping out half the nation, but I also can't tell you that it's healing half the nation either. Buying organic and/or local, though, is the one way you can ensure that you're not eating GMOs.

If You Can't Buy Organic

Sometimes, no matter how hard we try or how much we'd like to, it's just not possible to buy all-organic produce. In these instances, I recommend referring to the Environmental Working Group's Dirty Dozen, a list of the twelve fruits and vegetables that often have the highest amount of pesticide residue. Either do your best to buy organic versions of these items or consider not buying them if conventional is all that's available:

- Strawberries
- Spinach
- Kale/mustard/collard greens
- Nectarines
- Apples
- Grapes
- Cherries
- Peaches
- Pears
- Bell and hot peppers
- Celery
- Tomatoes

On the flip side, the EWG also lists the Clean 15, which are fruits and veggies with the lowest pesticide residue and therefore the safest bets for buying nonorganic. In 2021 these included:

- Avocados
- Sweet corn
- Pineapple
- Onions
- Papayas
- Sweet peas
- Eggplants
- Asparagus
- Broccoli
- Cabbage
- Kiwis
- Cauliflower
- Mushrooms
- Honeydew melons
- Cantaloupes

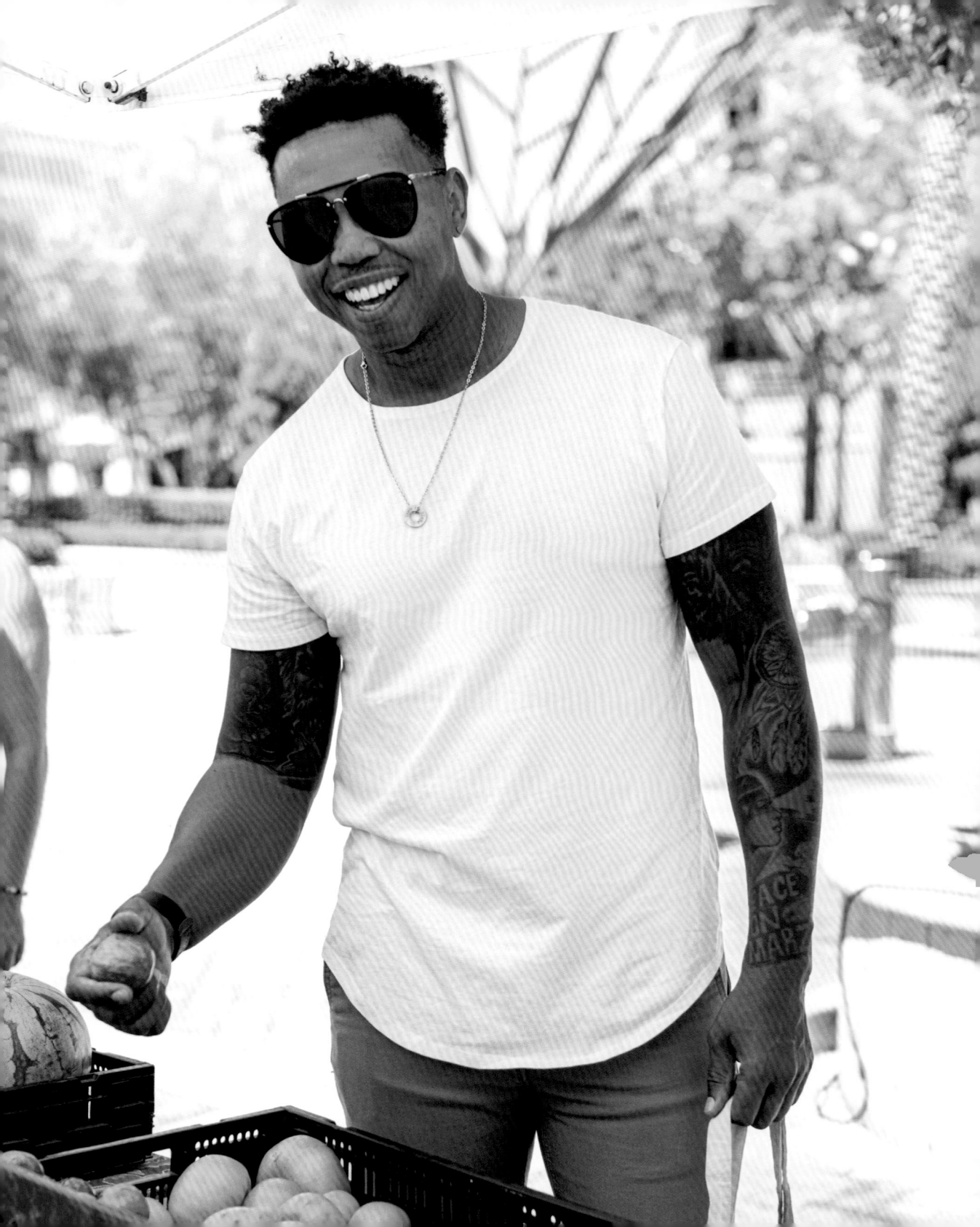

CHAPTER 8

THE GARDN' OF EATIN'
All the Fruits and Veggies

There's a wide, vibrant world of fruit and veg out there beyond the lettuce and tomatoes on that burger. Meet the players, fall in love. The first time I had a real, fresh-ass mango and not just "mango-flavored" juice, my life was changed forever. This is your new menu, from plantains to passion fruit, bok choy to broccoli. Now's not the time to get down on things just because you haven't tried them before. You dehydrated? Get some fucking celery juice then, bro. You never know what's going to change your life.

One thing you'll notice here is that I didn't include any "superfoods." That's because plants are innately superfoods. Fruits and vegetables are full of vitamins and minerals that are required for your body to function. They help to lower your cholesterol, lower your blood pressure, reduce your risk of heart disease, and maintain a healthy weight. They also contain phytochemicals, powerful compounds that actively protect you from type 2 diabetes, stroke, heart disease, and cancer. So while people love telling me that they eat all kinds of "superfoods" like Irish moss and camu camu and spirulina, I'm like, *Yeah, and you go home and have a pint of Hennessy.* If you're still eating the same bullshit that made you sick, not even a plant's superpowers can save you. When you go plant-based, you don't need the fancy stuff to unleash plant power, because they're all packin'.

You can use a few factors to figure out which fruits and vegetables you want to get down with: Type, Taste, and Color of the Rainbow.

HOT TAKES

Things you shouldn't be scared of anymore:

AVOCADOS: You're gonna want to make friends with these guys. They're creamy, filling, and so versatile. You can mash 'em up and add them to grain bowls, salads, and soups or just go at them with a spoon. Frozen avocado is also a great secret weapon for a creamy smoothie. General rule of thumb: The brighter the green of an avocado's skin, the less ripe it is. It should give slightly when you squeeze it gently but not be too squishy. There's a small window of time when it's ripe, and if you don't get to it, you just lost that 'cado. So if you're not planning to eat avocado for a few days, buy firmer ones at the store; they'll be ripe by the time you want to enjoy them.

BANANAS: If it has a spot on it, it's not spoiled. In stores, they try to put out only the perfect yellowish-green ones. These are not ripe; they're meant to get nice and brown. That's when they peak in nutrients and sweet banana flavor.

DATES: I didn't have a date until I'd been living in Florida for about eight years. At first I thought, I'm not eating that roach-looking thing. But then I realized, *Oh my God, it's nature's caramel.* They're also high in disease-fighting antioxidants and full of fiber. So even though they're sweet, they're actually helping you regulate your blood sugar.

JACKFRUIT: This is like the Swiss Army knife of plants. It can be sweet like Juicy Fruit gum—you remember the stuff in the yellow wrapper?—or mild tasting so you can pull it, toss it with BBQ sauce, and eat it like pulled pork because it's got great meaty texture. I like to eat it right out of the shell and add it to smoothies and fruit bowls.

KIWIS: I get it—they're hairy and green. But this tiny fruit that comes from New Zealand is packed with vitamins and antioxidants. They're like the Hulk of fruit; plus they're tasty and sweet. All you need to do is slice the things and eat the skin, cut them in half and scoop out the flesh with a spoon, or peel off the skin and eat the inside—no need to take out the seeds.

MUSHROOMS: These are some of the most powerful foods that grow on Earth, and there's a ton of variety. Shiitake, portobello, cremini, button, oyster, enoki, beech, maitake, lion's mane, just to name a few. I get that you think they're gross because they're fungus. But really they're earthy, meaty, delicious gems that are healthy as fuck. A lot of mushrooms are grown using pig waste, but there are now companies—like my friend's Wicked Healthy—that use wood and spores.

SWEET POTATOES: Did you know there are over four hundred different types of sweet potatoes out there? Some are more starchy and savory, while others are like baked candy. My favorite are the Japanese sweet potatoes, which are a beautiful purple color. Your relationship with sweet potatoes changes when you're plant-based because you realize how versatile and delicious these roots can be. You can slice 'em up and serve 'em with things like beans and enchilada sauce and feel like you're eating a piece of meat because they're so hearty, or drizzle them with maple syrup and feel like you're having the best pie in the world.

Types of Fruits and Vegetables at a Glance

Need a refresher or just some inspiration? Start here:

CITRUS: oranges, grapefruits, mandarins, lemons, limes

STONE FRUIT: nectarines, apricots, peaches, plums

BERRIES: strawberries, raspberries, blueberries, blackberries

POME FRUIT: apples and pears

TROPICAL AND EXOTIC: bananas, mangoes, kiwis, passion fruit, dragon fruit, jackfruit

SWITCH-HITTERS: tomatoes and avocados

LEAFY GREENS: lettuce, spinach, arugula, collard greens, kale, Swiss chard

CAPSICUM: chili peppers, sweet peppers/bell peppers

CRUCIFEROUS: cabbages, cauliflower, broccoli, Brussels sprouts

GOURDS: pumpkins, squashes, zucchini, cucumbers

ROOTS: potatoes, sweet potatoes, yams, carrots, beets, radishes

STEMS: celery and asparagus

ALLIUMS: onions, garlic, shallots

FUNGI: mushrooms

ALGAE: nori, hijiki, wakame, kelp

The Five Tastes

When you're trying to narrow down which plants to toss into your grocery cart or put together in a dish, another way to think about them is by their flavor. There are five receptors on your tongue that sense the flavors that we taste: bitter, sour, sweet, salty, and umami.* Each of these flavors can act on its own, but how they *interact* is essential to making food taste delicious. The more you activate any of these tastes, the more it enhances the other flavors. Bottom line: Variety across the spectrum is going to taste the best, while also keeping you healthy. That's because each of the flavors represents different nutrient profiles. So the more variety you get, the more well rounded the nutrition you're getting too. You'll also notice that as you stop eating processed foods pumped full of sugar and salt, the better your whole, plant-based foods will taste.

All five tastes can be found in the following fruits and vegetables:

BITTER: chilies, black pepper, parsley, chicory, arugula, coffee, hops, chocolate

SOUR: citrus fruits (lemons, limes, oranges, grapefruits)

SWEET: kiwis, blueberries, apples, watermelons, grapes, pears, carrots, sweet potatoes, beets

SALTY: celery, rhubarb, bok choy, sea vegetables

UMAMI*: leafy greens (arugula, kale), tomatoes, mushrooms, raw corn

*Umami is a Japanese word that describes a meaty or savory taste. Many times processed food gets its umami flavor from the chemical compound monosodium glutamate, or MSG, which is derived from naturally occurring glutamate. While the FDA says that there's nothing to worry about with MSG, some health experts are suspicious of the way it triggers nerve cells and overstimulates the brain, and many people report that they don't feel great after they eat it. Glutamate, on the other hand, provides that same savory sumptuousness but without the side of chemicals. Tomatoes and mushrooms are high in free-form glutamate, which gets intensified when you roast or saute them.

Color Me Tasty

Another way to make selections for your plate is to shop by color. That's because the plant rainbow is a code that tells us what unique set of vitamins, minerals, nutrients, and antioxidants a certain plant has. Fruit and veg with similar colors generally contain similar protective compounds, and the more colors you eat, the bigger dose of nutrients you're getting. Some examples:

RED = phytochemicals lycopene and anthocyanins (cherries, cranberries, red bell peppers, tomatoes, and beets)
Phytochemicals are thought to boost heart and circulatory health, improve memory, support urinary tract health, and decrease the risk of certain types of cancers.

ORANGE = vitamin C, carotenoids, bioflavonoids (carrots, oranges, sweet potatoes, and peaches)
These nutrients support skin and eye health, amplified immunity, a decreased risk of cancer, and a healthy heart.

YELLOW = alpha- and beta-carotenes (pineapples, yellow bell peppers, star fruit, and yellow beets)
Yellow foods increase immunity, decrease the risk of some cancers, promote healthy eyes and skin, and aid in digestion and brain function.

GREEN = phytochemicals lutein and indoles (broccoli, spinach, kiwis, leafy greens, peas, avocados, and green apples)
These phytochemicals are associated with eye health, reduce the risk of some cancers, promote muscle growth and strong bones, and also help with maintaining strong teeth.

BLUE/PURPLE = anthocyanins (blueberries, blackberries, plums, eggplants, figs, and purple potatoes)
These phytochemicals are known for their antioxidant and anti-aging properties. The nutrients in blue and purple fruits and vegetables promote bone health, reduce the risk of some cancers, improve memory, support urinary tract health, and increase circulation in the body—which is good for everyone at the party: heart, brain, organs, muscles, blood, and bones.

WHITE = anthoxanthins (cauliflower, garlic, mushrooms, and jicama)
It's not technically a color, but white veggies still bring it in the color department. They promote cellular recovery, strengthen the immune response, and lower the risk of disease. Also, many white foods contain the chemical allicin, which is believed to contribute to lower cholesterol and blood pressure.

CHAPTER 9

YOU WON'T GO HUNGRY
Fill Your Belly with Grains, Legumes, Protein, and Healthy Fats

Grains and legumes are two of the least expensive, most accessible, deliciously filling ingredients that are at the foundation of most of my meals, along with vegetables and fruits. You can fill your pantry with these dried goods for pennies on the dollar compared to fast food, and with a lot more variety. There's couscous, quinoa, amaranth, farro, all the different types of rice (brown, wild, jasmine, basmati, Carolina Gold), even oats. They're a grain too. We've been taught that oatmeal needs to be full of sugar and packed with flavorings, but I guarantee you that a steaming-hot bowl of naturally buttery oats with a little drizzle of maple syrup can go toe to toe with Quaker's any day—and there's no rule that you can eat that only for breakfast. Then there's beans (which are a category of legumes): adzuki, kidney, black, lima, navy, you name it. So many different flavors and textures that will make your meals more filling and exciting than they ever were with meat. And have you ever seen the highest-quality meat selling for two dollars a pound or eighty-nine cents for a can? Probably not. You can't expect to feel like a million bucks if you keep eating from the dollar menu.

The other undeniable feature about legumes and grains is that they are going to supply you with the nutrients that you need. Let's start with whole grains.

Grains

I know some folks who are on modern diets like paleo or some shit say that grains cause inflammation and chronic disease. I'd say that's half-true because *refined* grains like bread, pasta, pizza crust, cereal, and baked goods will do those things. But listen when I tell you that whole grains have been part of the human diet for *tens of thousands of years*, and nothing has changed in the good-for-you department.

This food group in particular is the one I recommend people start really loading up on when they switch to a plant-based diet, making it the foundation of their meals. Grains are super filling; they're neutral tasting, so you can dress them up with all kinds of other ingredients, sweet or savory; and they really do bring a whole lot of nutrition to your plate. In particular, whole grains:

○ **Lower your risk of heart disease.** A review of ten studies found that three 1-ounce (28-gram) servings of whole grains daily may lower your risk of heart disease by 22 percent. And a ten-year study in almost eighteen thousand adults observed that those who ate the highest proportion of whole grains in relation to their total carb intake had a 47 percent lower risk of heart disease.

○ **Lower your risk of stroke.** In an analysis of six studies of nearly 250,000 people, participants who ate the most whole grains had a 14 percent lower risk of stroke than those eating the fewest.

○ **Prevent obesity and help weight loss.** Eating three servings of whole grains daily was linked to lower body mass index (BMI) and less belly fat in a review of fifteen studies of almost 120,000 people. That's most likely because eating fiber-rich foods—like whole grains instead of refined grains—can help fill you up and prevent overeating.

○ **Lower your risk of type 2 diabetes.** Studies have linked whole-grain intake to lower fasting blood sugar levels and improved insulin sensitivity. And since losing weight can also decrease insulin resistance, that's another way whole grains can help.

- **Reduce chronic inflammation.** Some evidence suggests that whole grains can help reduce inflammation. In one study, women who ate the most whole grains were least likely to die from inflammation-related chronic conditions. In another recent study, people who replaced refined wheat products with whole wheat products saw a reduction in inflammatory markers.

Replacing Refined Grains with Whole Grains

As I said before, not all grains are the same. The kinds of stripped-down grains that you find in many breads, pastas, and baked goods aren't the kind that are doing you any favors. For now, during these first thirty days, you can give yourself some grace with the kinds of processed foods you're buying. But by next month, we'll be taking a harder look at why you should steer clear of pretty much refined anything. In the meantime, here are some easy ways to get more whole grains into your diet:

- Make large batches of cooked grains and store them in your fridge to top with vegetables, legumes, and sauces/dressings.

- You can do the same thing with porridges, such as oats or quinoa, that you can enjoy with fruit, chia seeds, and other sweet things.

- Sprinkle toasted buckwheat groats on cereal or vegan yogurt.

- Have air-popped popcorn as a snack.

- Swap out white rice with brown rice, or for a different whole grain like quinoa or farro.

- Stir cooked grains into stews and soups.

- Use stone-ground corn tortillas—or tortillas made out of whole-grain flours like cassava or chickpea—instead of white flour tortillas in tacos.

Grains Cheat Sheet

Hundreds of varieties of grains are grown all around the world, but here's a small sampling of what you can most likely find at your local grocery store:

AMARANTH: This gluten-free and protein-rich grain is native to Peru. It has a nutty, toasted flavor and is just as good enjoyed in grain bowls and soups as it is cooked down into a porridge.

BARLEY: Barley is a nutty cereal grain that's full of protein and fiber. You can buy it with bran intact (hulled) or removed (pearled), which cooks quicker. It's got a good, sturdy texture for adding to salads and soups. And no, throwing back a beer doesn't count as a serving of barley.

BULGUR WHEAT: Bulgur is made from the grains of parboiled or steamed wheat kernels or berries. It's then dried, with some of the bran removed, and then further ground. It's a neutral-tasting grain that cooks fairly quickly, depending on how finely it's ground. You often see it as the foundation of tabbouleh, a Middle Eastern salad.

FARRO: Farro is an ancient grain that is a solid source of fiber, protein, and iron. It has a nice, firm texture that makes it as satisfying as tucking into a big bowl of pasta.

FREEKEH: This grain is a little smoky, a little nutty, and made from immature durum wheat. It has three times more fiber and two times more protein than white rice, rivaling quinoa in its macronutrient profile. You can buy it whole or cracked and boil it until tender.

It's often eaten in eastern Mediterranean and North African dishes like salads and pilafs.

OATS: You'd have to be a real smart-ass to know that oats are actually a cereal grass, but for our purposes let's just call them a grain and move on. You probably know oats for their smooth, creamy goodness, but what you probably don't know is how rich they are in protein, fat, and carbohydrates, as well as beta-glucans. Beta-glucans are sugar compounds found in bacteria, yeast, some mushrooms, algae, and plants such as oats and barley. They're a source of soluble fiber. Unlike insoluble fiber, which is that great intestine-scrubbing stuff we get from fruits and vegetables, soluble fiber can be dissolved by water and then feeds the gut directly. Research has shown that beta-glucans may reduce high cholesterol, lower triglyceride levels, and improve skin conditions like eczema.

WHEN GRAINS MIGHT NOT BE FOR YOU

There are some people—granted, not a lot, but some—for whom whole grains may not be a good fit. If you have celiac disease or gluten sensitivity, then gluten-containing grains like wheat, barley, and rye are out. But buckwheat, rice, oats, quinoa, and amaranth are in. For those of you with IBS, whole grains may cause digestive distress. Know that this is because your digestive system isn't where it needs to be. Working with your health-care provider—ideally one who knows their way around a plant-based diet—to heal this condition will mean that you'll most likely get to enjoy whole grains eventually.

QUINOA: I remember walking into a Whole Foods once and asking for *keenawoo*. I'm holding up my phone trying to show the guy a picture of it, and he's like, "Oooh, quinoa." I've been there when it comes to making an ass of myself because I don't know how to pronounce this stuff. So now you don't have to; it's *keen-waah*. Say it with me now. *Keenwaaah*. Good.

Quinoa isn't technically a grain—it's a seed. It comes from the goosefoot plant from the Andes Mountains. But we embrace it with open arms into the grain family because texturally it's very similar to things like couscous and rice, and it's one of the few plant-based proteins that provide all nine essential amino acids, or the crucial compounds that help your body perform just about every important function. One thing to remember with quinoa

STORING AND COOKING YOUR GRAINS

STORING AND COOKING YOUR BEANS

Whole, intact grains can last as long as six months at room temperature (and even longer in the freezer). The best way to get the most mileage out of your shopping—especially if you're buying in bulk, which I encourage you to do because it'll save you money—is to store your grains in airtight containers with tight-fitting lids. Even a zip-top plastic bag can do the trick.

Because there are so many different types of grains, there's no universal way to cook them. But I can assure you that it's not rocket science and usually just involves a pot and some boiling salted water. The packaging for the grains will give you cooking instructions. Or if you're buying in bulk, go to the Whole Grains Council (wholegrainscouncil.org).

Oh, and I don't know why this is hard for some people to figure out, but cook your grains *while* you make the rest of your dinner; that way they're ready to go when it's time to eat. Or better yet, cook up enough to last you the week and store it in the fridge.

Like grains, the best way to buy beans is in bulk because you're getting the most bang for your buck (and also not wasting a ton of plastic packaging). You can store beans in an airtight container at room temperature for *up to a year*. Although, I do hope you're cooking beans more often than that.

As for cooking beans, you have a couple of options: You can buy them canned and just drain them, rinse them, and heat them up (totally fine with me); or you can cook them from dried. I always recommend soaking your beans first, usually overnight, which helps break down the starches that give beans the reputation of the musical fruit . . . After that, beans can be simmered on the stove or in an Instant Pot, if that's something you already have in the kitchen. A good resource for bean cook times is the Bean Institute (beaninstitute.com).

is that the seeds have a protective coating called saponins, which keep the seed from being absorbed by the body of the animals who eat it. That way their poop is like free fertilization and transportation for more quinoa plants. But we want to unlock that nutrition, so you should rinse your quinoa before cooking it. A few minutes under cold running water will do it.

RICE: Those little grains you see are actually the endosperm of the rice plant, where all the energy is held. That's what makes rice a carbohydrate- and protein-filled powerhouse. We're not talking about what you're getting at Panda Express, the stripped-down stuff that's had its nutrient-filled husk, bran, and germ removed. No, we're talking about the hundreds of varieties that exist—brown, black, jasmine, red, short, long, medium, just to name a few. Surprisingly to some, wild rice (like oats) is actually the grain of four different species of grass. Though technically it's not a rice, it's commonly referred to as one for practical purposes.

Legumes

Like whole grains, legumes are a no-bullshit way of loading up your plate with hearty, filling, nutrient-packed meals. And like whole grains, legumes are the real deal when it comes to how they can impact your health. Legumes are a rich source of plant protein, in addition to fiber and a wide array of vitamins, minerals—including iron—antioxidants, and phytochemicals. A number of studies and controlled trials suggest that replacing meat with legumes can have a positive impact on life span, blood sugar control, and cardiovascular disease risk. Eating legumes has also been associated with a reduced risk of colorectal cancer, and soybeans and soybean-based products in particular are linked to a reduction in LDL cholesterol levels.

Plus, like whole grains, you get a ton of variety—there are over four hundred different varieties of beans—and you don't have to have gone to culinary school to be able to prepare them. It doesn't require a lot of imagination to use them either—most would be at home tossed into salads, soups, stews, and pasta and rice dishes. Here are some that you might come across:

Legumes Cheat Sheet

ADZUKIS: Adzukis are a type of red bean that is traditionally used in both sweet and savory dishes because they're slightly sweet, but overall, pretty nutty and mild.

ANASAZIS: *Anasazi* is Navajo for "the ancient ones," and these beans come from the American Southwest. They turn pale pink when cooked and have a nice, meaty texture that makes them perfect for baked bean dishes, mixing with rice, and pretty much anything Tex-Mex.

BLACK BEANS: Black beans are some of the most common legumes you'll find in cooking, mostly because they're versatile and have a mild, not-too-beany flavor. They can be used in just about any bean dish that calls for legumes.

BLACK-EYED PEAS: These have an earthy taste and a dense texture that's similar to chickpeas and white beans.

CANNELLINI BEANS: Sometimes called white kidney beans, cannellini beans are one of the largest types of white bean, which makes them nice and meaty. They hold up well in soups and stews or when tossed into salads and, like other white beans, have a mild, nutty flavor.

CHICKPEAS (GARBANZOS): Chickpeas have a mild, slightly sweet flavor and a great meaty texture that holds its own in any dish you add them to. They're also great mashed (like in hummus) or roasted into crispy bites that you can use for texture in a salad or eat as a snack.

FAVA BEANS: You can buy these fresh if you see them at the farmers market or dried. They're a little bitter, a little sweet, and are great stirred into just about anything that you're cooking.

FAYOT (FLAGEOLET) BEANS: These dudes are small, tender, and creamy with a mild flavor. You most often see them in French cuisine, but there's no need to get fancy when you eat them.

GREAT NORTHERN BEANS: These are pretty much the mildest of the beans, which means they're great at taking on flavor. In addition to all the ways you'd normally eat a bean, smashed white beans with a little salt, maybe some garlic, and a drizzle of olive oil is a killer dip.

KIDNEY BEANS: You've probably had your fair share of kidney beans, since that's what you find in chili. In fact, thanks to the fact that they're big and beefy beans, you won't miss the meat if you make your favorite chili, omit the meat, and double up on beans.

LENTILS: These tiny guys can be prepared in various ways and come in a number of different varieties (French, black, brown, red, and so on). Each has its own unique flavor and texture, making some better for creamy stews (red) and others for salads (French, black, brown). They're also a great mild-tasting canvas for layering on spices, herbs, dressings, and other flavors.

LIMA BEANS: Sometimes also called butter beans, depending on where you live, lima beans are typically small light-green beans that look like seeds. You may have seen them tossed in with carrots and peas in succotash. They have a mild flavor and creamy texture.

MUNG BEANS: Mung beans are cultivated in East Asia, Southeast Asia, and the Indian subcontinent. They're small green beans that have a slightly sweet, nutty flavor.

NAVY BEANS: Navy beans are another type of white bean. They don't hold their shape as well as great northern beans but are still hearty and tender with a creamy texture and mild taste. They are commonly eaten in white beans and rice (a southern dish), navy bean chowder, and Boston-style baked beans. They also taste great in salads and pasta dishes.

PEAS: That's right, peas are beans too. But whether you want to eat them as a veggie or a bean, it doesn't matter so long as you enjoy them in all their nutritional glory. I like to keep a stash in the freezer and toss 'em into soups and pastas as they're cooking.

PINTO BEANS: Pinto beans are who you have to thank for refried beans, and they also make an appearance in chili. They're creamy, earthy, nutty, and a fan favorite.

RED BEANS: Often used in Caribbean, Latin, Cajun, and Creole cuisines, red beans are kind of the classic bean: earthy, mild, slightly sweet, nutty, and with a soft texture. They're great for soups, chilis, and, obviously, red beans and rice.

SOYBEANS: Soybeans get a lot of side-eye because soy itself has such a bad rep. But, as you'll read below, organic, minimally processed soy can be a healthy part of your diet. And soybeans, being the least processed of all, are great for eating alone (think edamame when you go out for Japanese food) or mixing into salads and soups.

To Soy or Not to Soy: Seitan, Tofu, and Tempeh

Like most plants that haven't been fucked with in a lab or food processing facility, soy in its whole form is actually good for you. It's high in nutrients that you find in most other legumes, like fiber, iron, magnesium, potassium, protein, and zinc. What usually gets people all worked up about soy is that it naturally contains a type of phytoestrogens called isoflavones. People hear "estrogen" and think soy is going to mess with their hormones. But soy contains a "selective estrogen receptor modulator" that helps estrogen do the good stuff (like make your bones stronger) and not the bad (increase your risk of breast cancer). In fact, researchers have found that women diagnosed with breast cancer who ate the most whole soy lived significantly longer and had a much lower risk of breast cancer recurrence than those who ate less.

Then there are fermented soy products like tempeh, miso, and fermented bean curd. Fermentation is an aging process that converts and breaks down amino acids in the soy. As a result, the health benefits of soy become even more bioavailable, or more easily absorbed by your body. Fermented soy proteins are associated with disease prevention and overall improved health. They can help reduce your risk of osteoporosis, support heart health (they contain essential nutrients like niacin, calcium, magnesium, folate, potassium, and copper), and may ease the symptoms of menopause.

Protein Alternatives: Tempeh, Tofu, and Seitan

Soy also deserves an honorable mention because it's the foundation of two of the three main protein alternatives: tofu and tempeh. These meat stand-ins, along with seitan, can get some eye rolls from meat-eating folks because they sound like some hippy-dippy shit. But I assure you, when you've got a case of the meats and want something filling and tasty to eat, you're gonna be thanking me for introducing you to these three clutch players.

TEMPEH

Tempeh is made from soybeans that have been fermented and cooked. It's then formed into a pressed cake, which has a nice, sturdy texture. That, in addition to its mild nutty flavor, is what makes it ideal for slicing up for sandwiches, throwing on the grill, or cutting up into cubes that can be roasted as nuggets or added to stews and salads.

TOFU

Tofu is what you get when soybeans get soaked in water, crushed, and boiled. Then the pulp is strained out, leaving behind the "milk." The soy-milk gets coagulated, and the curds get strained out and pressed into tofu. Depending on how long the curds are pressed, the tofu can be either nice and firm (great for tossing in some marinade and roasting or stir-frying) or soft and silky (perfect for blending into smoothies or making creamy dressings).

SEITAN

Meet seitan, aka "wheat meat." Although seitan is not a nutritious whole food like tempeh and tofu because it is technically a processed food (it's made out of wheat gluten), I wanted to give you a formal introduction because there's a time and a place for seitan in your diet—especially as you kick off your plant-based journey. Seitan is what a lot of processed vegan food is made from (chicken wings, cutlets, burgers) and comes in a ton of different flavors (bacon, chorizo, barbecue, and so on). So while it's not necessarily a health food, it is in bounds and is one way for you to enjoy your meals when you're missing meat.

Fats Make the Meal

As I mentioned in chapter 7, a little healthy fat is nothing to be afraid of. In fact, adding a little to your plate or bowl can be the difference between a meal that gets the job done and one that gets the job done *right*. They're not only loaded with good-for-you nutrients; they're also the ingredients that bring that little sump'n sump'n to the party. When it comes to whipping up a quick meal, think about how fat can make things a little bit more interesting.

Here are some fats to get familiar with:

Fats Cheat Sheet

AVOCADO: Creamy, rich avocados are like the butter of the plant world. I can't think of any dish that doesn't get better with a scoop. Luckily, avocados are also really good for you because they're packed with heart-healthy monounsaturated fat, specifically oleic acid. Oleic acid—also the main fat

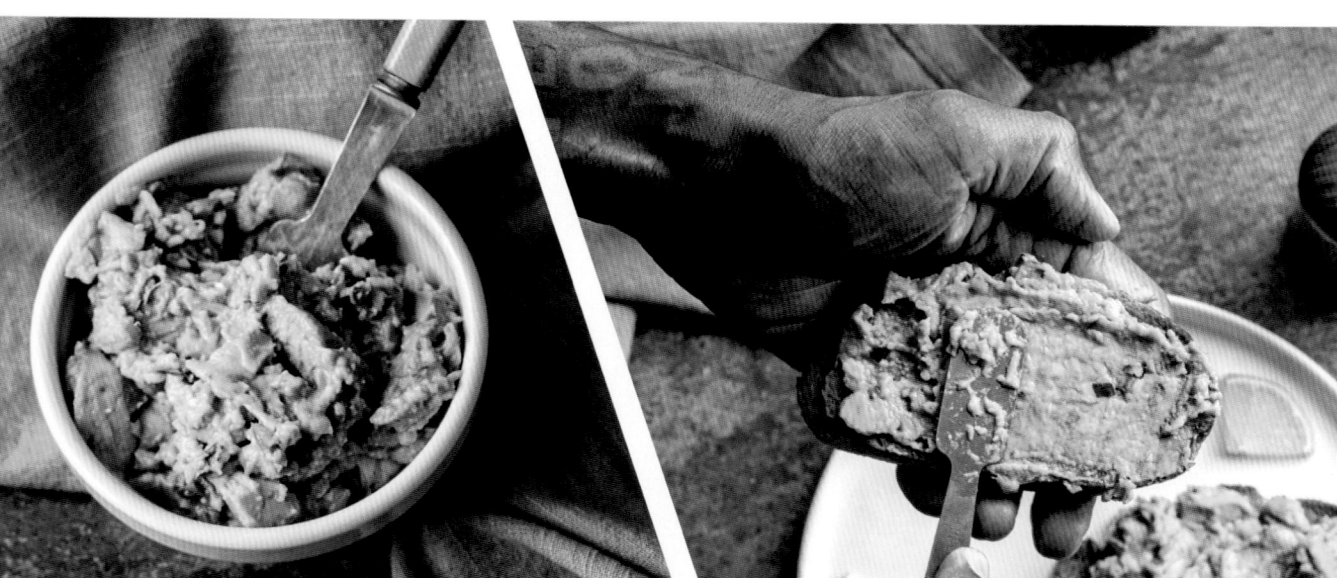

in olive oil—is anti-inflammatory; lowers unhealthy LDL cholesterol and increases healthy HDL cholesterol; and reduces your risk of stroke and coronary heart disease. And here's another fun fact of the day: Avocados have twice the potassium of bananas.

CACAO: We're not talking about the sad sack of cocoa powder that you bought for banana bread five years ago and haven't used since. And we're definitely not talking about a packet of Swiss Miss. Cacao comes from South America, where it was domesticated five thousand years ago. Ever since, the beans from the trees have been harvested to make both cocoa and cacao. The difference between them is in the processing: Cocoa is heated at high temperatures to create a smooth, sweet taste. Cacao, on the other hand, is processed at a low temperature before being milled into a powder or crushed into nibs. As a result, it retains its original nutritional value, which is off the charts. It's particularly rich in flavonoids, which are nutrients that have been shown to help lower blood pressure, improve blood flow to the brain and heart, and help prevent blood clots. Cacao also helps increase insulin sensitivity, decrease the risk of heart disease, and reduce inflammation throughout the body. But what I'm most excited about is the intense, rich, chocolaty flavor you get when you add a scoop of powdered cacao or cacao nibs to your oats, granola, or smoothies.

CHIA SEEDS: These little black seeds are originally from Mexico and were eaten by Aztec warriors for energy and endurance. Chia seeds are a good source of calcium as well as potassium and magnesium, and they're also hydrophilic, meaning they absorb water—almost twelve times their weight's worth. When they do, they take on a gel-like texture. In your body, that retained water helps you feel full and also helps hydrate the beneficial bacteria in your gut. In the kitchen, that cool texture is what makes chia great for puddings and smoothie bowls.

COCONUT: Some jerks might tell you that coconut is high in saturated fat and should therefore be avoided. While it's technically true, the type of saturated fat in coconut is in the form of medium-chain triglycerides. That's different than saturated fat from animals, which comes in the form of long-chain triglycerides. The long-chain triglycerides come into the body ready to be stored up, as in, in your ass. Medium-chain, on the other hand, show up in your liver ready to be used as energy. So when you're looking for new products to play with as a badass vegan, check out coconut milk and yogurt, and add coconut flakes or sprinkles to your meals.

NUTS: Nuts are one of the healthiest foods and one of the healthiest sources of fat. They're a plant-based source of protein, and they contain fiber, which keeps your belly full and your gut happy. There are also tons of varieties, each of which has its own unique flavor—cashews, almonds, walnuts, macadamia nuts, pecans, hazelnuts, just to name a few. You can eat them by the handful, sprinkle them over your meals for texture, soak them and blend them into milks, or grind them into butters.

OLIVE OIL: Those Greeks got it right with this one—thousands of studies have proven that olive oil is associated with minimizing the risk of cardiovascular disease, type 2 diabetes, cancer, and Alzheimer's disease, while also lowering inflammation. Which, as you remember, is the root of pretty much all disease. Do yourself a favor and buy an organic bottle that's not the shittiest but also not the most expensive. You'll end up with one that tastes good and can be what you reach for to make salad dressings and marinades or to drizzle over salads, grains, soups, and roasted vegetables.

OLIVES: These tasty, salty little bites are a great flavor weapon in the vegan kitchen. Not only are they rich in healthy fat, they're also high in antioxidants. You can't go wrong with any kind you find at the store, except for the ones stuffed with blue cheese.

TAHINI: This seed butter, commonly used in Middle Eastern cuisine, is made from ground sesame seeds. If you've ever had hummus, then you've had tahini. On its own, it's full of healthy fats and protein and has a deep sesame flavor. I like to use it in dressings, when I'm making my own hummus, and drizzled straight up over just about everything.

To view the references cited in this chapter, please visit badassvegan.com/citations.

CHAPTER 10

JUMP-START MEAL IDEAS AND QUICK HITTERS

There's just one more tool left for me to give you before you go out into the world and start living your best plant-based life: meal ideas. Some books will give you a week's worth of recipes as a menu for you to kick things off. I can see how that would be helpful in terms of providing guidelines for a new way of eating, but what really ends up happening is that you go to the grocery store, spend a ton of money, and then feel either pressure to make yourself a different recipe for every single meal or like you're captive to these meals. That's not exactly a winning argument for plant-based eating being inexpensive, simple, and fun.

Instead, what I'd like to do is two things: First, I want to give you permission to eat the same thing every day. I know I just got done telling you that there's so much variety in the plant world that you'll never get bored—and that's true—but here's the thing: Don't feel like you *have* to change it up every single day. Actually, it's easier if you don't. Once you find a meal that you love, you don't have to leave it behind just because you feel like you should. Have those oats every morning. Eat that rice and beans every night. Change it up with different fruits, veggies, and dressings. Throw some hot sauce on that shit. The consistency can be really helpful, not only because it takes some of the heavy lifting out of meal planning in the beginning but also because that's how people tend to like to eat. If you think about it, before the industrialized world, that's how people had to eat. You ate what was around. If you grew up under a mango tree, you ate damn mangoes every day. So now we're spoiled. But I know that I personally do better when I eat the same thing every day. The consistency helps me keep track of how I'm doing with my macros (which you don't have to worry about just yet; we'll be getting to that in part III), and also, it's just one less thing to think about. And you know what? I'm never bored, and I *always* enjoy what I eat.

Second, I want you to understand that you can change things up on a weekly basis instead of a daily one. Eat the same thing every day for one week, and hey, if you have an all-time favorite, don't feel bad about carrying it over to the next week. By eating the same things that you love every day, you dispel not only the myth that vegan is boring, but also the myth that eating vegan is expensive . . . imagine how much "bread" you are saving.

So flip ahead to the recipes (see part IV, page 160), and find one or maybe two that speak to you. Then eat those things all week. You'll not only be eating what you enjoy but also be saving a shitload of money and time. Maybe it's the Berrylicious or Chocolate Smoothie (page 172 and page 177) in the morning. Double up batches of my Badass Sweet Potato Soup (page 193), Smoky Spicy Mountain Chili (page 232), or Pasta al Pesto (page 230) for easy lunches and dinners to have on hand. Then the next week, change it up. You'll still be getting in some variety in terms of the plants you're eating; it will just be week to week instead of day to day. So long as you're enjoying what you're eating, you're doing it right. And if the kitchen is your happy place and you love to try new recipes, that's what they are there for! Go crazy.

Quick-Hit Meals and Snacks

The other secret to meal-planning success is knowing how to put together simple ingredients quickly so you always feel like you have something to eat. Something you *want* to eat. These days, everybody knows how to pop something in the microwave, but few people know how to make a meal with just a few simple steps. These are some mini "recipes" that you can reach for—and no, you're not gonna mess them up. They're also cheap and don't require a lot of ingredients because most of 'em came from when I was broke and would need to figure out what I could eat from the few groceries I had.

BANANAS ON A DATE: Add 4 to 5 dates to a blender (or, if you're greedy like me, make that 6 or 7). Add about ¼ cup of water with a pinch of cinnamon, nutmeg, and allspice. Blend it up until it's nice and smooth, adding more water if you need it. Slice 3 bananas and toss 'em in a bowl. Top with the date mixture, some shredded coconut, and sliced almonds.

CARAMEL APPLE: Make some date caramel as you do above and dip some sliced apple in there.

BAKED APPLE: Preheat your oven to 350°F. Slice an apple and toss with a pinch of cinnamon and nutmeg. Bake for 15 minutes, just long enough to get that apple pie flavor. Better yet, make a whole tray so you can get an even quicker hit later.

GRILLED PEACH WITH MAPLE SYRUP: Halve a peach and discard the pit. Pour a little maple syrup into the "well" where the pit was. Put the peach skin side down on the grill until you see the syrup start to bubble. Have this for dessert, or if you want to eat a grilled maple peach for breakfast, it won't stop the continuum of time.

GRANOLA: Preheat your oven to 350°F. In a big bowl, toss together 2 cups rolled oats and 1 cup dried fruit, plus any nuts and seeds you like. Spread it out over a pan. Drizzle it all with about ¼ cup maple syrup and bake it until it's golden brown, about 20 minutes.

FRUIT SALAD: Grab 4 or 5 of your favorite fruits, slice them up, and toss them with some shredded coconut, maybe even some granola. Makes a great breakfast or a snack.

QUINOA OATMEAL: Fuck those little maple brown sugar instant oatmeal packets; make your own oatmeal and swap in quinoa for the oats. Rinse and drain 1 cup of quinoa and put it in a medium pot. For extra credit, toast it over medium heat until it smells nutty. Otherwise, skip to pouring in 2 cups of nut milk and 1 tablespoon of maple syrup. Cook until the liquid has absorbed and the quinoa is tender, about 15 minutes. Throw on some fresh fruit and call it breakfast.

CAULIFLOWER RICE PILAF: Instead of using rice, use riced cauliflower. Simmer it in a pan until it's tender, along with veggies like snow peas and diced carrots. Or if you're looking to really make a bang, add some tofu or tempeh.

PEANUT BUTTER CHOCOLATE MELT: Put some vegan chocolate chips in a small pot and pour a little agave in there plus a little nut milk to help loosen everything up. Heat it over medium-low for about 15 seconds, until it's a melty sauce. Pour it over some peanut butter and try to figure out what took you so long to become a vegan.

BROKE-AS-HELL SPECIAL: This was my go-to bowl that I'd make when I had barely any money for groceries, but you better believe I still eat this even though I'm no longer broke. I batch-cook and then assemble quinoa or other grains, baked or fried sweet plantains, grilled onions, and guacamole or sliced avo.

HUMMUS POPS: I got the idea for this when I didn't feel like hummus but wanted something similar. All you do is add drained, rinsed, and dried canned chickpeas and a

ADD A SHAKE

Most days, especially if I'm really busy or I know I'll be spending a long stretch at the gym, I like adding a shake into my rotation for some instant nutrition. I even developed my own brand of them, Badass Vegan. You don't necessarily need to buy my formula; so long as you're getting one that's 100 percent plant-based (i.e., casein-free), you're heading in the right direction. Then you can count your shake toward one of your carbohydrate or protein blocks.

little olive oil to a pan, plus a pinch of cumin, turmeric, and salt (the seasonings in hummus). Heat until the chickpeas start to crisp up.

SPICY CHEESE DIP: I learned this recipe almost ten years ago and people who eat it don't believe that it's vegan. I've seriously won cooking competitions with this no-cheese cheese, serving it without telling anyone it was vegan. Then after the judges were done losing their minds, I'd let them in on the little secret. In a blender, combine 1 cup cashews, 1 chopped red bell pepper, 1 chopped jalapeño, a pinch of sea salt, and ½ cup of water. Blend it up, adding more water if necessary to loosen the sauce. Dip veggies, chips, your fingers, you name it.

NAUGHTY BUT NICE CREAM: Add 2 to 3 frozen bananas (or more, if you're feeling frisky) and ¼ cup of water to a blender and blend until it's smooth like soft serve. Eat it as is, or blend in flavorings like cacao, fresh mint, even grapes. More people should understand the amazing combo that is grapes and bananas.

AVOCADO MOUSSE: In a blender, combine 6 pitted dates, 1 peeled and pitted Hass avocado, 3 teaspoons cocoa or cacao powder, and ½ cup plus 2 tablespoons water. Blend until smooth. Serve over fresh berries, maybe with some maple syrup.

CHIA PUDDING: The basic ratio here is 2 tablespoons of chia seeds for every ½ cup of water or nut milk. All you do is stir the two together by hand (not in a blender) and then let it set in the fridge for a couple of hours or overnight. You can add everything from chopped dates to your favorite fruit to maple syrup or agave to coconut flakes. Choose your own adventure.

EATING
FOR LIF
THE NEXT
THIRTY DAYS
AND BEYOND

PART III

You did it—**YOU MADE IT TO THIRTY DAYS** eating all the plants you can possibly eat. Maybe you had a couple of slips and some animal food just *happened* to make it into your mouth, but the important thing is that you got back on track and added a few more days of eating plants to the bank. And now you're cashing that check and taking things to the next level.

That's right, **IT'S TIME TO LEVEL UP**—but you've done a lot of the hard work already. Now we're going to take everything you learned during the previous four weeks and fine-tune it just a little bit so that you can really **START MOVING THE NEEDLE.** What that needle is could be anything, depending on your personal goals. Is it getting cut? Losing weight? Having more endurance? Being able to keep up with your grandkids? Decreasing the amount of medication that you're taking? Whatever it is, the information you learn in this part is going to get you there. You'll still be getting your plant buffet on, but now you're going to go a little deeper into how food works in your body, and more importantly, how it can *work for you*.

These next few chapters are leading up to a plan I created called the Building Block Plan. This is a simple—seriously, it's **HELLA EASY**—way to figure out not just how many calories you should be eating a day (for the body you *want*, not the body you *have*), but more importantly, how to move around your macronutrients like a game of *Tetris* in order to burn fat, gain energy, lose weight, put on muscle, or maintain whatever gains you've made. My Building Block Plan conceives of macronutrients as blocks to put together throughout the day (or doses, if you want to keep thinking of your food in terms of medicine, which is a true story). It was extremely helpful to me when I first started eating a plant-based diet because it took the mystery out of what to eat and how much. I knew I needed so many blocks, or doses, of carbohydrates, fats, and proteins a day. And by manipulating how many of them I was eating and in what ratios, I saw the effects in how my body looked and felt.

The Building Block Plan consists of three phases, or "Floors," each lasting one month: **THE BURNER, THE BOOST,** and **THE BUILDER**. During these time frames, the number and types of blocks you'll be playing around with will change. That's because the ratio of blocks you eat produces different results. During the first month, you'll be eating fewer blocks of carbohydrates and fat, and more blocks of protein. By month two, you'll have more blocks of carbohydrates and a few less of protein. And by month three, you'll be eating mostly carbohydrate blocks, with blocks of protein and fat in supporting roles.

This approach is designed to **KICK-START** the process of burning off any extra fat stores you've been lugging around, then shift your body into high gear making lean muscle, and then finally get to a solid, healthy place for your body to stay at—in theory—for the rest of your life.

CHAPTER 11

DAILY DOSAGE
Carbohydrates, Fats, and Proteins

Macro- and micronutrients are literally what your food is made out of and what give your body the energy and nourishment it needs to run right. Your macros are the biggies: carbohydrates, protein, and fat. I like to think of these groups as doses, like you'd get with medicine—after all, we're doing right by Hippocrates and letting your medicine be your food and your food be your medicine. Each of these macronutrients delivers unique benefits, so it's up to us to figure out how many doses you need of each to maximize what we want out of your body's performance. What's surprising to a lot of people is how much *less* protein you need than you've been programmed to believe and, on the flip side, how much more carbohydrates and healthy fats you can eat and still look and feel the way you want to.

Micronutrients, on the other hand, are the vitamins and minerals your body needs to both function and fend off chronic ailments. Luckily, you can hit most of your micronutrient targets without breaking a sweat if you're eating a varied whole food, plant-based diet (translation: a shitload of different kinds of unprocessed plants). There are some micronutrients you can't get from food, but meat eaters and vegans are both in that same boat, and in chapter 15 we'll talk more about how to get what you need with supplements. Just remember that getting in your macros and micros doesn't just keep you powered up and healthy; it also keeps you feeling satisfied and happy—which to me is what it's all about.

Carbohydrates: The Queen Bey

Macronutrients are like Destiny's Child—you need all three members to make good music. But no shade to Kelly and Michelle, it was Beyoncé who made it a *show*. All the macronutrients are important, and you want to hit all three in every meal, but the one that should get prime real estate on your plate—and for good reason—is carbohydrates.

Unlike protein and fat, carbohydrates are what your body, including your brain, naturally uses as fuel. When you eat carbohydrates, they're first converted into glucose, then stored in your liver and your muscles as glycogen until they're used as energy down the road. When you move your body, that stored glycogen is what gets used as fuel. And if you burn through that glycogen, then your body moves on to using stored fat. Protein, contrary to popular opinion, barely figures into that equation.

But before you go thinking that you can cheat the system by skipping the glycogen step just to burn fat—something low-carb diets like keto argue you can do—keep in mind that your most important muscle, the brain, is not designed to run on anything other than glycogen. Keeping your body in a constant state of ketosis (what it's called when your liver is forced to start making ketone bodies as emergency fuel because it's out of glycogen) can have negative effects on your long-term health. Eating a carbohydrate-rich diet, on the other hand, is the best way to kick your body into a safe, sustainable fat-burning mode. But beyond that—and much more importantly—we *need* carbohydrates. They don't just power your tissues and cells; they're also necessary for the health of your cardiovascular system, central nervous system, and digestive system.

Which brings me to: the gut. Not your beer belly but the trillions of microorganisms that live in this part of your digestive system. Some of these bacteria are good for you, but some are inflammation causing. The goal is to keep the good guys healthy and fed so that they're not overrun by the bad guys. What feeds the bad guys? Meat, dairy, and processed sugar. What do the good guys eat? Fiber, fiber, and more fiber. The soluble kind that comes from plant-based carbohydrates. When they're feeling good, you do too. When there is more good bacteria than bad bacteria present, it leads to decreased inflammation, decreased digestive issues like IBS and diverticulitis, a decreased risk of colon cancer, a decrease in bloating, and an increase in energy. And because your gut talks to all of your body—including your brain, hormones, and immune system—a healthy gut also means keeping your stress at healthy levels, your metabolism revved up, and your moods balanced, not to mention that you'll be sick less often. That all starts with carbohydrates.

Carbohydrates are also one of the most nutritious macros because high-carbohydrate foods are like tiny micronutrient powerhouses. Board-certified family physician Dr. Joel Fuhrman developed the Aggregate Nutrient Density Index (or ANDI) score to grade foods based on the micronutrition they provide. The grades range from 1 (least nutrient dense) to 1,000 (most nutrient dense). I won't leave you in suspense about which foods get the top scores—that's right, carbohydrates from whole plants (not Little Debbie snack cakes and apple juice).

Which foods get the top scores? That's right, carbohydrates from **WHOLE PLANTS**.

Protein: Your Overhype Man

Okay, fine, it's not completely overrated, because protein is crucial for things like building muscle, repairing muscle tissues, making essential hormones and enzymes, and even keeping your immune system functioning. But when it comes to eating to be healthy and strong, protein just isn't at the top of the list of recommendations. That's not because protein is inherently bad; it's just because (1) you don't actually need that much protein for peak function, and (2) you get plenty of the stuff by eating whole food, plant-based carbohydrates like grains, beans, lentils, and some vegetables. Nutrition experts, dietitians, and sports scientists agree that it's ideal for all people to consume 0.8 grams of protein per kilogram (0.36 pounds) of body weight. That comes out to 56 grams per day for the average man and 46 grams per day for the average woman. Now consider the fact that just 1 cup of lentils has 18 grams of protein, a serving of seitan has 25 grams, and 1 cup of most beans has 15. That right there is 58 grams in one meal, and you haven't even counted in any other naturally protein-containing foods you've had that day (which is most of them).

Then there's the important point about where plant protein really stacks up against animal-based sources: It's no consolation prize. Protein is made up of twenty amino acids, and your body needs to collect the whole set of them to make a "complete protein." We make eleven of those amino acids, which means we need to get the other nine from our food. Well, all nine are found in plant foods. A recent study published in the *American Journal of Clinical Nutrition* compared the muscle and strength of men and women who ate a plant-based diet with that of omnivores. The researchers found that so long as people were eating enough protein, it didn't matter whether it was plant- or animal-based. There's no specific nutritional requirement that we need our protein to come from animals or animal-based food. We just need protein, and not too much of it.

But really, the funniest part of the protein myth is that people don't even understand what protein is. When people ask me the age-old question of "Where do you get your protein?," that's when I come back with this mind-boggling response: "I'm not worried about my protein; I'm focused on my amino acids." And if I'm feeling nice, I'll explain what an amino acid is. Then I hit them with this follow-up question: "Since you are so worried about my protein, can you name any of the essential amino acids that we need?" Ten out of ten times, the answer is . . . no. The next time you find yourself in this position, feel free to rattle these off: histidine, iso-leucine, leucine, lysine, methionine, phenylalanine, threonine, tryptophan, and valine.

You can also let them know that you can get all nine by eating foods like quinoa, buckwheat, hempseeds, chia seeds, and spirulina; or by enjoying a variety of nuts and nut butters, seeds, grains, legumes, and tofu.

Fat: The Backup Generator

When I first introduced you to healthy fat in chapter 7, we talked about how it's a surprising but necessary part of your diet. That's because fat helps absorb nutrients, produces hormones, supports cell growth, and is the second-preferred source of fuel for your body (after carbohydrates). Hear that, protein?! If you run out of carbohydrate energy, your body dips into the fat reserve. That said, you do need to be smart about how you're harnessing fat's powers. Fat packs a lot of calories per gram, or is what's known as "calorie dense." Basically, if you're trying to hit a caloric goal in order to lose weight or not gain weight, then you want to be mindful of how many calories you're taking in versus burning up as energy. Foods rich in healthy fats, like nuts, oil, coconut, and avocado, will max you out on calories more quickly than, say, carbohydrate-rich foods. They're also not as filling, and more importantly, they're not as rich in nutrients and fiber. Think of it this way: A tablespoon of olive oil has 119 calories. You'd have to eat about 4 cups of kale just to hit that. For now, understand that fat doesn't necessarily make you fat if you (1) eat it in moderation and (2) eat the best possible sources of it, which will always be minimally processed and plant-based.

////

Minimally processed and plant-based is going to be the name of the game not just for fats but for carbohydrates and protein too. That's because not all plant foods are created equal; not all plant foods are necessarily good for you or your goals. This isn't me going back on my promise that plant foods are superior—it's just that like the humans we are, we've found a way to fuck things up for ourselves, and our food is included in that. In the next chapter, we'll take a closer look at the details of building a plant-based diet that will do you and your health a favor in the long run.

To view the references cited in this chapter, please visit badassvegan.com/citations.

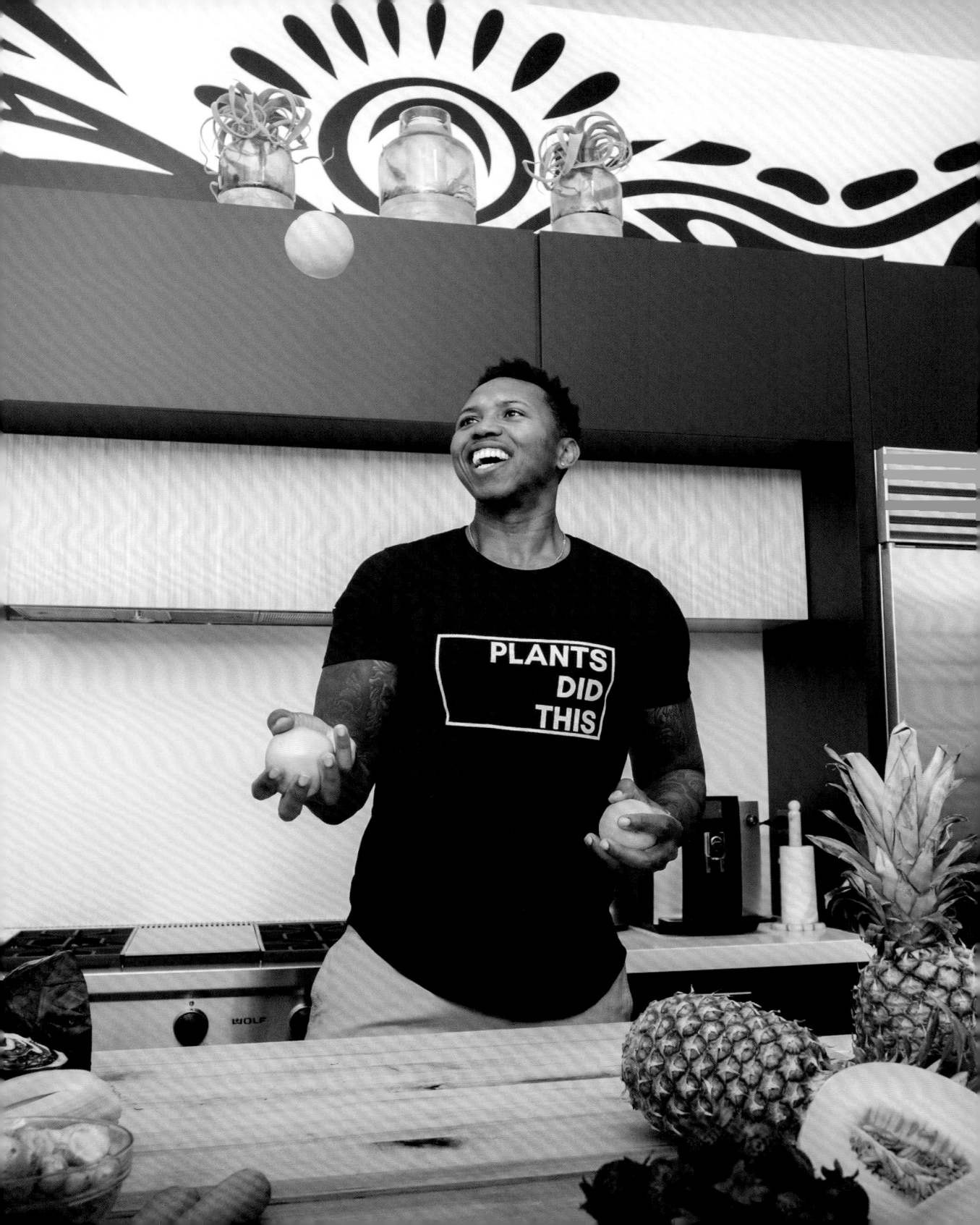

CHAPTER 12

NOT ALL PLANT FOODS ARE CREATED EQUAL

During the first thirty days, I didn't want you to have any restrictions on what you were eating so long as it was plant-based. But now that we're getting down to the nitty-gritty, it's time to talk about the fact that just because a food is plant-based doesn't mean it's good for you. I like vegan birthday cake as much as the next guy, but if I'm really trying to do right by my health and my body, I'm going to do my best to go for plant foods that come out of the ground and not out of a factory. In this chapter, I'll break down how things like processed sugar, certain types of fat, and additives can stand in the way of you achieving your health goals, even if you're following a plant-based diet. Are processed plant-based foods still preferable to animal foods? Damn straight. Is there still a time and place for your favorite treats? Hell yes. This isn't about talking you out of processed food *completely* but giving you an idea of how these choices stack up when it comes to keeping your ass out of the doctor's office.

Sugar: The Other White Powder

I think it's safe to say that if processed food companies were dealers, then we'd all be junkies because sugar is one of the most addicting substances in our food. Actually, researchers now know that sugar is just as addictive as heroin because of how it lights up our brain's pleasure centers and leaves it jonesing for more. So don't go underestimating sugar—it's a completely legal drug that our food system allows to be pumped into just about anything packaged you can buy. Food manufacturers know that if they give us the sweet goods, then we're going to come back for more. The problem with this is that sugar doesn't just manipulate our brains; it can also increase your risk for heart disease, type 2 diabetes, fatty liver, depression, and cancer. And it accelerates how quickly your body ages (i.e., degrades) and decreases your energy and drive. Sugar is literally sucking the life out of you. Luckily, when you kick sugar, you'll see the effects in days. You'll sleep better, think more clearly, and feel more balanced; get fewer headaches, migraines, and menstrual cramps; and most likely see a drop in your blood pressure.

The easiest way to "Just Say No" to sugar is to stick with whole-plant foods. And no, you don't have to be worried about the naturally occurring sugar in fruit because that sugar is bound to fiber, which changes the way your body can use that sugar for fuel. Processed sugar, or sugar that's been separated from its original plant source, is what we're talking about here. Food that comes in packaging is most likely going to be the biggest offender, especially if you see ingredients that

- end in *-ose*, for example, dextrose, fructose, glucose, maltose, and sucrose;

- end in *-trin* or *-tran*, such as maltodextrin and dextran;

- include *syrup* in their name, such as corn syrup, high-fructose corn syrup, brown rice syrup, fructose syrup, carob syrup, and sorghum syrup;

- include fruit juice, fruit juice concentrate, sorbitol, barley malt, or caramel.

Also, highly refined carbohydrates like bread, bagels, and pasta act like sugars in the body, so try to limit these foods as much as possible. And don't even get me started on artificial sweeteners like NutraSweet or Equal. These substances ('cause they're definitely not food) can disrupt your microbiome, have neurotoxic properties (meaning they fuck with your brain and nervous system), and will trigger sugar cravings just like the real deal.

Then there are more "natural" sources like maple syrup, monk fruit, agave, and coconut sugar. These sources are better, but they're still sugar. So think of it this way: You have X number of calories to eat in a day—how do you want to spend them? On foods that aren't actively building health, or those that are? Don't get me wrong, there are some recipes in this book that have sugar in them, but it is minimally used. We just don't want the basis of our nutrients coming from processed sugar.

When Fat Isn't All That

In chapter 9 I got you to change your mind about fat and see how it can sometimes be good for you. Now it's time to read the fine print and understand how the type of fat you're eating makes a difference. There are four main types of dietary fat:

Monounsaturated fats are the good guys. Getting these from food isn't essential to our survival (because our bodies can make omega-9 essential fatty acids, or EFAs), but there are still benefits to eating sources of omega-9 EFAs. Monounsaturated fats have been proven to decrease inflammation, improve insulin sensitivity, increase "good" HDL cholesterol, decrease "bad" LDL cholesterol, and help eliminate the heart attack– and stroke-causing plaque in the arteries. You'll find monounsaturated fat in nuts (almonds, cashews, walnuts), avocados, chia seeds, and coconuts. Some vegetable oils, such as sunflower and olive oil, contain omega-9 EFAs, but the whole-food versions of these foods are going to deliver more nutrition and contain more micronutrients. Because believe it or not, oils are technically a processed food—the oil has been pressed from the original plant source.

Polyunsaturated fats are the other good-guy squad. Unlike monounsaturated fats, they *are* essential to our health because they contain omega-3s, which we can't make ourselves but need in order to function optimally. Omega-3s are the building blocks for our cell membranes and can improve heart health, boost mental health and mood stability, aid weight loss, and contribute to brain development. They also fight inflammation, prevent dementia, reduce the symptoms of asthma, promote bone health, and decrease liver fat. Omega-3s are harder to come by through our food and therefore are deficient in most people's diets. But you can get what you need by eating walnuts, hempseeds, chia seeds, and flaxseeds. You could also supplement omega-3s as an insurance policy, which we'll talk more about in chapter 15. But for now, challenge yourself to get as much as you can from your food.

Saturated fats are like the people in your life who you like running into once in a while—but not that often and not for too long. You don't want too many saturated fats in your diet because they can raise the level of harmful LDL cholesterol in your blood, which increases your risk of heart attack and stroke. And they're usually coming from not-so-great sources, even if you're eating plant-based. Because while saturated fats are frequently found in things like butter, lard, cheese, ice cream, and other dairy products, some baked goods or even energy bars can contain saturated fats in the form of processed oils. But a *small* amount of saturated fat in your diet—roughly 5 percent of your total intake—is not only acceptable but also recommended. A healthy source of saturated fat is coconut, which also delivers medium-chain triglycerides (MCT). These shorter chains of fats are easily digested and deliver many health benefits such as improving brain and memory function, increasing energy and endurance, lowering blood sugar levels and cholesterol, and promoting weight loss.

Trans fats are a no-go. You'll know why when I tell you where you find them: animal foods, especially processed meats and dairy, and artificial foods, like hydrogenated vegetable oils. There's not a whole plant to be seen here. Studies have linked consumption of trans fats to heart disease, inflammation, high LDL cholesterol, and lower HDL cholesterol. Eating trans fats also leads to an increase in triglycerides, which can cause stroke and heart disease. Luckily, when you're eating a whole food, plant-based diet, it's easy to avoid the pizza, chips, cookies, and other heavily processed foods where trans fats lurk.

Just 'Cause It's Vegan Doesn't Mean It's Healthy

One sign that the vegan movement has really picked up momentum is that food manufacturers are all hustling to get our money. It's awesome that you can go to the grocery store and have tons of choices, whether it's meat substitutes, dairy substitutes, baked goods, or dressings. But you probably know what I'm going to say next: These things ain't plants. They were at one point but not anymore. Processing changes a plant and the nutrients it can give you. Also, things like coloring and flavor additives have been tossed into the mix in order to make the product visually appealing, tasty, and shelf-stable. Case in point: Look at the label of your favorite vegan pancakes/buffalo wings/ranch dressing. I'm willing to bet there are at least two ingredients that wouldn't grow out of the ground. That's nothing new in the packaged food game. Since the 1800s, additives have been used to make food more appealing: chalk in flour, hayseeds in jam, bleach added to corn, coal-tar dyes to berries. Ironically, the more manufacturers tried to make food look "natural," the more unnatural it became. Now you can find a toxic flame-retardant chemical called brominated vegetable oil, or BVO, in things like sodas, sports drinks, and juices to keep the artificial-flavoring chemicals from separating from the rest of the liquids. BVO causes skin lesions, memory loss, and nerve disorders. There's also titanium dioxide, a mined substance that's sometimes contaminated with toxic lead and commonly used in paint and sunscreen, which Big Food also sneaks into processed salad dressing, coffee creamers, and icing. L-cysteine, a dough conditioner added to industrially produced bread and baked goods, is derived from human hair and feathers and can be contaminated with heavy metals (and is just straight-up nasty). And don't even get me started about castoreum, which is secretions from a beaver's anal glands and can be added to food as part of artificial raspberry or vanilla flavoring.

///

Moral of the story: Just because a food is marketed as "vegan" or "healthy" doesn't mean it is. The best way to know if food is healthy is to buy whole-plant ingredients instead of prepared or packaged food. Always read the label and buy only foods that have ingredients you'd reach for in your pantry.

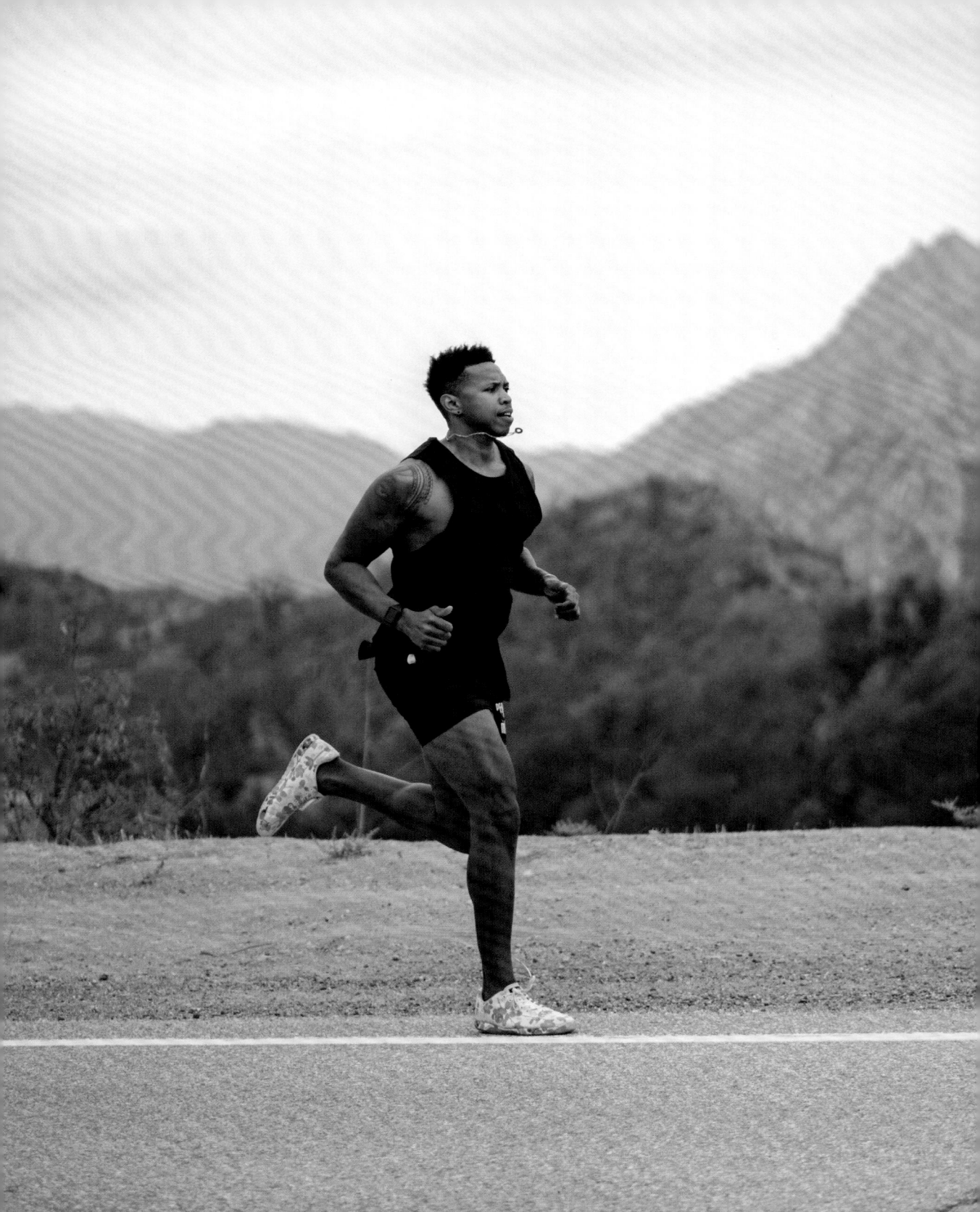

CHAPTER 13

TURNING DREAMS TO REALITY
Losing Weight, Gaining Muscle, or Maintaining Progress

Alright, you've made it through the first thirty days. You're feeling good, you're looking better, and hopefully, you're feeling satisfied. So what's next? For some of you, it might be staying the course—and that's fine. There's no shame in this plant-based game, tempeh chorizo nachos and all. But for others, if you're like me, you want more. You wanna dream bigger. You want to finally lose that extra weight that's been holding you back, or you want to start making muscle gains at the gym. Maybe you want to start training for a sport again—or for the very first time. Maybe that 5K race is calling your name. Or maybe you just want to feel sexy. As I've said before, the plants will get you there every time—if you're making the right choices.

By "the right choices" I mean:

1. You're eating the number of calories for the body you want, not the body you have.

2. You're getting the right number of daily doses of the right kinds of foods.

3. You're moving your body every damn day—and in a way that supports your goal. There's no Arnold Schwarzenegger body with a Richard Simmons workout. But more on that later.

We're going to get into all the specifics of this new plan, but first, let's get clear on your goal and what that will entail:

If You Want to Lose Weight

Let's get something said straight out: I am not advocating that you lose weight. That's for you to know and want. I don't think there's some magical weight for you that is the key to ultimate health. I do, however, believe that your body will let you know when it's carrying too much weight. Maybe your joints hurt or you're huffing and puffing through your day with a fraction of the stamina that you actually need. That's your body saying that it needs its load lightened. I like to remind people that— unless they're Shaq—they have the same size organs as everyone else. Whether you're six seven or five seven, we all basically have almost the same size brains, kidneys, livers, and hearts. The problem is that the more weight you put on (as fat weight, not muscle weight), the more fat those organs and joints and ligaments have to carry around. It's like putting the engine of a Ford Escort into a Ford F-150. So if you and I are going to be talking about weight loss over these next thirty days, know that I'm coming from a place of no longer putting an unnecessary toll on your body's machine, not making you feel bad about what size you are or the way you look.

If this is the route you'd like to go, the recommendation you're going to see here is to create a calorie deficit. That means eating fewer calories combined with moving more. BUT remember what we talked about earlier in this section? Just because you'll be operating on a tighter caloric budget does not mean you'll be going hungry. The beauty of eating only plant-based foods is that you'll most likely be eating *more* than when you were relying on animal foods to keep you feeling satisfied.

If You Want to Gain Muscle

This is one of my favorite conversations to have because it means I can get all up in the face of anyone who wants to tell me that you can't get abs without eating meat. As I covered in chapter 11, it's *carbohydrates*, not protein, that make up the perfect fuel for your body. When you work out, your body isn't reaching for that steak or that chicken breast. It's reaching for those greens, those grains, and those legumes. To refresh: Carbohydrates get converted into glucose, which then gets stored in your muscles as glycogen for energy. When you work out, your body uses that glycogen. And when the glycogen stores run low, your body switches to its backup generator, stored fat. That's exactly what you want when you're trying to build muscle and also lean out to show off those hard-earned abs.

I like to say: "You build the body in the gym, but you show it off in the kitchen." You could be doing eight hundred curls a day, but if you're going home and eating those Twinkies and Philly cheesesteaks, you're only going to be hiding that bicep under a layer of fat. Now if it were me and I was doing those eight hundred curls? I'm pretty sure I'd want to show off that bicep. That's when good, clean fuel comes into play. On this particular plan, you'll actually be eating a surplus of calories in order to put on that muscle weight. But you'll be doing it through extra doses of plant-based carbohydrates, healthy fats, and proteins.

Just one thing to note here: This muscle-gain plan is for the everyday person looking to get a little more jacked. If you're looking to go into professional bodybuilding or enter a hardbody contest, then you'd need to go deeper into the details with balancing your calories and macros along with your workouts. But if you're just starting out, this plan is the first step toward getting there.

There's No Such Thing as "Good Genes"

I don't post as many thirst-trap shirtless photos on social media as I used to, but when I do, I always hear from people that I must just be lucky to have "good genes." A lot of my friends in the fitness industry hear the same thing—as though their success in building their incredible bodies were just an ability they were born with, rather than something they had to work very, very hard at doing. I definitely take issue with that. For one thing, I bust my ass to keep this body in shape. I may have been blessed with a six-six frame, but I still have to get up and work hard to be in the kind of shape that I want to be in. And I wasn't lying about loving me some vegan cake. But more than that, I really don't like that people think my kind of success isn't available to them. Nobody's born obese. Nobody's born with lifestyle diseases. These are the results of a lot of things—our diet, our environment, our stress levels—but they're not written in stone. I say that until you put your DNA to the test, you have no idea what it can do.

The Building Block Plan

Regardless of your goals, this is the plan you're going to follow over the next few months. I'm recommending it here for a few reasons:

1. It really helped me look at my food in a way that was simpler than just counting calories.

2. It takes away some of the nervousness people feel when they're just starting out. I always hear, "Am I doing it right?" This plan will help you think through that.

3. It will also help you figure out the best balance of macronutrients for your particular body, which nothing but experience can tell you.

I gave the Building Block Plan its name for two reasons. First, because it's going to get you thinking about your macronutrients in terms of "blocks" (or "doses," as you know I also like to call them). Every day, you'll get a recommended number of blocks for each macronutrient. And all you need to do is eat those blocks! As I said before, it's like a game of *Tetris*—you can put those blocks wherever you want to put 'em in your day, and it makes no difference to me so long as you're eating them.

The second reason why I like calling this approach the Building Block Plan is because it's a good reminder for how real progress gets made. If you wanted to build a wall and had never built a wall before, you wouldn't wake up one morning and say, "I'm going to build the biggest, strongest wall today." No, you'd get overwhelmed. You'd want to give up. And most likely, you wouldn't even do it right. Instead, if you said "Every day I'm going to put a few more bricks in place" and focused on doing it perfectly each time, then eventually you'd have that wall. Rome wasn't built in a day, and neither was your body. Every perfect building block that you put into it is one step closer to getting the health and the body that you deserve.

When I first started out on a plant-based diet, this approach was huge because I wasn't getting too hung up on how many calories I was taking in. Instead I could just say to myself, "You've got one block of protein left today, one block of fat, and three blocks of carbohydrates—that's dinner." Or if I was going out to a restaurant and I knew I had to get in those last few doses, it helped me decide what to order. To help you out even more, I've included not just nutritional information with each of the recipes in this book but also the number of blocks for each macro that you're getting in.

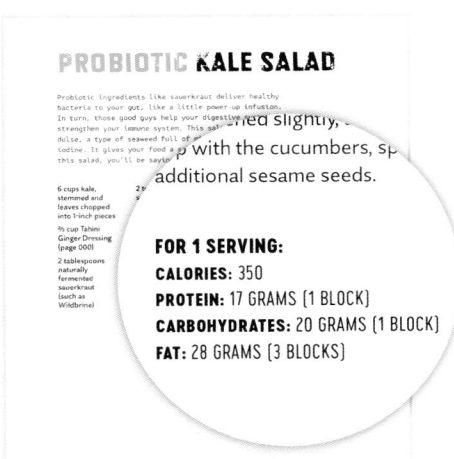

PROBIOTIC KALE SALAD

Probiotic ingredients like sauerkraut deliver healthy bacteria to your gut, like a little power-up infusion. In turn, those good guys help your digestive infusion. strengthen your immune system. This sal... red slightly, dulse, a type of seaweed full of iodine. It gives your food a p with the cucumbers, sp this salad, you'll be sayi... additional sesame seeds.

6 cups kale, stemmed and leaves chopped into 1-inch pieces

½ cup Tahini Ginger Dressing (page 000)

2 tablespoons naturally fermented sauerkraut (such as Wildbrine)

FOR 1 SERVING:
CALORIES: 350
PROTEIN: 17 GRAMS (1 BLOCK)
CARBOHYDRATES: 20 GRAMS (1 BLOCK)
FAT: 28 GRAMS (3 BLOCKS)

The number of blocks that you get in a day will be determined by your goals. If you're on the weight-loss tip, you'll have fewer than if you are looking to gain muscle. And if you've been at this a little while and are feeling good with how things are going, you're going to have a number of blocks dictated by your current weight and caloric needs.

The other factor in what your blocks will look like will be which *floor* you're on. The Building Block Plan has three floors, one for each month of the plan. Each floor is calibrated to make a shift in how your body's machinery is working. By shifting the ratio of *types* of blocks you're eating on each floor, you're also adjusting how your food is being used as fuel. Check it out:

Month 1, Floor 1: The Burner

This month will help kick off the leaning-down process and get some of the extra weight off your joints and surrounding your organs, whether or not you're looking to ultimately bulk back up with muscle. The ratio of blocks that you'll see in this phase is heavier on the proteins than on the carbohydrates and fats (40 percent protein—35 percent carbohydates—25 percent fat). This is to keep you in a low-glycemic state, which is ideal for fat loss.

Month 2, Floor 2: The Boost

Now we're bringing up the carbs and taking down the proteins but keeping the fat the same (35 percent protein—45 percent carbohydrates—20 percent fat). You'll likely notice during this time that your weight loss tapers a bit as you start to form more lean muscle. If your primary goal is weight loss, so long as you're still within your target caloric range (eating the suggested number of blocks for your level), you'll still be on track, even though there's been a shift in your nutrition that supports muscle development. The biggest reason for doing this is that while you can get results by taking the carbohydrates down temporarily (which you've just done for four weeks), if you go without carbs for too long, you start losing energy and drive. Don't worry about seeing a slight slowdown in how much weight you're losing; as long as you're not overshooting that number of blocks, you aren't going to bulk up.

Month 3 and Beyond, Floor 3: The Builder

This is the phase where you bring it all home and set yourself up for success for . . . well, the rest of your life. You're going to be shifting into the most sustainable ratio of blocks, which will mean getting a majority of your nutrition from carbohydrates followed by an equal split of protein and fat (20 percent protein—60 percent carbohydrates—20 percent fat). You're also going to be recalibrating how many calories you're eating in a day, adding slightly more based on whether you've met your goal by this point. I'll have you recalculate your ideal caloric intake so that this final floor is perfectly suited for where you are and where you're going. Ideally, you'd hang out on this floor for at least three months to make sure you're really sealing in those results that you've earned on the previous two floors.

Using the Building Block Plan Every Day

You can without a doubt use this plan for the rest of your life. I've been at this plant-based thing for almost twenty years, and I still use it. Sometimes

I go back through the floors if I feel like I've been slippin' or I want to get another jump start on looking lean and cut. Other times, I'm just hanging out on Floor 3, maintaining what's worked for me.

That said, not every body is the same. I could tell you to do exactly what I do, but unless you're six-foot-six and 240 pounds, it won't be accurate. You may find that one of the floors works better for you in terms of how your body looks and feels—your energy levels, stamina, weight, symptoms of any chronic ailment. While I do recommend getting a majority of your nutrition from carbohydrate blocks, feel free to play around with how protein and fat figure in and the results you get. As long as you're being honest with yourself, sticking with more unprocessed food than processed, and keeping your body moving, you're going to end up where you want to be.

If the Building Block Plan Is Too Much for You Right Now

I get it—here I am, telling you that all you need to do is eat more plants to get healthy, and now I'm all up in your business about floors and blocks. What I'm *not* saying is that you have to do all these things to get healthier. This is a foolproof plan for making lasting changes to your body. These changes also lead to better health, but granted, are more ambitious than taking plant-based baby steps. If right now your focus is on eating more plants, go with that. Maybe see if you can also challenge yourself to eat fewer processed foods, more carbs (especially vegetables), and fewer unhealthy fats. Play with the recipes in the book. Celebrate all the delicious food that's making you feel better. Whatever you do, do you (vegan-style).

///

That's it. There's nothing else standing between you and a seriously life-changing, and potentially life-saving, evolution. The next chapter begins your next three months of fueling right, moving right, and getting your mind right. I'll come along for the ride and support you every step of the way, but I can't do the work for you. So take a minute to reconnect with your why, get clear on what's riding on this process, and turn the page like a fuckin' beast.

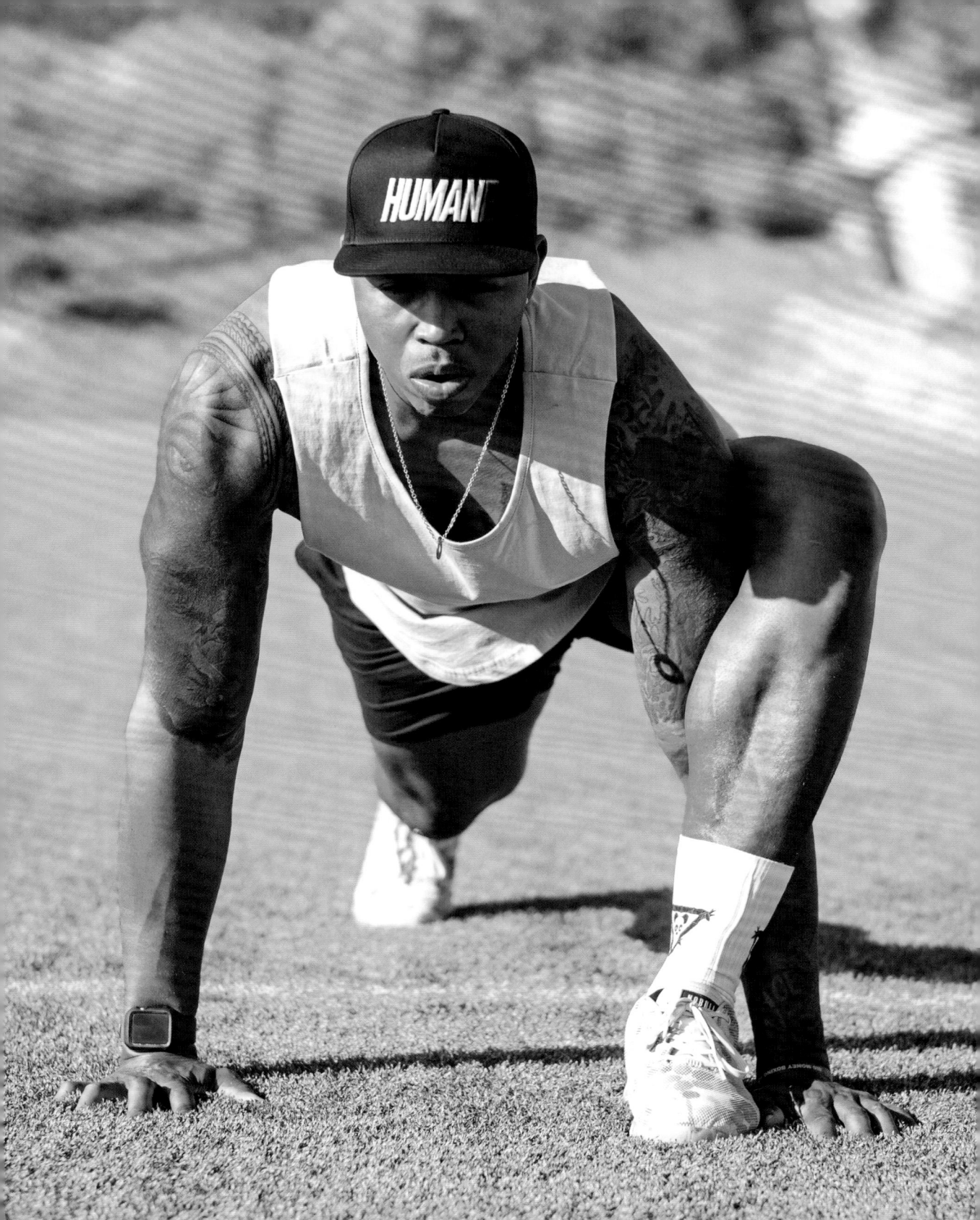

CHAPTER 14

THE BUILDING BLOCK PLAN
Eat Right, Move Right, and Get Your Mind Right

Here's a refresher for how this is going to go down: Over the next three months, you're going to move through three phases, or *floors*. For each floor, you'll have a set number of blocks, or doses, of macros that you'll want to hit every day (hence the Building Block Plan). That's it. That's the key to burning some fat, building some muscle, and bringing your health to a better, stronger place. All you need to do is work the steps, one block, one floor, one month at a time.

But before you do anything, before you even read this chapter, I want you to take a deep breath. In. Out. Let it go. Good. I don't want you to get overwhelmed here. The plan itself is really simple, but in the beginning, it might feel like rocket science. So take a minute to chill out, stop worrying, and definitely stop overthinking things—that's only going to make things feel way harder than they need to be. It's all going to work out. I got you.

Step 1: Pick Your Floor

Unless you have been at the plant-based game for a while and are in solid shape in terms of your health and your goals, I strongly suggest that you start at the beginning on Floor 1. Remember, this isn't a race. This process is setting you up for lifelong wellness. So no, you can't game the system and jump in at Floor 2 or 3 and expect quicker results. I also recommend that you stick with each floor for at least one month. This will give your body time to adjust to the new balance of macronutrients it's using as fuel, and it will give you time to adjust your meals according to that phase's suggested block breakdown. Here's a reminder of what that will look like for each floor:

PHASE	GOAL	PROTEIN	CARBOHYDRATES	FAT
Floor 1: The Burner	Strengthen muscle and shed excess body fat	40%	35%	25%
Floor 2: The Boost	Continue your positive transformation and gain more energy	35%	45%	20%
Floor 3: The Builder	Long-term, sustainable maintenance	20%	60%	20%

Step 2: Calculate Your Fuel Level

To figure out how many blocks you get each day, we have to first figure out how much fuel your body needs in order to run right. It will ensure that you're eating enough to give your body sufficient energy but not so much that you're storing energy for later (aka gaining weight). We're going to talk about this in terms of calories, but don't freak out. This is not so you can get obsessed with a number, because (1) no one needs that in their life, and (2) the quality of calories that you're eating on a plant-based diet is way different than when you're an omnivore. Instead, I want you to think of your food as fuel because calories are, at the end of the day, just a unit of energy. I suggest recalculating your Fuel Level before you advance to the next floor, or every thirty days.

I suggest recalculating your Fuel Level before you advance to the next floor, or every thirty days.

1. **CALCULATE YOUR RESTING METABOLIC RATE (RMR).** This is the bare minimum number of calories you need for your body's factory to keep you alive—to pump your blood, grow hair, breathe, and so on.

    Your Body Weight × 10 = RMR (in calories)

2. **CALCULATE YOUR DAILY ACTIVITY BURN.** This is how many calories you need just to move your body around during the day, aside from exercise, e.g., getting out of bed, walking to the fridge, running errands.

    Your RMR × 1.2 = Daily Activity Burn

3. **FIND YOUR FUEL LEVEL.** Use your Daily Activity Burn to find your level on this table:

YOUR ENERGY AMOUNT	FUEL LEVEL
1,800–2,399	Level I
2,400–2,499	Level II
3,000+	Level III

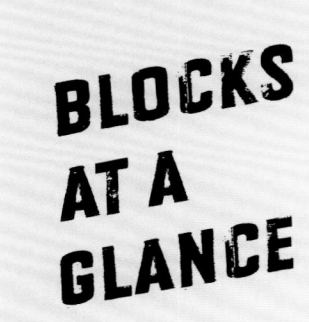

BLOCKS AT A GLANCE

The key to making the Building Block Plan work for you is to not overcomplicate it or overthink it. Here's a key for what makes up the blocks.

PROTEIN BLOCK = 20 GRAMS

CARB BLOCK = 20 GRAMS

FAT BLOCK = 10 GRAMS

Step 3: Get Your Blocks

Again, the reason you're going to look at your food servings as blocks is because that won't require you to think too much about calories or portions,

FLOOR 1: THE BURNER

FUEL LEVEL I:

Protein
Carbohydrates
Fat

(aim for 1 block of fruit and 2 blocks of vegetables)

FUEL LEVEL II:

Protein
Carbohydrates
Fat

(aim for 1 block of fruit and 4 blocks of vegetables)

FUEL LEVEL III:

Protein
Carbohydrates
Fat

(aim for 2 blocks of fruit and 4 blocks of vegetables)

FLOOR 2: THE BOOST

FUEL LEVEL I:

Protein
Carbohydrates
Fat

(aim for 1 block of fruit and 2 blocks of vegetables)

FUEL LEVEL II:

Protein
Carbohydrates
Fat

(aim for 1 block of fruit and 3 blocks of vegetables)

FUEL LEVEL III:

Protein
Carbohydrates
Fat

(aim for 2 blocks of fruit and 2 blocks of vegetables)

FLOOR 3: THE BUILDER

FUEL LEVEL I:

Protein
Carbohydrates
Fat

(aim for 2 blocks of fruit and 2 blocks of vegetables)

FUEL LEVEL II:

Protein
Carbohydrates
Fat

(aim for 3 blocks of fruit and 3 blocks of vegetables)

FUEL LEVEL III:

Protein
Carbohydrates
Fat

(aim for 3 blocks of fruit and 4 blocks of vegetables)

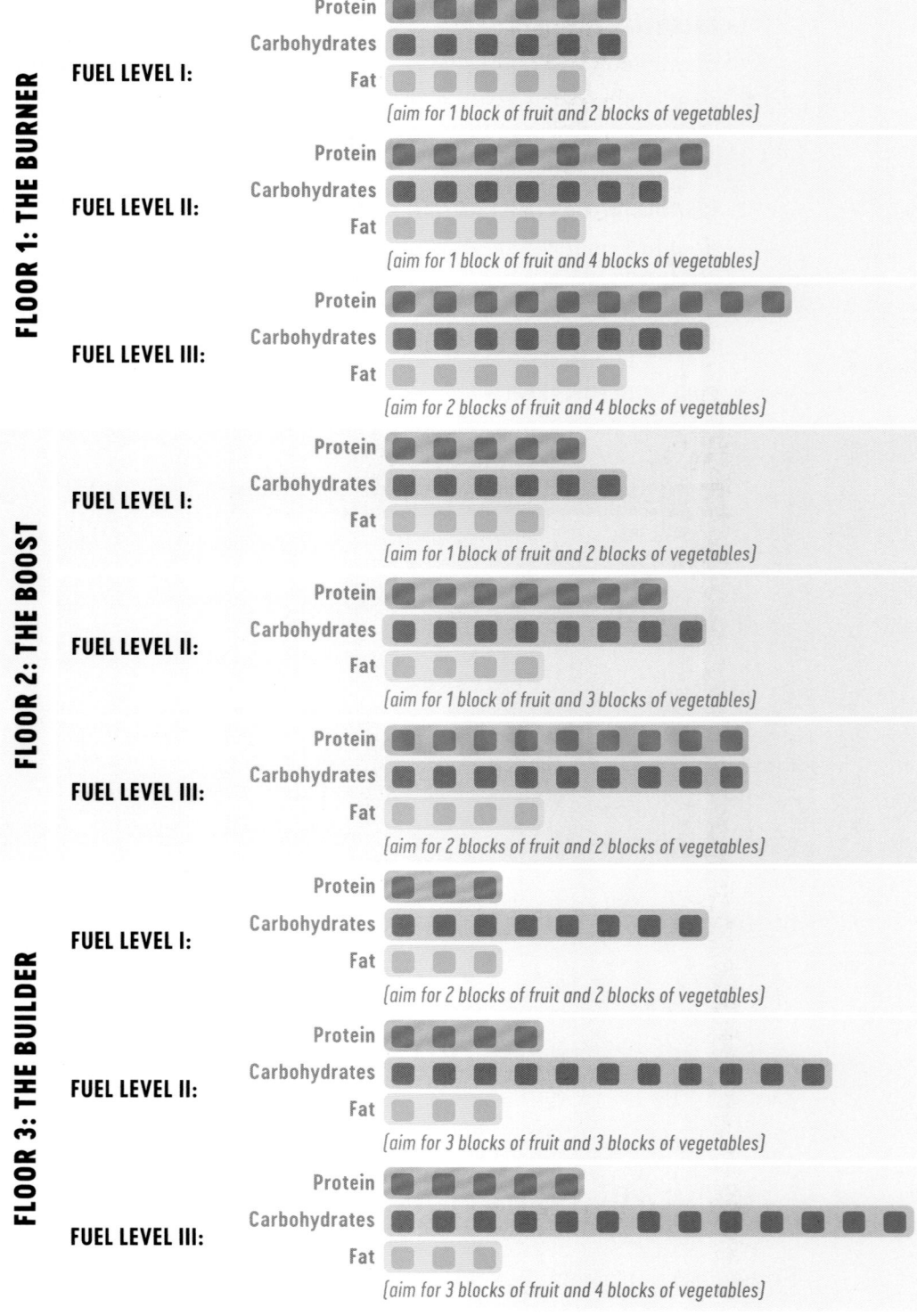

or to make complicated recipes. You just need to think about what plants you want to eat and how much of them you want to eat to feel satisfied. That's a much healthier and more sustainable way to look at food than counting every last calorie and not understanding the underlying nutrition.

One block is equal to one serving of that food. For example, 1 block of fat could be one-third of a medium avocado, 1 tablespoon of olive oil, or 18 cashews. A block of vegetables would be 2 cups of raw spinach, 1 cup of chopped cauliflower, or 1 cup of green beans. While you're getting the hang of this whole block thing, I recommend using a food tracking app like My-FitnessPal or Cronometer. Again, not to get hung up on calories necessarily, just to have a gauge of how much you're eating and make sure you're hitting those blocks, no more and no less.

Here's a sample of what 2,000 calories a day will look like:

THE BURNER

10 blocks of protein = 200 grams of protein = 800 calories

8.75 blocks of carbs = 175 grams of carbs = 700 calories

5.5 blocks of fat = 55 grams of fat = 500 calories

THE BOOST

8.75 blocks of protein = 175 grams of protein = 700 calories

11.25 blocks of carbs = 225 grams of carbs = 900 calories

4.4 blocks of fat = 44 grams of fat = 400 calories

THE BUILDER

5 blocks of protein = 100 grams of protein = 400 calories

15 blocks of carbs = 300 grams of carbs = 1,200 calories

4.4 blocks of fat = 44 grams of fat = 400 calories

What Counts as What?

More deep breaths, please. I can feel you starting to get amped up about these blocks; I know you want to make things more complicated, and I love you for that. But chill the fuck out. The beauty of a plant-based diet is that most of your food gives you multiple macronutrients at once. Your quinoa is a grain, but it's also got a nice amount of protein; seeds and nuts have fat but also protein; tofu has protein, but it's also gonna have carbs. So at the end of the day, if you're eating a balanced diet, then you're also going to get a balanced amount of macronutrients. So your designations of "fat," "protein," and "carbohydrate" could vary from day to day—and that's fine.

Dessert and Snacks

No matter which floor you're on or what your goals are, I want you eating all day (unless you're fasting, but we'll talk about that more in chapter 16). That includes snacks, and that definitely includes dessert. The beauty of the Building Block Plan is that you can eat whatever you want—so long as it's

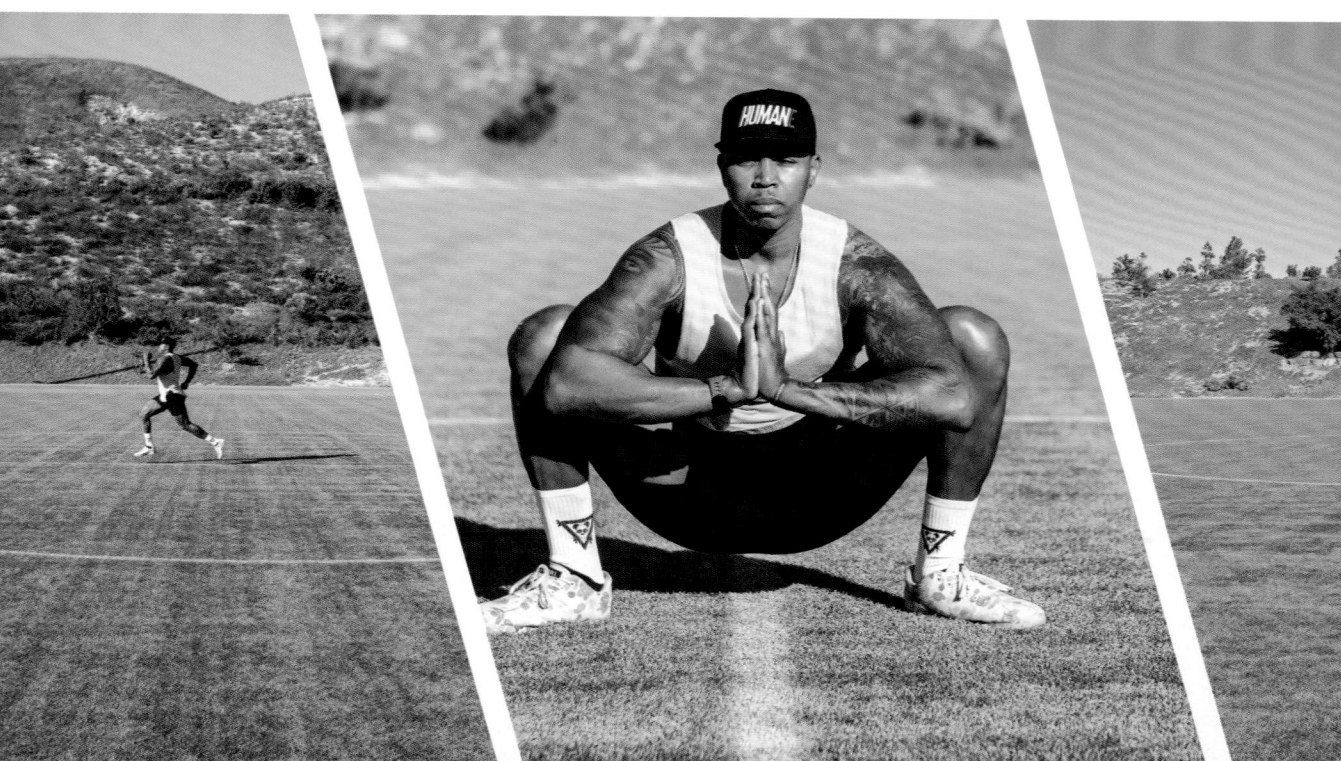

plant-based and so long as you're being honest about what you're eating in terms of counting the number of blocks. You can have that nut butter as a snack; just make sure you're counting that fat and then maybe not including that extra dollop of hummus at dinner in order to stay within your total recommended fat blocks for the day. Same goes for dessert—it's just food. Especially if you're making the recipes from this book, which don't include things like processed sugar and simple carbohydrates. Have a portion, count it, and continue living your life.

Exercise Your Right to Move That Body

I always say that the human body was the first piece of machinery put on Earth. And we've all forgotten that in order for any machine to work, you gotta use it. We don't use our bodies the way we should—we get out of bed, sit down and watch TV while we eat breakfast, sit in the car, sit at a desk, sit down to eat dinner, lie down for bed. We have joints for a reason! We have muscles for a reason! But if you don't use 'em, you lose 'em.

A place that I like to start with is 10,000 steps a day. We now know that

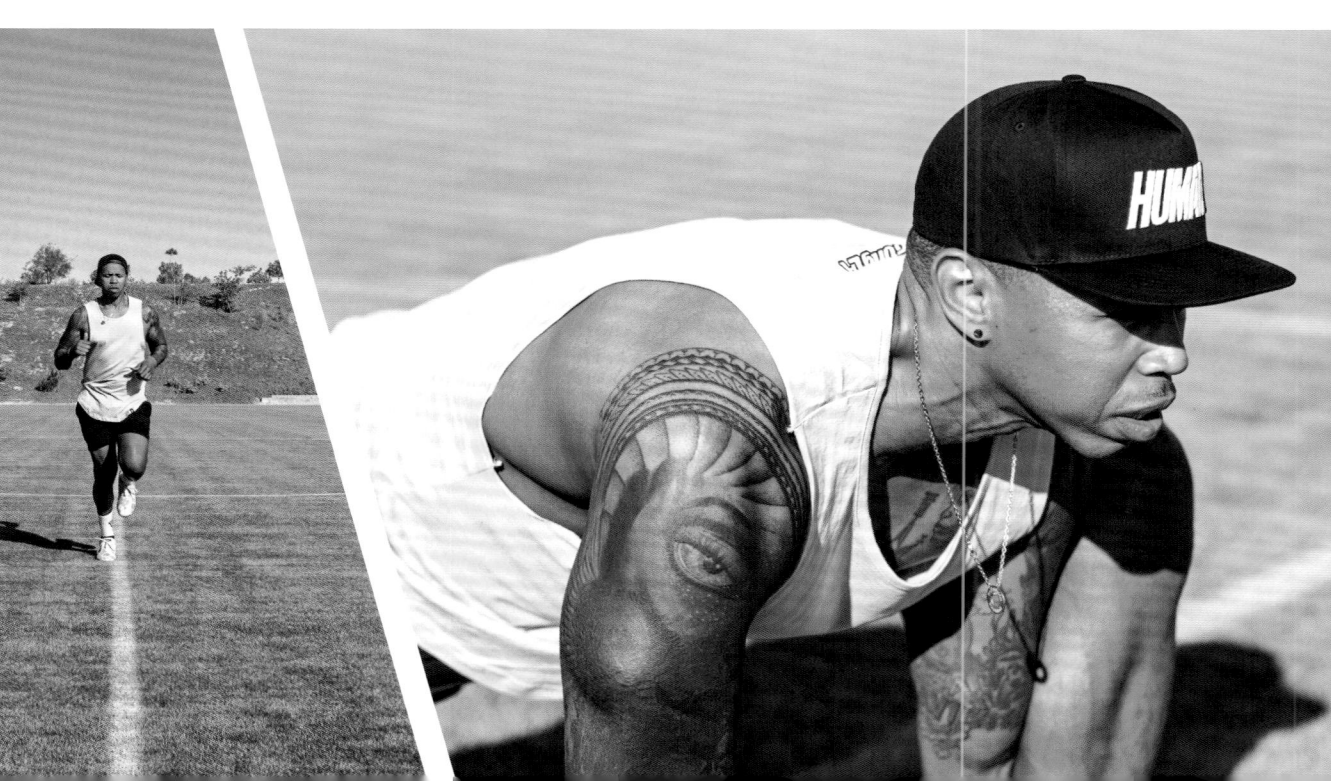

if you walk between 2,000 and 3,000 steps a day, then your mortality rate is around 75 percent—which isn't so great. (Meaning you're 75 percent more likely to die than someone who gets all their steps in.) But if you increase those steps from 3,000 to 6,000 a day, then you drop that mortality rate all the way down to 25 percent. And if you increase to 10,000, that rate goes down even more, to just 6 percent. It doesn't matter if you're walking, crawling, skipping, or jumping rope, your mortality rate gets much, much better. And if your mortality rate is that low, imagine how the rest of you will feel. Imagine combining that with your food. That's the kind of health I'm talking about. It's not about being able to lift up a truck or run a marathon; it's the consistent, daily movement that's important. So if you're looking to lose weight and are feeling overwhelmed about adding exercise, just start by walking every day. Then, little by little, move your body more and more.

Now, if you're trying to get the kinds of results that really make a dramatic difference, that's another story. You're going to need consistent movement, too, but you're also going to have to get real about the effort you're putting in. Like I said before—a lot of people want the Arnold Schwarzenegger body but are doing the Richard Simmons workout. They want the fifteen-minute burn, but the body that they're admiring is the product of one to two hours in the gym minimum. The food's an important part of getting there, but you also gotta put in the work.

CHAPTER 15

CYA

Cover Your Assets
(with Vitamins and Supplements)

When you're eating a plant-based diet, your food pretty much has you covered when it comes to getting all the good, nutritious stuff you need to stay healthy. So don't go thinking that a plant-based diet isn't where it's at just because of what I'm going to say next: You still need to supplement your diet with a few essential nutrients. No matter how healthily you eat, there are some things you can't get from your diet—and no, meat eaters aren't any better off. Because of changes in our food system, our environment, and even the natural limitations of plants themselves, we're not able to get every nutrient we need from our food. Our fruits and veggies don't have the same nutrient level they did a thousand years ago. Just think, the foods come from the earth, and the earth is depleted now. And just like any living organism (yes, the earth is alive), if the organism is depleted, then anything that comes from it will be depleted as well. So even though we get many of our vital nutrients from our food, there are a few that are so essential we need to be topping them off in the tank. I'm talking specifically about vitamins B_{12} and D, zinc, iodine, K_2, and omega-3s. These nutrients are very important when it comes to things like making healthy DNA, influencing the function of all your major systems (immune, neurological, cardiovascular), helping your brain work optimally, and balancing your hormones.

As far as how much of these supplements to take, I recommend working with your health-care provider to determine the dosage that's right for you. In particular, I strongly suggest finding a provider who regularly works with plant-based folks (and is maybe plant-based themselves), so they understand how you're getting your nutrition primarily from your food.

Vitamin B$_{12}$

This vitamin is actually made by *microbes*, the kind you normally find in our soil and water. But in this Clorox-wipe-everything day and age, our daily dose of microbes has gone way down. So unless you're eating what our ancestors ate (bugs, dirt), it's a good idea to supplement. Vitamin B$_{12}$ is crucial to the very foundation of your health because it helps make DNA, or the set of instructions that your body uses to make new cells. Insufficient B$_{12}$ can lead to fatigue, weakness, constipation, brain fog, difficulty with coordination and balance, depression, and neurological issues. It can be hard to know if you're deficient in B$_{12}$, so it's a good bet to go ahead and supplement it for guaranteed protection.

You'll see two primary sources of vitamin B$_{12}$ listed on supplement bottles: cyanocobalamin and methylcobalamin. They're virtually the same, except methylocabalamin is naturally occurring and cyanocobalamin is synthetic. It's currently understood that neither form is better than the other, so long as you're getting your daily dose of B$_{12}$.

Vitamin D

For whatever reason, we call this a vitamin, but it's actually a hormonelike steroid that plays a big role in all of your major systems, including immune, neurological, and cardiovascular. Vitamin D deficiency can lead to getting sick more often and more severely, depression, fatigue, muscle pain and weakness, bone loss, heart disease, high blood pressure, diabetes, and multiple sclerosis. Your body can actually produce its own vitamin D when it's exposed to sunlight, but now that most of us have lifestyles that keep us indoors more often than not, we don't get enough "vitamin sun" to make vitamin D. And we can't get vitamin D from our food, unless it's been forti-

BADASS VEGAN

fied with it (which only really happens in dairy products). Basically, if you spend most of your day under artificial light, live somewhere other than a tropical climate, or live in an area that's mildly polluted, then you need to supplement vitamin D. Yeah, so all of you. You are going to get this "D," and your body is going to love it!

Omega-3 Fatty Acids

Omega-3s are basically brain food—they fuel brain function, ease depression and anxiety, and contribute to better mental focus. They're also powerful anti-inflammatories, so they can reduce risk factors for heart disease and metabolic syndromes. We can get some omega-3s through a plant-based diet but not all. See, omegas are made up of the fatty acids DHA, EPA, and ALA. We get ALA from things like nuts and seeds, but DHA and EPA are harder to come by. People who eat fish tend to get a sufficient amount, but those sources also tend to be high in contaminants that come from water pollution—not exactly a compelling argument for eating fish. It's also worth mentioning that some individuals have a difficult time converting ALA to DHA/EPA, just based on their biology. Bottom line: Err on the side of caution and take a plant-based omega-3 supplement.

Iodine

Your body relies on iodine to create essential thyroid hormones, which are what help you regulate your metabolism in addition to other vital functions. Iodine is similar to the omega-3s in that you can get this mineral from certain plants (namely seaweeds like kelp, hijiki, kombu, and wakame), but my guess is that most of you aren't exactly shoveling these in as part of our Western plant-based diet. And that's okay! You can get some iodine from potatoes and cranberries, but how much you're getting isn't a sure thing and depends on soil quality. There's also iodized salt, or table salt, that's fortified with iodine, but too much sodium isn't great for blood pressure or cardiovascular health, so that's not a viable source either. Plus, iodized salt tends to contain other not-great things like anticaking agents.

Vitamin K$_2$

Vitamin K, like omegas, comes in multiple forms. There's K$_1$, which is easy to get on a plant-based diet thanks to leafy greens, and then there's also K$_2$, which is more commonly found in animal sources like butter and egg yolks. You do get a small hit from fermented sources like natto, miso, and tempeh (all forms of fermented soybeans) but not enough to call it a day. Especially when you consider that K$_2$ is essential for getting calcium to your bones and teeth and away from places it shouldn't be, like your brain and heart. It also helps combat chronic inflammation.

Zinc

Zinc plays a number of different important roles in the body. It stimulates the activity of more than one hundred enzymes, supports immune function and gene regulation, and helps neurons communicate, which contributes to memory formation and learning. There have also been studies linking zinc with decreased age-related chronic illness thanks to less systemic inflammation. The good news is that we get zinc from many of the foods that we eat, especially legumes, tempeh, and tofu, along with many nuts, seeds, and grains. The bad news is that we don't always absorb it properly. Long story short, some of the vegan foods we eat that are rich in zinc also contain phytates, which block the body's ability to absorb zinc. You can decrease phytates by soaking and sprouting your nuts, seeds, and legumes before cooking them, but just to play it safe, it's recommended to supplement.

STFU About Iron

Iron is just one of those things that people who eat meat love to harp on. *But what about iron?* I can practically hear the trolling now. That's because someone somewhere pulled off one of the greatest scams of all time: convincing us that meat is the best source of iron. Is that true? No. Not even close.

To understand why, you have to understand iron. There are two types: heme, which is found in animal foods, and nonheme, which is found in plants. It is a fact that heme is better absorbed than nonheme iron, and that vegetarians and vegans may have lower iron stores than omnivores. But—hear me when I say this—VEGANS DO NOT HAVE HIGHER RATES OF ANEMIA. Studies have shown that just because your iron reading is "low-normal" does not mean that's bad. Actually, there's some evidence that slightly lower iron stores can be beneficial and contribute to better insulin function and lower rates of heart disease and cancer. And it's all a wash anyway because while meat eaters are filling up on animal foods like eggs and dairy products, which have virtually no iron, we vegans are getting doses with many of the plants we eat, especially tofu, tempeh, legumes, grains, nuts and seeds, and vegetables like Swiss chard, collard greens, kale, broccoli, Brussels sprouts, and spinach. In fact, your body can absorb a higher percentage of iron when your meal contains only a few milligrams, versus trying to cram a whole bunch onto your plate as a one-shot deal. But no matter how much iron you suspect you're getting from your diet, I still suggest working with your health-care provider to figure out whether you're within a healthy range.

Vegans DO NOT have higher rates of anemia.

To view the references cited in this chapter, please visit badassvegan.com/citations.

CYA

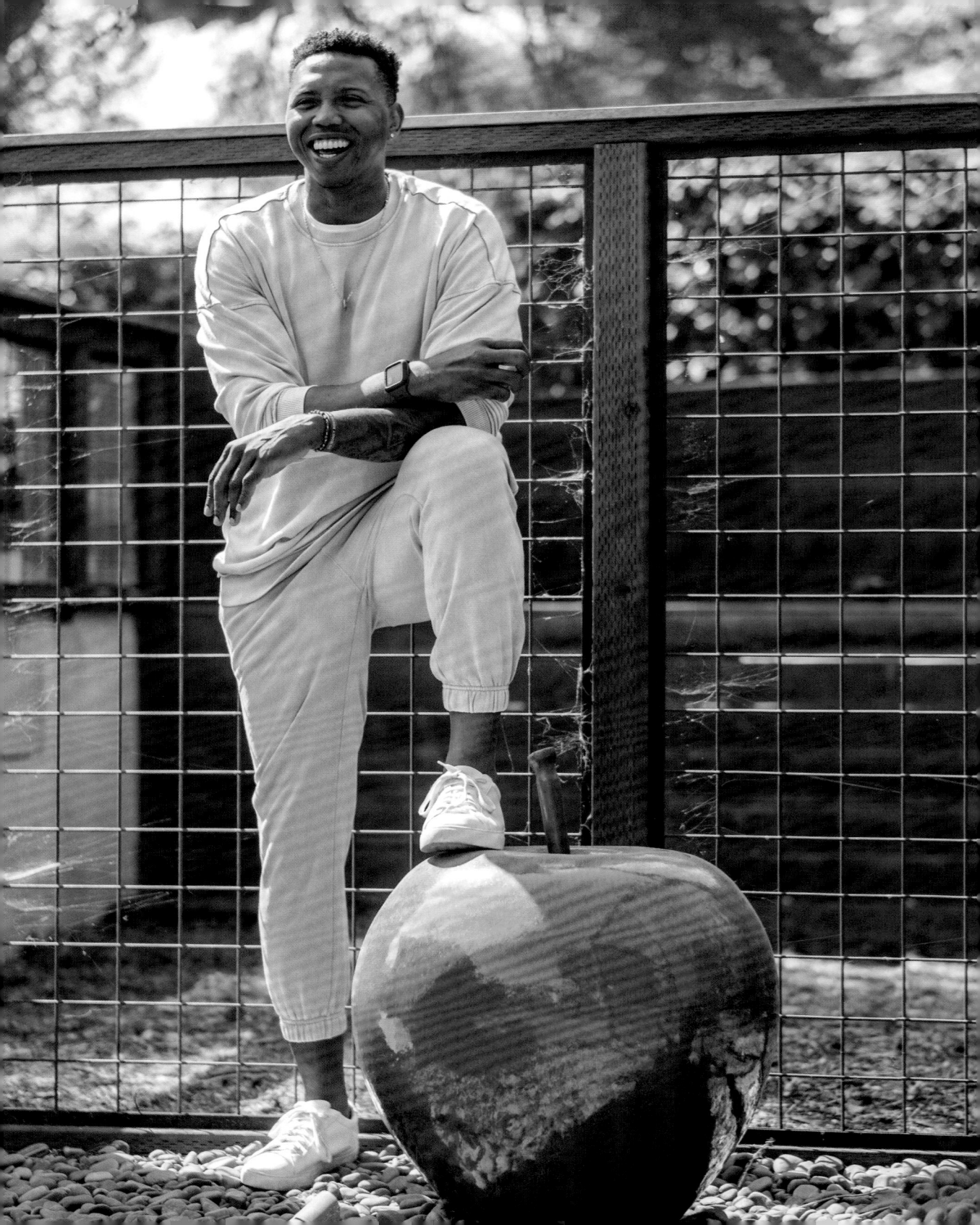

CHAPTER 16

START F***ING
Intermittent Fasting

I love telling people they should be f***ing at least twice a week, that f***ing properly relaxes your mind and body, and that f***ing can even help with metabolic regulation, stabilization of blood sugar, decreasing blood pressure, weight loss, and both looking and feeling younger. That's right, fasting is great for your health. Did you think we were talking about something else?

Fasting for part of the day, or intermittent fasting, has roots that go way back to ancient history (in Buddhism it was believed that it was the key to achieving Nirvana). Brief, periodic fasts are actually the norm for our human make and model because it wasn't like we always had food on demand. For over two million years, our ancestors were pretty much all hunter-gatherers. They spent the majority of their time gathering mainly low-calorie foods, like wild grains, roots, and berries. In order to survive long periods of time without access to food, these early humans would fast, sometimes up to ten days at a time. It turns out that this cycle of feasting and fasting changed us on a biochemical level. We had to adapt to this situation, so those who couldn't hack it . . . well, they died. And the early humans who could go without food during those times passed on their genes, which meant that over time, humans became capable of not only fasting for extended periods of time but benefiting from it.

Another way to think about fasting is that animals rarely eat until they're full. Why? Because a full animal is useless and defenseless. An animal that's stuffed until it hurts all the time can't do shit, least of all defend itself from predators. Plus, its digestive system isn't meant to handle all that food. Well, remember, we're animals too. And yet, we've ignored our natural instincts to eat until we're satisfied only every once in a while, until it's become our own man-made nature to eat until we're full multiple times a day, 365 days a year. That means our digestive system is constantly working to process more food than it's meant to handle. Then, what can't move through the system gets stored. But what can start as storing can easily turn into hoarding. Ever seen *Hoarding: Buried Alive*? Those houses filled with garbage bags and piles of stuff to the ceiling and those little paths to get to the bathroom—that's your digestive system. Sure, your body can turn some of that into energy, but not all of it. And again, what's not burned off ends up clogging the system. Because your body is a larger system made up of smaller systems, if one of these systems starts to fuck up? You guessed it—it'll eventually negatively affect the other systems until your entire body is affected by the simple, but unnecessary, act of eating all the time.

On the other hand, thousands of research teams have investigated how calorie restriction can benefit the body, so we now know that:

○ Your digestive system works better when it can have the occasional rest.

○ Your metabolism and hormones can resync to their factory settings.

○ Your metabolism has a chance to burn fat that is stored in the body.

○ There's a longer-than-normal period of low insulin in the blood, which tells your body to burn energy to keep insulin low. This is the opposite of what happens when you're continuously eating food.

○ It activates a process called autophagy, a fancy way of saying "taking out the trash." When your body can take a break from digesting, it can use that energy to do things like remove waste material from cells and fuel the factories in your cells that make energy.

There are a few ways you can incorporate fasting into your routine:

○ **THE SIXTEEN-HOUR FAST:** No eating for sixteen hours. This might sound intense, but you naturally fast for eight hours at night. If you fast between dinner and a late breakfast the next day, that's sixteen hours right there.

○ **ALTERNATE-DAY FASTING:** Eat only every other day.

○ **ONCE-A-WEEK TWENTY-FOUR-HOUR INTERMITTENT FAST:** This is what I usually go with—you fast for twenty-four hours once per week on the same day every week.

In terms of finding the right fit for you, you just have to be willing to experiment to see what works best. It's like a bikini—it's not one size fits all. You might work a night shift and can't fast all day and eat at night, or you might not be able to fast for twenty-four hours because you have a job that doesn't allow you to take a break and rest if you need it. (Being able to pause and take a nap is crucial for me on fasting days.) When choosing a plan, go with one that works for your work schedule, family schedule, workout schedule, and lifestyle. Or maybe you don't want to fast at all, and that's totally fine. If you do choose to fast and have any conditions that you take medication for, you may want to consult your health-care practitioner first, just to be cautious.

TIPS FOR MAKING IT THROUGH A FAST:

○ **Drink lots of water.** It will not only keep you feeling hydrated, which will make it less likely that you'll feel discomfort like headaches, but it also helps scratch that satiety itch when food's not available. When your stomach feels food, it sends a signal to your brain, which can take the edge off your hunger. An easy way to get in plenty of water is to buy a half-gallon or gallon-size reusable water bottle and make sure you're downing a lot of that during your fasting window (or even when you're not fasting so you stay nice and hydrated). Herbal teas can be nice here, too, because the flavor makes it feel like you're eating something. And some people choose to have black coffee (meaning nothing added to it) during their fasting window.

○ **Get busy.** Find something to distract you from fasting. Run errands, take a nap, focus on work—the less you think about the fact that you're not eating, the less you'll even notice it. Over time, it won't even register.

○ **Have good food waiting for you.** In the beginning, as your body gets used to fasting, you might come out of a fast and want to dive head-first into a bag of chips. Instead, have some good whole food, plant-based meal options available so that the food you do eat is in line with your health goals.

///

I know this chapter might be a stretch for some of you—and that's okay. The main goal of this book is to get you eating plants, plain and simple. If that means that all you do is swap out your animal foods for plant-based ones and call it a day, that's a win. If you decide to give up processed plant foods for whole ones, then that's another win. And if you decide to go even further and start experimenting with your macros and intermittent fasting, then again, that's a win too. There's no such thing as being the "best" vegan—it's not a competition (although some people definitely haven't gotten that memo). As far as I'm concerned, anything you do above and beyond eating plants is (mushroom) gravy. If you want to level up, I'm here for you and so is this information. But if not, no shame in that either. You've already won.

To view the references cited in this chapter, please visit badassvegan.com/citations.

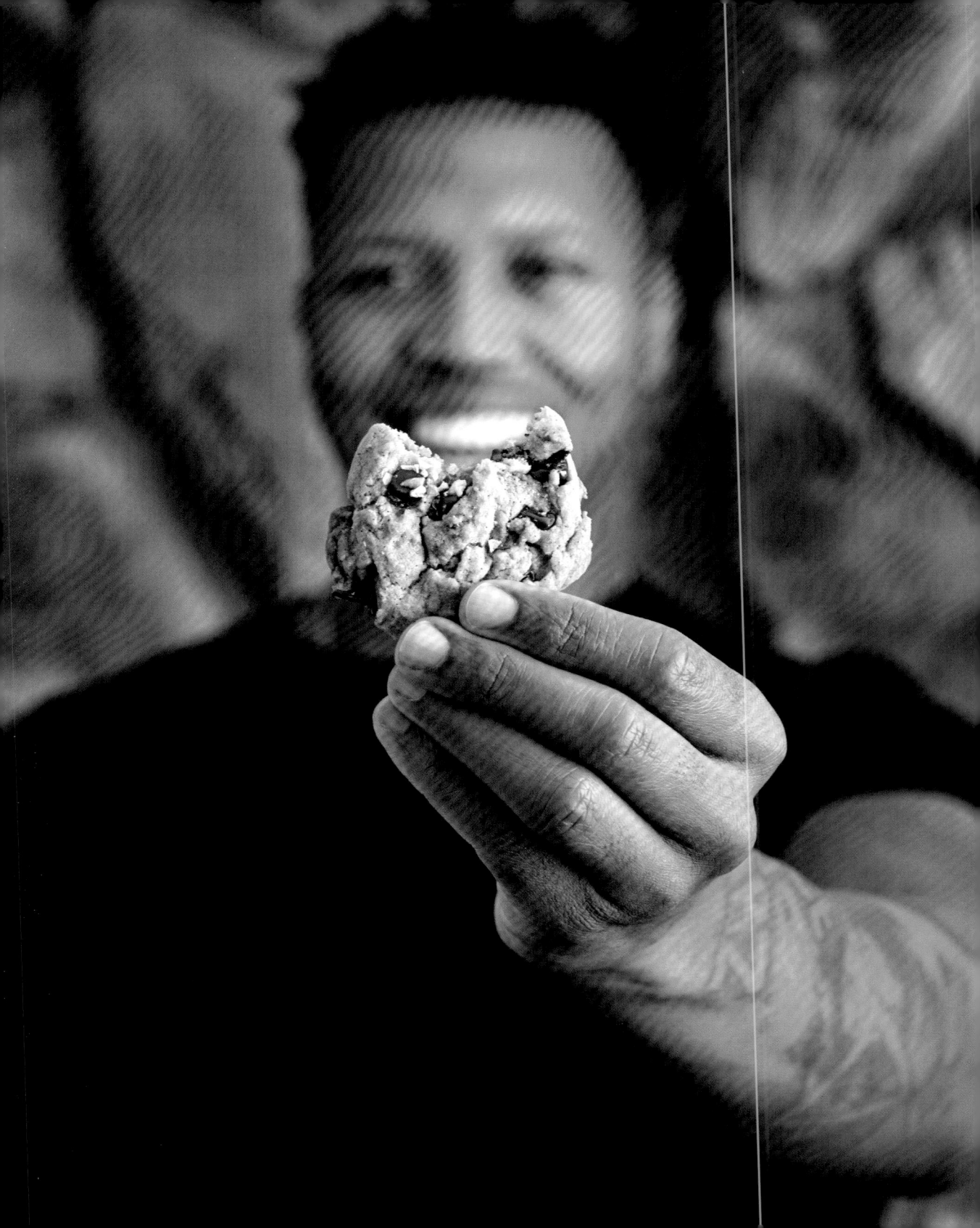

BADASS
RECIPE

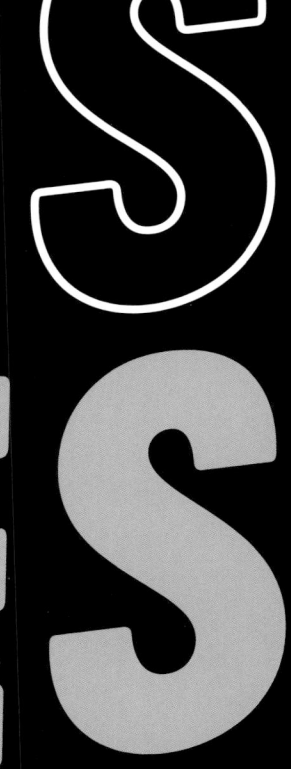

Alright, alright—you did it. You are almost at the end of the book, **BUT FIRST: FOOD. YOU GOTTA EAT,** after all. So no matter what point you are in your veganhood, you're in the right place. If you're just starting out, these recipes are going to show you just how tasty plant-based food can be, and how **EASY, INEXPENSIVE,** and **CROWD-PLEASING** it can be to make it in your own kitchen. If you've been at this for a while, the recipes will be like hitting the refresh button on your usual rotation. You might not recognize some ingredients, and some steps might feel a little more complicated than punching buttons on the microwave, but I promise you, from the bottom of my heart, that if **YOU GIVE ME YOUR TRUST,** then **I'LL GIVE YOU SOME DAMN GOOD MEALS** in return. My good friend and personal chef Tara Punzone and I put a lot of work into these recipes so that you wouldn't have to.

A NOTE ON SALT

A lot of people think they can't have salt or that they need to cut down on their salt for health reasons, especially people with hypertension, heart disease, and diabetes. The thing is, the salt that doctors are referring to when they tell you that is table salt—you know, the stuff in the shakers when you sit down at a restaurant. Table salt comes from natural underground salt deposits, but it's heavily processed to strip out minerals, and an anticlumping agent is added to it. And like any other processed food, we want to avoid that. Sea salt, on the other hand, comes straight from the ocean or saltwater lakes, with little to no processing, so it has all its minerals and trace elements still intact. That's why all the recipes here call for sea salt, which you can easily find at the grocery store.

CHAPTER 17

BREAKFAST AND SMOOTHIES

COCONUT ANTIOXIDANT YOGURT BOWLS

I didn't throw "antioxidants" into the name of this dish just to look impressive (even though it is pretty impressive). Our body needs these amazing compounds to prevent some bad business from going down. It also benefits from probiotics, or beneficial bacteria, that strengthen your digestive and immune systems. That's why you'll see the addition of probiotic powder—it's easy to throw into pretty much any bowl or smoothie.

Note: You can find cleaned and frozen young coconut meat in specialty food stores. **SERVES 4**

FOR THE COCONUT YOGURT

½ pound young coconut meat, thawed but still cold

½ cup raw cashews, soaked for 6 hours and rinsed

1 Medjool date, pitted

2 tablespoons fresh lime juice

2 teaspoons vanilla paste or extract

2 teaspoons vegan probiotic powder

Pinch of sea salt

FOR THE BOWLS

¼ cup blueberries

¼ cup strawberries

¼ cup raspberries

¼ cup cacao nibs

¼ cup dried goji berries

1 **MAKE THE COCONUT YOGURT:** In a high-speed blender, add the coconut meat, cashews, date, lime juice, vanilla, probiotic powder, and salt and blend until completely smooth. If making in advance, store the yogurt in an airtight container in the refrigerator for up to 6 days.

2 **MAKE THE YOGURT BOWLS:** Divide the yogurt between four bowls and top with the blueberries, strawberries, raspberries, cacao nibs, and goji berries.

FOR 1 SERVING:
CALORIES: 375
PROTEIN: 7 GRAMS (0.5 BLOCK)
CARBOHYDRATES: 26 GRAMS (1.5 BLOCKS)
FAT: 32 GRAMS (3 BLOCKS)

BREAKFAST AND SMOOTHIES

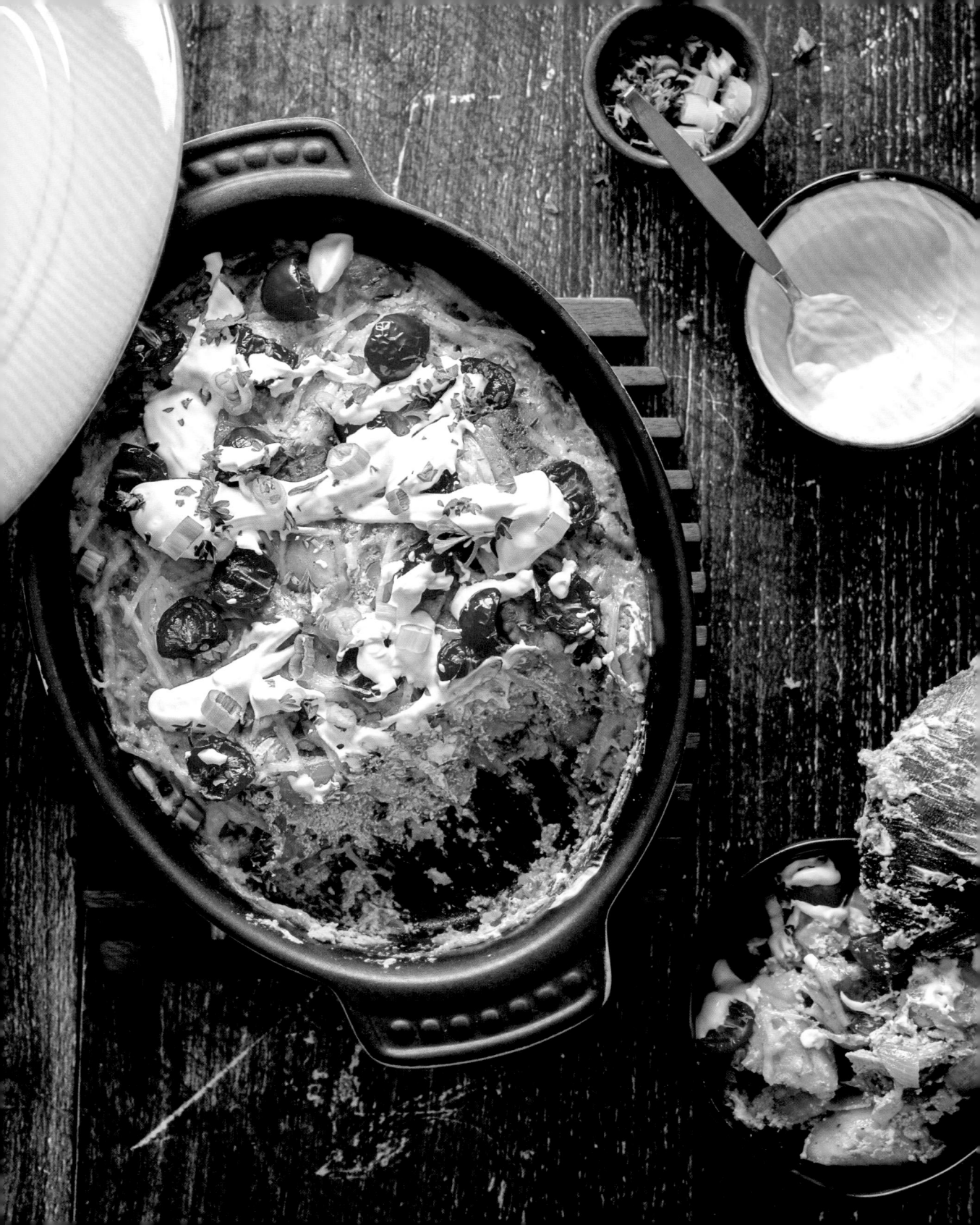

LOADED POTATO CASEROLE

Breakfast can be boring and bland. All those cereals for adults like Special K and Cheerios—what's that about? I say if you're gonna carb out, carb out on something you actually like. Why not have a loaded baked potato for breakfast? Because that's what this casserole essentially is; you got your sour cream, you got your chives, you got your cheese, and you got your tomatoes—everything you need for something warm and hearty in the morning. This recipe is perfect for those first thirty days when you're just having fun with things, but you can definitely work it into your Building Block Plan down the road by portioning for your goals.

Note: This recipe calls for black sea salt. It can be a little bit of a dance to find it, but it lasts a long time and gives the "eggs" that magic savory flavor that makes them taste like the real thing. Just do yourself a favor and buy a damn jar, okay? **SERVES 6**

FOR THE FILLING

5 medium Yukon Gold potatoes

2 tablespoons extra-virgin olive oil

1 medium onion, chopped

Sea salt and ground black pepper, to taste

2 teaspoons paprika

1 (5-ounce) block tempeh, sliced into 1-inch pieces

1 tablespoon store-bought BBQ sauce

1 teaspoon tamari soy sauce

FOR THE VEGAN EGG MIXTURE

1 (10-ounce) package silken tofu

1½ tablespoons extra-virgin olive oil

1 tablespoon cornstarch

1 teaspoon ground turmeric

½ teaspoon paprika

Pinch of black sea salt

½ cup vegan cheese, plus more for sprinkling

1 tablespoon chopped fresh or frozen chives

½ cup chopped cherry tomatoes

FOR ASSEMBLY

Chopped scallions (optional)

Chopped fresh parsley (optional)

Vegan sour cream (optional)

RECIPE CONTINUES >>

1 MAKE THE FILLING: In a medium pot, add enough cold water to cover the potatoes by about an inch. Bring the water to a boil over high heat, reduce the heat to a simmer, and cook the potatoes until you can easily pierce them with a fork or knife, about 20 minutes. Drain and let the potatoes cool slightly before peeling them and slicing them into bite-size cubes.

2 Heat 1 tablespoon of the olive oil in a large pan over medium heat. Add half the chopped onion and cook until soft and translucent, about 2 minutes. Add the potatoes and season with salt, pepper, and 1 teaspoon of the paprika. Cook until the potatoes are browned and crispy on the outside, about 5 minutes. Transfer the mixture to a bowl and set aside.

3 In the same pan, add the remaining tablespoon of oil and cook the remaining onion until tender and translucent, about 2 minutes. Add the tempeh and stir in the BBQ sauce, the remaining teaspoon of paprika, and the tamari. Season with salt and pepper to taste and cook for 5 minutes. Remove the pan from the heat and set aside.

4 MAKE THE VEGAN EGG MIXTURE: In a medium bowl, combine the tofu, oil, cornstarch, turmeric, paprika, and black salt. Whisk until smooth. Stir in the vegan cheese and chives.

5 ASSEMBLE: Preheat the oven to 350°F.

6 Combine the crispy potatoes and BBQ tempeh in the bottom of a casserole dish. Stir in the vegan egg mixture. Top with a sprinkling of cheese and the cherry tomatoes. Bake until the casserole is bubbling at the edges and cooked through, 15 to 20 minutes. Serve with the toppings of your choice, such as scallions, fresh parsley, or vegan sour cream, if using.

FOR 1 SERVING:
CALORIES: 270
PROTEIN: 13 GRAMS (0.5 BLOCK)
CARBOHYDRATES: 31 GRAMS (1.5 BLOCKS)
FAT: 14 GRAMS (1.5 BLOCKS)

BADASS
BEAUTIFUL MESS

This dish is dear to my heart because I came up with this recipe (and many other recipes) when I only had twenty-two dollars in my bank account. It's not flashy, it's not fancy, but it is f*cking delicious. **SERVES 2**

2 teaspoons extra-virgin olive oil

2 very ripe plantains

1 large white onion, sliced into ½-inch rounds

Sea salt, to taste

2 cups cooked quinoa

¼ cup Holy Moly Guacamole (page 262) or store-bought

1 Preheat the oven to 400°F. Line a baking sheet with foil and brush with a teaspoon of the olive oil.

2 Using a sharp knife, trim both ends of the plantains and cut a shallow slit down the length of the peel. Peel the plantains starting from the seam— it should come off in one big piece. Chop the plantains into 1-inch pieces.

3 Set the plantains on the prepared baking sheet and bake for 15 minutes. Turn the plantains and bake for 15 more minutes, until very tender and fragrant.

4 Heat a grill or grill pan to medium-high heat. Brush the onion rounds on both sides with the remaining teaspoon of oil and season with salt. Carefully place the onion rounds on the grill and cook, undisturbed, until nicely charred, 3 to 5 minutes.

RECIPE CONTINUES >>

Flip, doing your best to keep the rounds intact (it's okay if they separate a bit), and cook for another 3 to 5 minutes. Transfer the grilled onions to a cutting board and chop them roughly.

5 Divide the quinoa between two bowls and top each with half the baked sweet plantains, about ½ cup of the chopped grilled onion, and 2 tablespoons of the guacamole.

FOR 1 SERVING:
CALORIES: 470
PROTEIN: 12 GRAMS (0.5 BLOCK)
CARBOHYDRATES: 83 GRAMS (4 BLOCKS)
FAT: 14 GRAMS (1.5 BLOCKS)

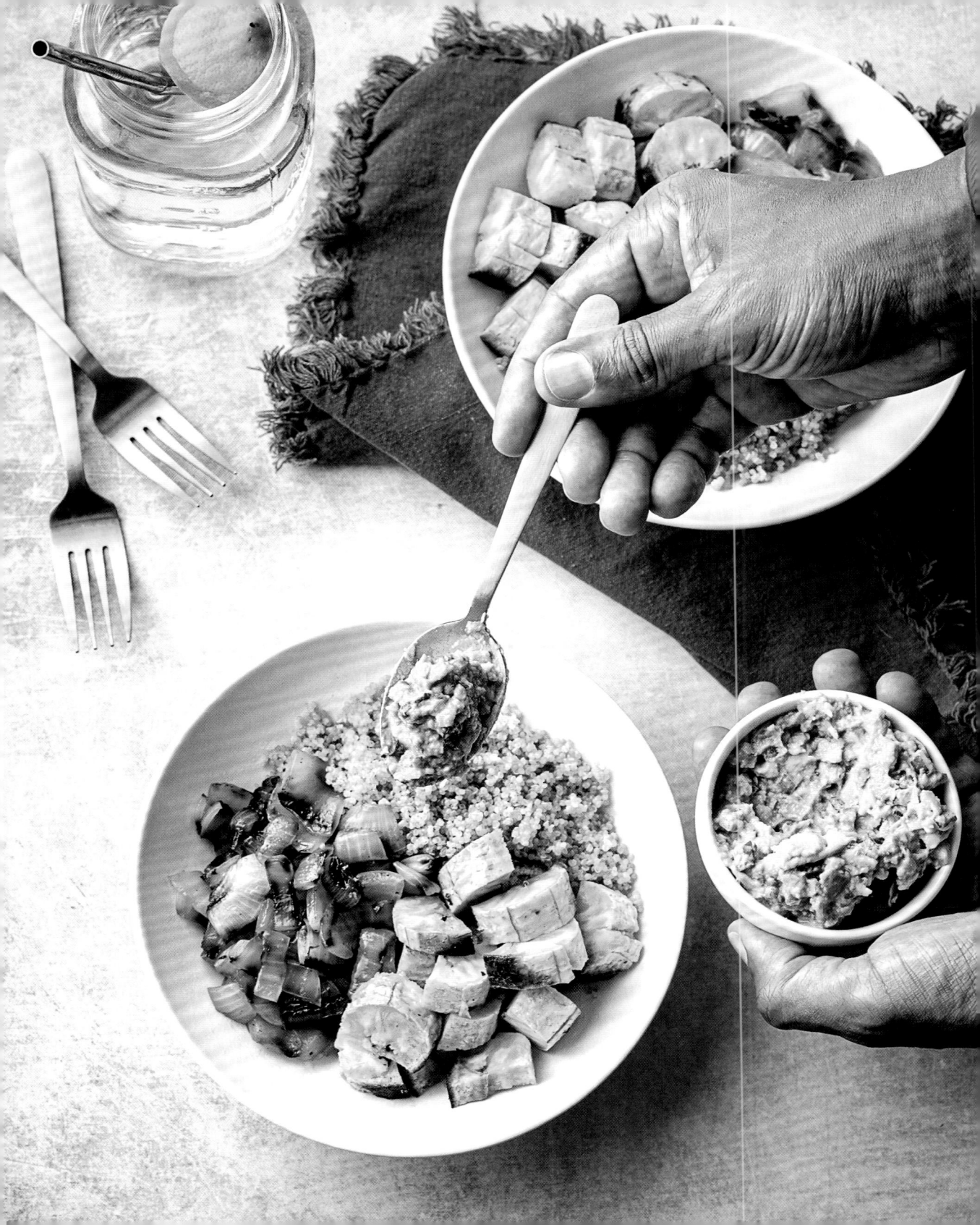

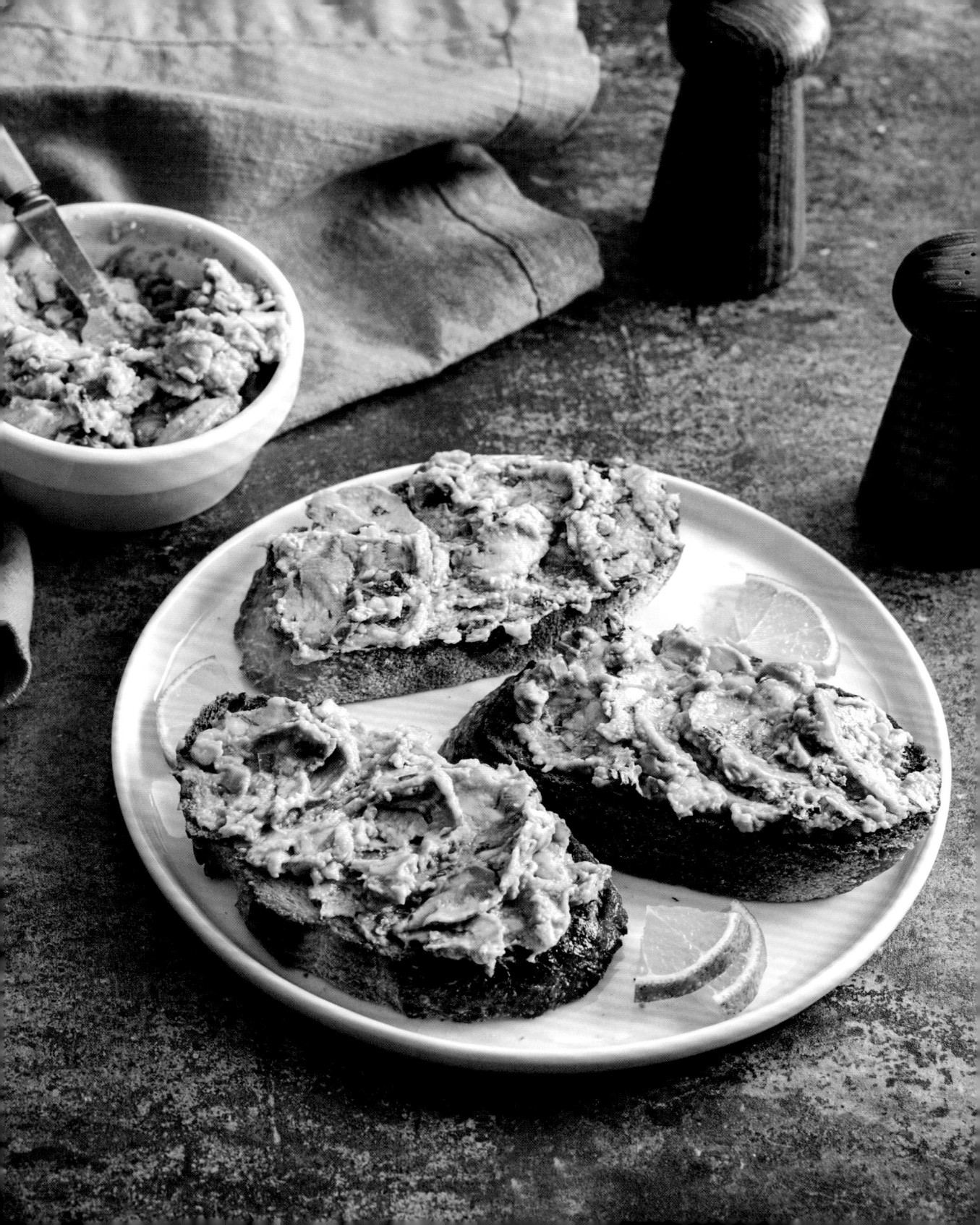

AVOCADOÉ TOAST

There's a big difference between avocado toast and badass
avocado toast . . . okay, maybe not huge, but by using
guacamole instead of straight-up avocado, you're packing in a
lot more flavor. **SERVES 2**

**4 thick slices
bread (I like
fresh-ass
sourdough or
Dave's Killer
Bread)**

**½ cup Holy Moly
Guacamole
(page 262) or
store-bought**

In a toaster or under the broiler, toast
the bread to your liking. Top each slice
of toast with about 2 tablespoons of the
guacamole and serve.

FOR 1 SERVING:
CALORIES: 490
PROTEIN: 18 GRAMS (1 BLOCK)
CARBOHYDRATES: 87 GRAMS (4.5 BLOCKS)
FAT: 10 GRAMS (1 BLOCK)

SMOOTHIES

What can I say? I love me a smoothie, which is why I'm giving you a whole bunch of my favorite combinations. They're quick to throw together and are perfect for breakfast, lunch, snacks, desserts, late-night quickies, you name it. And the best part is that they always bring it with both the nutrition and the flavor.

GRAPE APE SMOOTHIE

MAKES 1 SMOOTHIE

1 banana

1 cup red or green seedless grapes

1 cup strawberries, hulled

In a high-speed blender, add the banana, grapes, and strawberries and blend until completely smooth.

CALORIES: 240
PROTEIN: 3 GRAMS (0 BLOCKS)
CARBOHYDRATES: 63 GRAMS (3 BLOCKS)
FAT: 1 GRAM (0 BLOCKS)

BERRYLICIOUS SMOOTHIE

MAKES 1 SMOOTHIE

1¼ cups coconut water

½ cup frozen strawberries

⅓ cup frozen sliced banana

¼ cup frozen acai puree

¼ cup frozen blueberries

In a high-speed blender, add the coconut water, strawberries, banana, acai, and blueberries and blend until completely smooth.

CALORIES: 160
PROTEIN: 3 GRAMS (0 BLOCKS)
CARBOHYDRATES: 46 GRAMS (2.5 BLOCKS)
FAT: 2 GRAMS (0 BLOCKS)

RECIPES CONTINUE >>

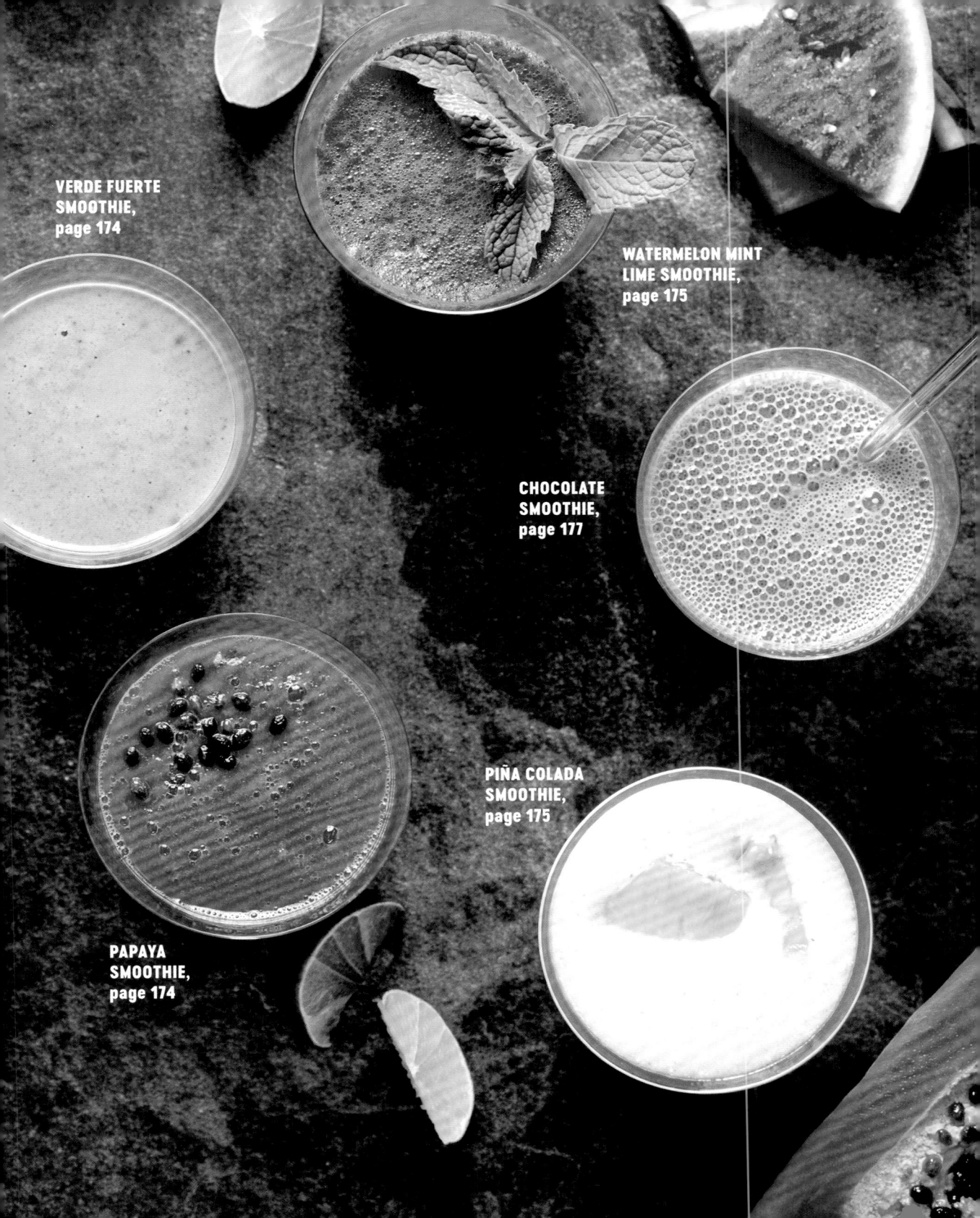

VERDE FUERTE
SMOOTHIE,
page 174

WATERMELON MINT
LIME SMOOTHIE,
page 175

CHOCOLATE
SMOOTHIE,
page 177

PIÑA COLADA
SMOOTHIE,
page 175

PAPAYA
SMOOTHIE,
page 174

PIKA-CHEW SMOOTHIE

MAKES 1 SMOOTHIE

1¼ cups frozen sliced banana

½ cup cold-brewed coffee

⅓ cup oat milk

2 pitted dates

1 tablespoon chia seeds

1 tablespoon cacao nibs

In a high-speed blender, add the sliced banana, coffee, oat milk, dates, chia seeds, and cacao nibs and blend until completely smooth.

CALORIES: 370
PROTEIN: 8 GRAMS (0.5 BLOCK)
CARBOHYDRATES: 67 GRAMS (3.5 BLOCKS)
FAT: 12 GRAMS (1 BLOCK)

VERDE FUERTE SMOOTHIE

MAKES 1 SMOOTHIE

1 cup hemp milk

1 cup frozen sliced banana

1 serving of protein powder of your choice

1 teaspoon spirulina powder

1 pitted date

In a high-speed blender, add the hemp milk, banana, protein powder, spirulina, and date and blend until completely smooth.

CALORIES: 370
PROTEIN: 31 GRAMS (1.5 BLOCKS)
CARBOHYDRATES: 45 GRAMS (2.5 BLOCKS)
FAT: 9 GRAMS (1 BLOCK)

PAPAYA SMOOTHIE

MAKES 1 SMOOTHIE

½ ripe papaya, peeled and seeded

2 tablespoons fresh lime juice

In a high-speed blender, add the papaya, lime juice, and 1 cup of water and blend until completely smooth.

CALORIES: 80
PROTEIN: 1 GRAM (0 BLOCKS)
CARBOHYDRATES: 23 GRAMS (1 BLOCK)
FAT: 0 GRAMS (0 BLOCKS)

CUCUMBER WATERMELON SMOOTHIE

MAKES 1 SMOOTHIE

1¾ cups roughly chopped fresh watermelon, seeds removed

1 cup roughly chopped fresh cucumber

2 to 3 fresh mint leaves

2 tablespoons fresh lime juice

In a high-speed blender, add the watermelon, cucumber, mint, lime juice, and 1 cup of water and blend until completely smooth.

CALORIES: 110
PROTEIN: 3 GRAMS (0 BLOCKS)
CARBOHYDRATES: 22 GRAMS (1 BLOCK)
FAT: 1.5 GRAMS (0 BLOCKS)

WATERMELON CILANTRO LIME SMOOTHIE

MAKES 1 SMOOTHIE

2¼ cups roughly chopped fresh watermelon, seeds removed

2 tablespoons fresh lime juice

2 to 3 sprigs fresh cilantro

In a high-speed blender, add the watermelon, lime juice, cilantro, and ½ cup of water and blend until completely smooth.

CALORIES: 120
PROTEIN: 2 GRAMS (0 BLOCKS)
CARBOHYDRATES: 25 GRAMS (1.5 BLOCKS)
FAT: 1 GRAM (0 BLOCKS)

WATERMELON MINT LIME SMOOTHIE

MAKES 1 SMOOTHIE

2½ cups roughly chopped fresh watermelon, seeds removed

2 tablespoons fresh lime juice

2 to 3 large fresh mint leaves

In a high-speed blender, add the watermelon, lime juice, mint, and ½ cup of water and blend until completely smooth.

CALORIES: 130
PROTEIN: 2 GRAMS (0 BLOCKS)
CARBOHYDRATES: 28 GRAMS (1.5 BLOCKS)
FAT: 1 GRAM (0 BLOCKS)

COCONUT SMOOTHIE

MAKES 1 SMOOTHIE

1 cup young coconut meat

1 cup coconut water (such as Harmless Harvest)

½ cup unsweetened shredded dried coconut or coconut flakes

In a high-speed blender, add the coconut meat, coconut water, dried coconut, and ½ cup of water and blend until completely smooth.

CALORIES: 600
PROTEIN: 6 GRAMS (0.5 BLOCK)
CARBOHYDRATES: 41 GRAMS (2 BLOCKS)
FAT: 56 GRAMS (5.5 BLOCKS)

PIÑA COLADA SMOOTHIE

MAKES 1 SMOOTHIE

1 cup Coconut Smoothie (above)

1 cup roughly chopped fresh pineapple

In a high-speed blender, add the coconut smoothie and pineapple and blend until completely smooth.

CALORIES: 580
PROTEIN: 5 GRAMS (0.5 BLOCK)
CARBOHYDRATES: 55 GRAMS (3 BLOCKS)
FAT: 48 GRAMS (5 BLOCKS)

RECIPES CONTINUE >>

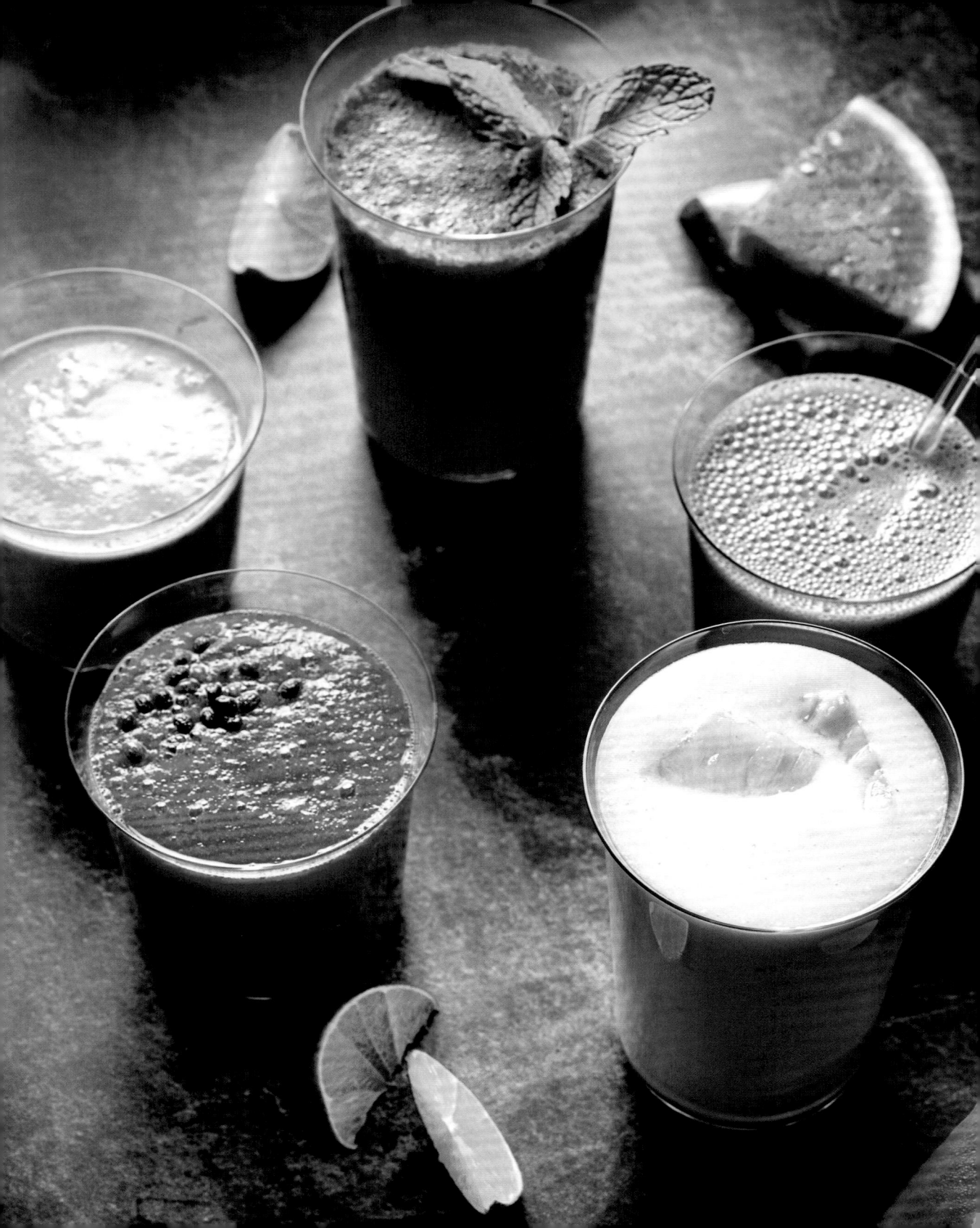

CHOCOLATE SMOOTHIE

MAKES 1 SMOOTHIE

2 cups Almond Milk (page 179)

2 tablespoons cacao powder

⅓ cup raw cashews, soaked overnight

⅓ cup young coconut meat

In a high-speed blender, add the almond milk, cacao, cashews, and coconut and blend until completely smooth.

CALORIES: 450
PROTEIN: 14 GRAMS (0.5 BLOCK)
CARBOHYDRATES: 21 GRAMS (1 BLOCK)
FAT: 39 GRAMS (4 BLOCKS)

CHOCOLATE ALMOND BUTTER SMOOTHIE

MAKES 1 SMOOTHIE

1 cup Chocolate Smoothie (above)

1 tablespoon almond butter

In a high-speed blender, add the chocolate smoothie and almond butter and blend until completely smooth.

CALORIES: 340
PROTEIN: 11 GRAMS (0.5 BLOCK)
CARBOHYDRATES: 15 GRAMS (1 BLOCK)
FAT: 30 GRAMS (3 BLOCKS)

CHOCOLATE BANANA SMOOTHIE

MAKES 1 SMOOTHIE

1 cup Chocolate Smoothie (opposite)

½ small banana

In a high-speed blender, add the chocolate smoothie and banana and blend until completely smooth.

CALORIES: 260
PROTEIN: 7 GRAMS (0.5 BLOCK)
CARBOHYDRATES: 19 GRAMS (1 BLOCK)
FAT: 20 GRAMS (2 BLOCKS)

VANILLA SMOOTHIE

MAKES 1 SMOOTHIE

2 cups Almond Milk (page 179)

⅓ cup raw cashews, soaked overnight

⅓ cup young coconut meat

1 teaspoon vanilla extract

Scraped seeds from ½ vanilla bean

In a high-speed blender, add the almond milk, cashews, coconut, vanilla extract, and vanilla seeds and blend until completely smooth.

CALORIES: 400
PROTEIN: 11 GRAMS (0.5 BLOCK)
CARBOHYDRATES: 14 GRAMS (0.5 BLOCK)
FAT: 36 GRAMS (3.5 BLOCKS)

BREAKFAST AND SMOOTHIES

RECIPES CONTINUE >>

GREEN SMOOTHIE

MAKES 1 SMOOTHIE

1 cup Almond Milk (page 179)

1 cup kale, stems removed and leaves roughly torn

1 banana

1 Medjool date, pitted

In a high-speed blender, add the almond milk, kale, banana, date, and ½ cup of water and blend until completely smooth.

CALORIES: 180
PROTEIN: 3 GRAMS (0 BLOCKS)
CARBOHYDRATES: 38 GRAMS (2 BLOCKS)
FAT: 3 GRAMS (0.5 BLOCK)

ALTERNATIVE MILKS

Just because you're off the dairy tip doesn't mean you can't have "milk." Milks made from nuts and seeds are not only more biologically appropriate (because the only thing cow's milk is for is a baby cow) but easy to make and store in the fridge for all your milk needs. You can also use them as a base, and flavor them with things like chocolate and chai.

These recipes call for a nut milk bag, which is similar to a cheesecloth and is used to filter any nut solids from the milks. They make it easier to squeeze out every last drop of milk, are inexpensive, and can be found online or in most large stores that sell housewares.

ALMOND MILK

MAKES 8 CUPS

4 cups raw almonds, soaked for 6 hours, drained, and rinsed

2 Medjool dates, pitted

In a high-speed blender, add the soaked almonds, dates, and 8 cups of water and blend until completely smooth. Over a large bowl or container, pour the nut mixture into a nut milk bag. Let the milk drain, squeezing all remaining liquid out of the bag until the sediment feels dry. Refrigerate the milk immediately and store in the fridge for up to 5 days.

FOR 1 CUP:
CALORIES: 50
PROTEIN: 1 GRAM (0 BLOCKS)
CARBOHYDRATES: 5 GRAMS (0.5 BLOCK)
FAT: 3 GRAMS (0.5 BLOCK)

MACADAMIA NUT MILK

MAKES 8 CUPS

2 cups macadamia nuts, soaked for 6 hours, drained, and rinsed

2 Medjool dates, pitted

In a high-speed blender, add the soaked macadamias, dates, and 5 cups of water and blend until completely smooth. Over a large bowl or container, pour the nut mixture into a nut milk bag. Let the milk drain, squeezing all remaining liquid out of the bag until the sediment feels dry. Refrigerate the milk immediately and store in the fridge for up to 5 days.

FOR 1 CUP:
CALORIES: 110
PROTEIN: 1 GRAM (0 BLOCKS)
CARBOHYDRATES: 12 GRAMS (0.5 BLOCK)
FAT: 7 GRAMS (0.5 BLOCK)

RECIPES CONTINUE >>

CHAI MILK

MAKES 1 CUP

1 cup Almond Milk (page 179) or Macadamia Nut Milk (page 179)

1 teaspoon Chai Spice Mix (recipe follows)

In a high-speed blender, add the nut milk and chai spice mix and blend until the spices are evenly incorporated.

FOR 1 CUP:
CALORIES: 60
PROTEIN: 1 GRAM (0 BLOCKS)
CARBOHYDRATES: 8 GRAMS (0.5 BLOCK)
FAT: 3 GRAMS (0.5 BLOCK)

CHAI SPICE MIX

MAKES ABOUT ½ CUP

¼ cup ground cinnamon

1 tablespoon ground cardamom

2 teaspoons ground ginger

1 teaspoon ground cloves

1 teaspoon ground nutmeg

½ teaspoon ground black pepper

In a jar, combine the cinnamon, cardamom, ginger, cloves, nutmeg, and pepper, and stir or cover and shake to combine. Store in a cool, dark place for up to 4 months.

CHOCOLATE ALMOND MILK

MAKES 1 CUP

1 cup Almond Milk (page 179)

1 tablespoon cacao powder

In a high-speed blender, add the almond milk and cacao and blend until completely smooth.

FOR 1 CUP:
CALORIES: 70
PROTEIN: 3 GRAMS (0 BLOCKS)
CARBOHYDRATES: 9 GRAMS (0.5 BLOCK)
FAT: 4.5 GRAMS (0.5 BLOCK)

CACAO CHAI MILK

MAKES 1 CUP

1 cup Almond Milk (page 179) or Macadamia Nut Milk (page 179)

1 tablespoon cacao powder

1 teaspoon Chai Spice Mix (opposite)

In a high-speed blender, add the nut milk, cacao, and chai spice mix and blend until the spices are evenly incorporated.

FOR 1 CUP:
CALORIES: 80
PROTEIN: 3 GRAMS (0 BLOCKS)
CARBOHYDRATES: 11 GRAMS (0.5 BLOCK)
FAT: 4.5 GRAMS (0.5 BLOCK)

CACAO CINNAMON MILK

MAKES 1 CUP

1 cup Almond
Milk (page 179) or
Macadamia Nut
Milk (page 179)

1 tablespoon
cacao powder

1 teaspoon
ground cinnamon

In a high-speed blender, add the nut
milk, cacao, and cinnamon and blend
until the spices are evenly
incorporated.

FOR 1 CUP:
CALORIES: 70
PROTEIN: 3 GRAMS (0 BLOCKS)
CARBOHYDRATES: 10 GRAMS (0.5 BLOCK)
FAT: 4.5 GRAMS (0.5 BLOCK)

CHAPTER 18

LUNCH

PROBIOTIC KALE SALAD

Probiotic ingredients like sauerkraut deliver healthy bacteria to your gut, like a little power-up infusion. In turn, those good guys help your digestive system and strengthen your immune system. This salad also features dulse, a type of seaweed full of minerals like potassium and iodine. It gives your food a salty, umami flavor. After eating this salad, you'll be saying, "Kale yeah." **SERVES 2**

6 cups kale, stemmed and leaves chopped into 1-inch pieces

⅔ cup Tahini Ginger Dressing (page 269)

2 tablespoons naturally fermented sauerkraut (such as Wildbrine)

2 teaspoons black sesame seeds, plus more for serving

1 teaspoon dulse granules (I like Sea Seasonings brand)

½ cucumber, sliced thin

½ cup sunflower sprouts

In a medium bowl, toss together the kale, dressing, sauerkraut, sesame seeds, and dulse. Using clean hands, massage the dressing into the mixture until it is evenly distributed and the kale has softened slightly, about 2 minutes. Top with the cucumber, sprouts, and additional sesame seeds.

FOR 1 SERVING:
CALORIES: 350
PROTEIN: 17 GRAMS (1 BLOCK)
CARBOHYDRATES: 20 GRAMS (1 BLOCK)
FAT: 28 GRAMS (3 BLOCKS)

LUNCH

PINEAPPLE CHIPOTLE TEMPEH PO' BOY WRAPS

What I love the most about this wrap (or sandwich, if you prefer to use bread) is how many vegetables it packs in, but you don't feel like you're eating some kind of wimpy salad. With its sweet-smoky flavor and "meaty" tempeh, you won't feel po' after eating this baby here. That sweetness comes from coconut nectar, which is the sap from the flowers of the coconut tree. Many grocery stores now carry it in the sweetener section. **MAKES ABOUT 3 WRAPS**

FOR THE TEMPEH

1 cup diced tempeh

¾ cup diced fresh pineapple

½ cup Pineapple Chipotle Sauce (page 267)

½ cup finely chopped red onion

½ cup halved cherry tomatoes

½ cup chopped baby bok choy

½ cup chopped red bell pepper

1 tablespoon sesame seeds

FOR THE MARINATED CABBAGE SALAD

¼ cup brown rice vinegar

2 tablespoons tamari soy sauce

1 tablespoon coconut nectar

1¾ cups very thinly sliced green cabbage

¾ cup julienned carrots

1 tablespoon minced yellow onion

1 tablespoon black sesame seeds

FOR THE WRAPS

3 whole-grain wraps, warmed, or 1 whole-grain baguette, toasted and cut into three sections

Pineapple Chipotle Sauce (page 267), for drizzling

¼ cup fresh cilantro leaves (optional)

½ Hass avocado, peeled, pitted, and sliced (optional)

RECIPE CONTINUES >>

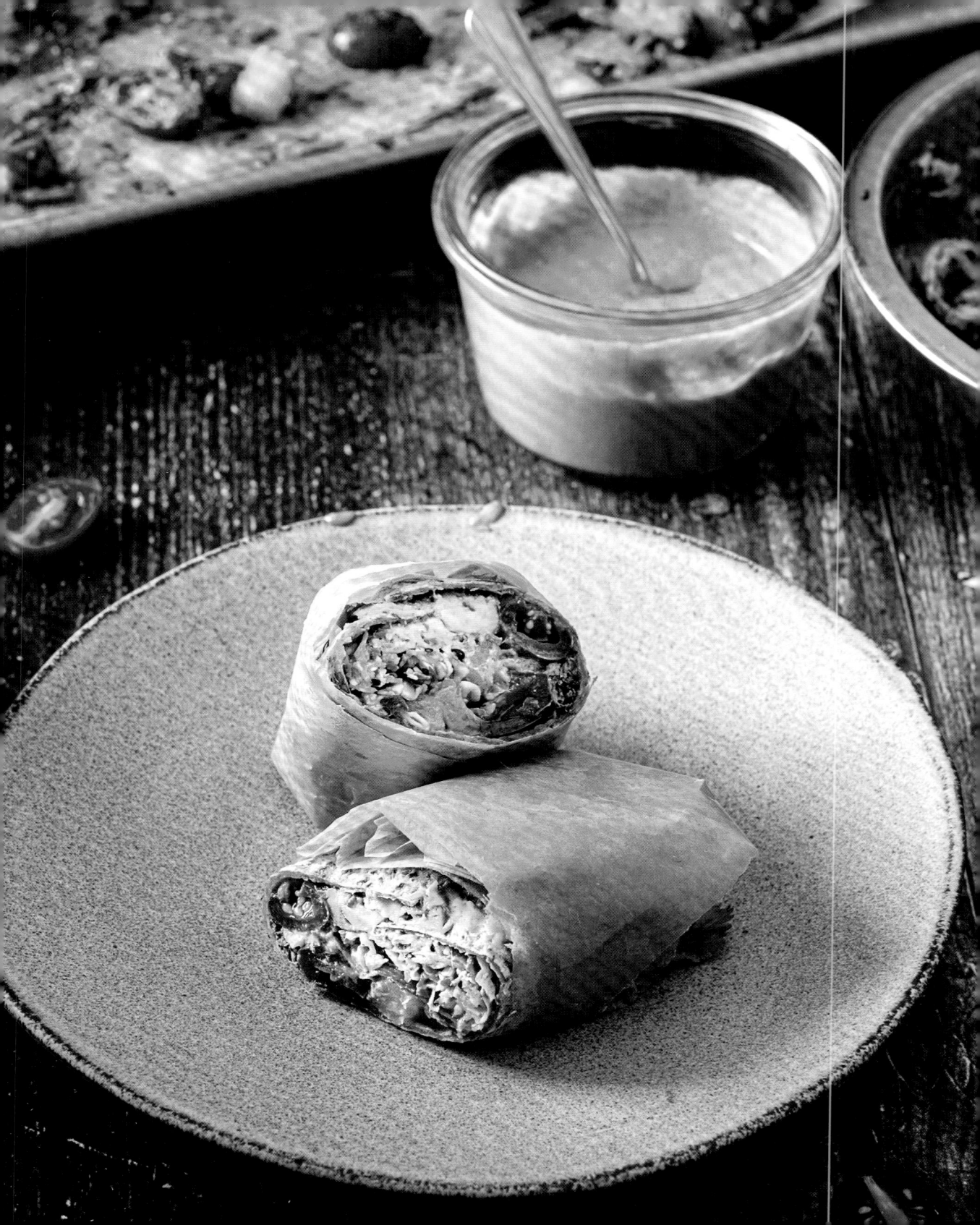

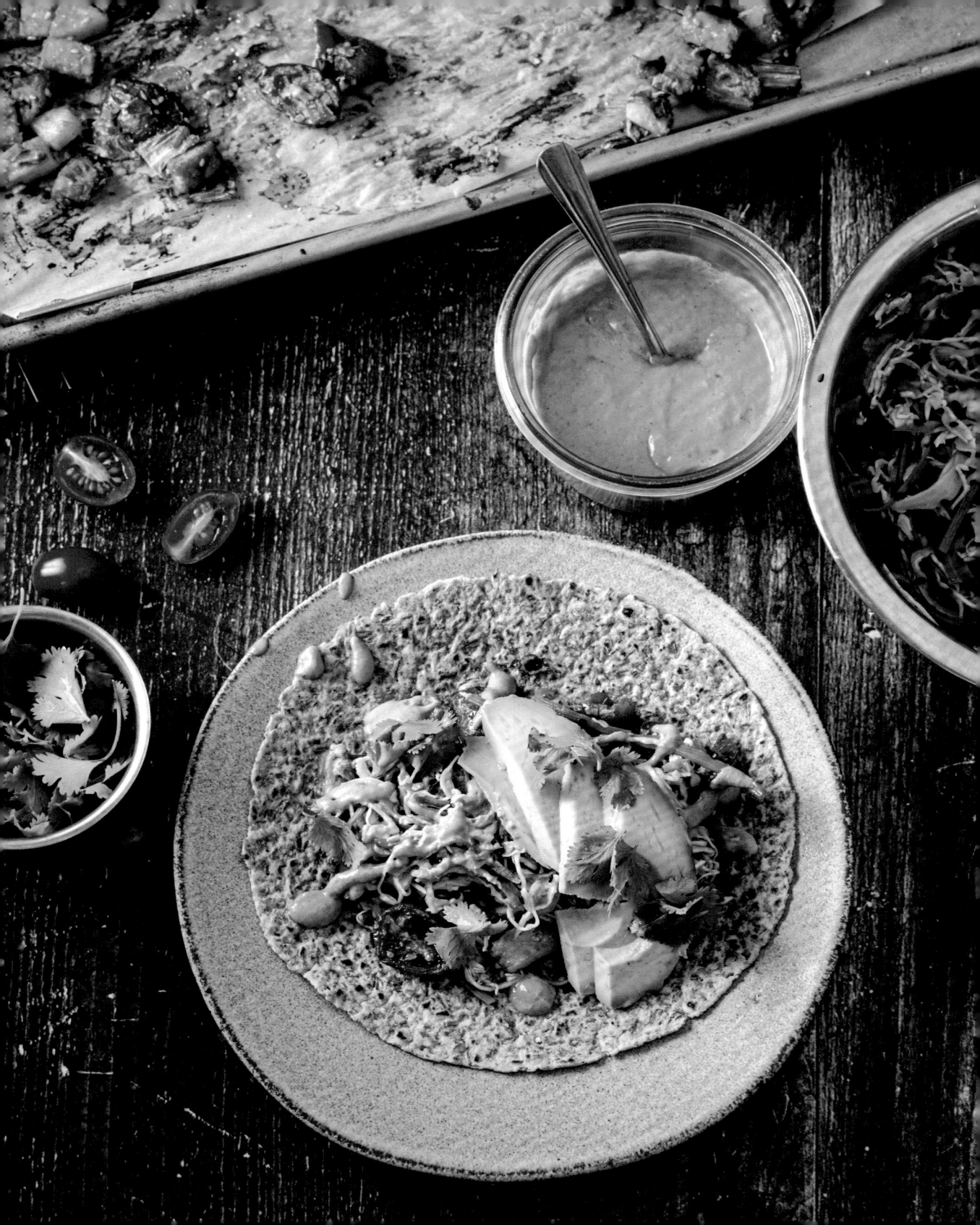

1 **MAKE THE TEMPEH:** Preheat the oven to 350°F. Line a baking sheet with parchment paper.

2 In a large bowl, toss together the tempeh, pineapple, pineapple chipotle sauce, onion, tomatoes, bok choy, bell pepper, and sesame seeds until thoroughly combined. Spread the mixture in an even layer on the prepared baking sheet and bake for 30 minutes, or until the mixture looks like it is drying out, stirring halfway through.

3 **MAKE THE MARINATED CABBAGE SALAD:** In a small bowl, whisk together the vinegar, tamari, and coconut nectar.

4 In a large bowl, add the cabbage, carrots, onion, and sesame seeds. Add the vinegar mixture and toss to coat. Let the cabbage sit for at least 10 minutes before using.

5 **ASSEMBLE THE WRAPS:** Fill each wrap with about ¾ cup of the tempeh mixture, ¼ cup of the marinated cabbage salad, and a drizzle of the pineapple chipotle sauce. If you like, add fresh cilantro and avocado.

FOR 1 WRAP:
CALORIES: 730
PROTEIN: 34 GRAMS (1.5 BLOCKS)
CARBOHYDRATES: 76 GRAMS (4 BLOCKS)
FAT: 43 GRAMS (4 BLOCKS)

KIMCHI NORI MAKI ROLL

Warning! Before you bite into these rolls, remember that they bite back. If you can't source a jade pearl rice, white sushi rice will do just fine. **SERVES 4**

FOR THE SUSHI RICE

2 cups jade pearl rice

½ teaspoon sea salt

2 tablespoons brown rice vinegar

1 tablespoon mirin

FOR THE KIMCHI MAKI ROLLS

4 large sheets toasted nori

24 pea shoots

¾ cup drained kimchi (I like Wildbrine), chopped if needed

8 asparagus spears, grilled with extra-virgin olive oil and sea salt

1 firm but ripe Hass avocado, peeled, pitted, and sliced thin

1 red bell pepper, stemmed, seeded, and julienned

2 scallions, cut lengthwise into ¼-inch strips

2 tablespoons sesame seeds

Sweet Miso Dipping Sauce (page 281), for serving

1 **MAKE THE SUSHI RICE:** In a large pot or rice cooker, combine the rice, salt, and 3 cups of water. Follow the package instructions to cook the rice.

2 Transfer the rice to a large bowl. Drizzle the vinegar and mirin over the rice and gently toss to coat. Let the rice cool completely.

3 **MAKE THE KIMCHI MAKI ROLLS:** Place one nori sheet shiny side down on a bamboo mat with one long side positioned closest to you. Spread 1 cup of the cooled rice in an even layer over the nori sheet, leaving a ½-inch border on the top long side.

4 Place 3 pea shoots facing out on each side, allowing the leafy tips to stick out each end of the nori. Arrange a quarter of the kimchi in an even line across the rice.

RECIPE CONTINUES >>

BADASS VEGAN

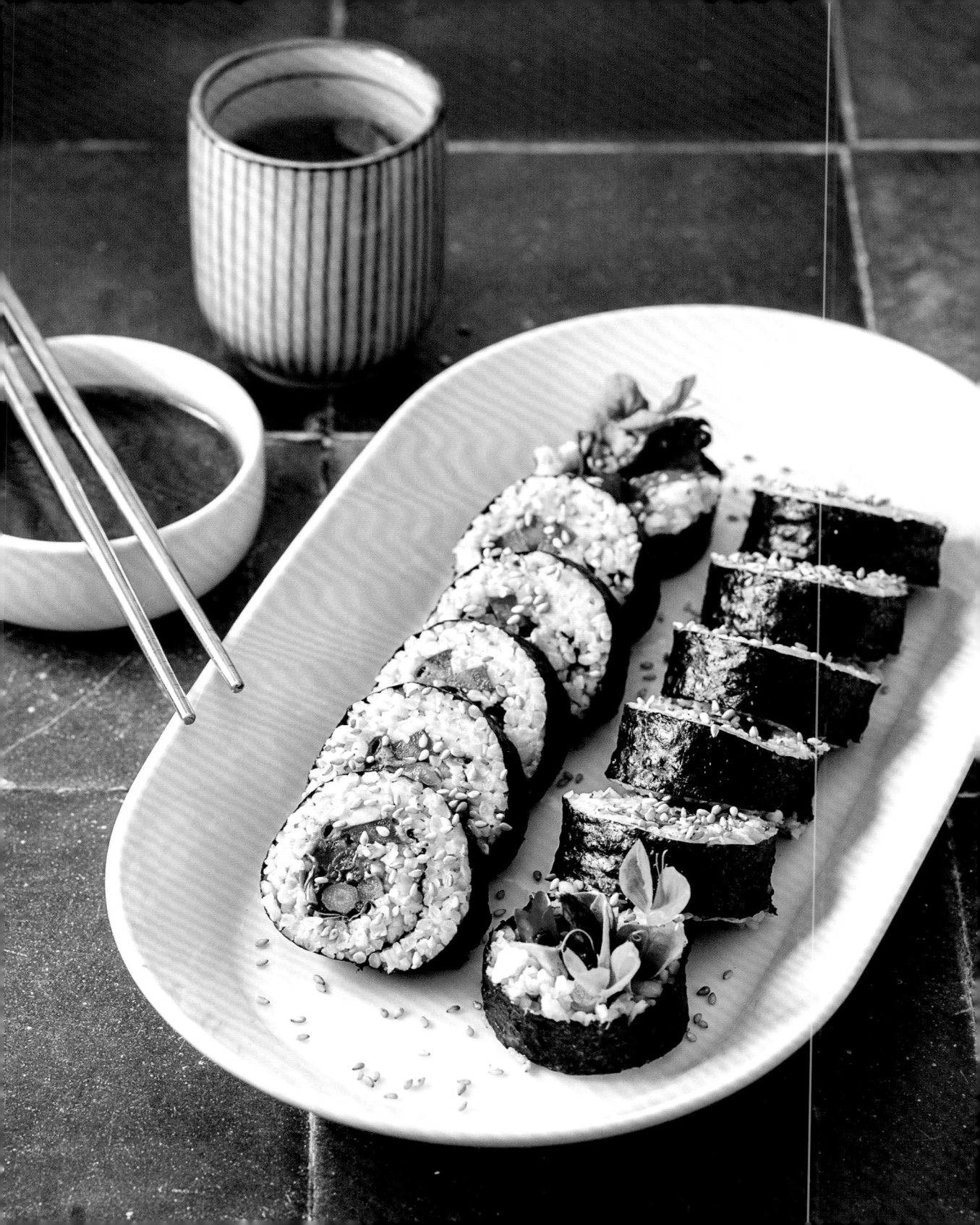

5 Just below the kimchi, arrange 2 asparagus spears facing out, with the tips slightly sticking out of the nori. Next, arrange a quarter each of the avocado slices, pepper strips, and scallions on top of the rice.

6 Starting with the side closest to you and using the mat as an aid, roll up the nori tightly, just like you would roll a joint. Moisten the opposite long edge with water and seal the roll. Repeat this process to make 4 rolls total.

7 Using a very sharp knife, cut each roll into 8 pieces about ½ inch thick. Arrange the slices cut side up on a platter, except for the two end pieces, which should be cut side down. Sprinkle with the sesame seeds and serve with the sweet miso dipping sauce.

FOR 1 ROLL:
CALORIES: 440
PROTEIN: 11 GRAMS (0.5 BLOCK)
CARBOHYDRATES: 78 GRAMS (4 BLOCKS)
FAT: 11 GRAMS (1 BLOCK)

GINGERED BLACK LENTIL SOUP

You'll notice that I'm a huge fan of ginger. That's not just because it's awesome for your health with all of its anti-inflammatory properties; it's also got a great kick and a little spice in the flavor department. Once you try this soup, you'll feel the ginger love too. **MAKES ABOUT 6 CUPS**

¼ cup sesame oil

½ cup diced onions

½ cup diced celery

½ cup diced carrot

½ cup diced kabocha squash

¼ cup minced fresh ginger

1 teaspoon sea salt, plus more to taste

2 teaspoons ground black pepper

2 teaspoons ground coriander

1 teaspoon ground turmeric

4 cups filtered water

1 cup dried black lentils, sorted, rinsed, and any small stones discarded

¼ cup tamari soy sauce

Thinly sliced scallions, for serving

Chopped fresh cilantro, for serving

1 In a large pot over medium heat, heat the sesame oil. Add the onions, celery, carrot, squash, ginger, salt, pepper, coriander, and turmeric and cook, stirring occasionally, until the onions are translucent, 8 to 10 minutes. Add the water and increase the heat to medium-high. Bring the mixture to a boil and add the lentils and tamari. Reduce the heat to medium and cook, stirring occasionally, until the lentils are tender, 10 to 15 minutes.

2 Taste and add more salt if desired. Divide the soup between bowls and top with the scallions and cilantro.

FOR 1 CUP:
CALORIES: 200
PROTEIN: 10 GRAMS (0.5 BLOCK)
CARBOHYDRATES: 25 GRAMS (1.5 BLOCKS)
FAT: 9 GRAMS (1 BLOCK)

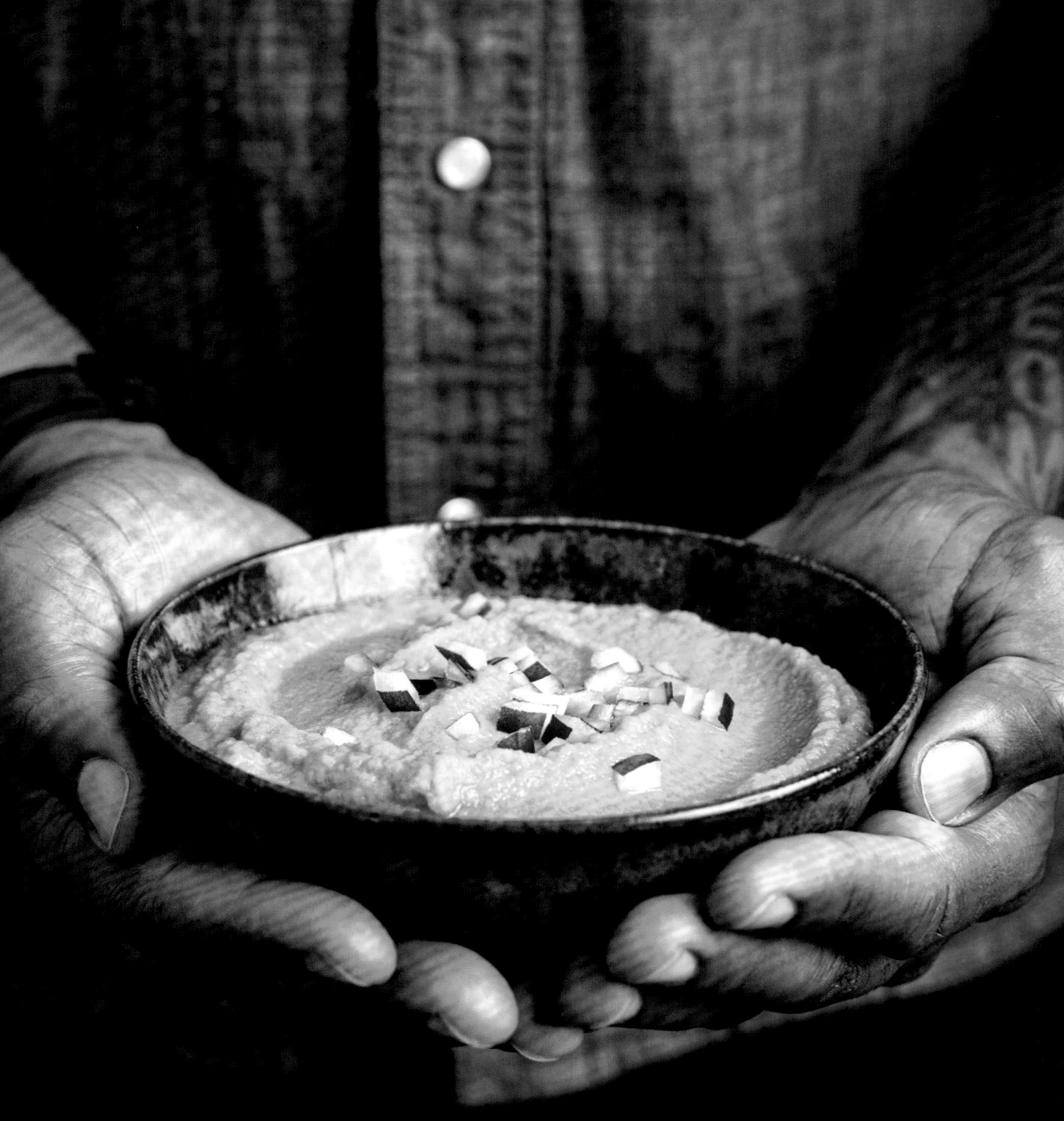

BADASS SWEET POTATO SOUP

This was one of my staples when I first went vegan and didn't really know what to make until I looked around the kitchen, saw these ingredients, and bam . . . badass sweet potato soup. Because you're chopping and blending the ingredients before cooking them, this dish takes minutes to come together. **SERVES 4**

1 large sweet potato, peeled and chopped

1 large carrot, sliced

3 Medjool dates, pitted

½ Hass avocado, peeled and pitted

2 garlic cloves

⅓ small jalapeño

⅓ medium red onion, diced

1 In a high-speed blender, add the sweet potato, carrot, dates, avocado, garlic, jalapeño, and 2 cups of water and blend on low speed for about 1 minute. Gradually increase the speed to medium-high and blend for 2 to 4 more minutes, until completely smooth.

2 Transfer the mixture to a medium saucepan and set over medium-high heat. Cook, stirring, until the soup is heated through, 5 to 7 minutes. (Alternatively, if your blender heats soups well, you can keep the soup in the blender and complete this step there.)

3 Garnish with the onion and serve.

FOR 1 SERVING:
CALORIES: 200
PROTEIN: 2 GRAMS (0 BLOCKS)
CARBOHYDRATES: 45 GRAMS (2.5 BLOCKS)
FAT: 4 GRAMS (0.5 BLOCK)

PEANUT HOISIN SEITAN SANDWICHES (OR WRAPS)

I'm all for a meal that comes together in minutes and is handheld or, in this case, a whole handful. The peanut hoisin sauce gives the seitan flavor that makes the whole thing pop with every bite. **MAKES 4 SANDWICHES**

FOR THE PEANUT HOISIN SEITAN

2 cups seitan, cut into ½-inch pieces

1 cup Peanut Hoisin Sauce (page 264), plus more for drizzling

1 cup diced red bell pepper

1 cup halved cherry tomatoes

1 cup chopped baby bok choy

¼ cup minced red onion

2 tablespoons sesame seeds

FOR THE SANDWICHES

4 whole wheat wraps or mini baguettes, toasted

½ cup Marinated Cabbage Salad (page 184)

8 leaves fresh Thai basil

4 sprigs fresh cilantro

Lime wedges (optional)

1 MAKE THE SEITAN: Preheat the oven to 350°F. Line a baking sheet with parchment paper.

2 In a large bowl, toss together the seitan, peanut hoisin sauce, bell pepper, tomatoes, bok choy, onion, and sesame seeds until thoroughly combined. Spread the mixture in an even layer on the prepared baking sheet and bake for 30 minutes, stirring halfway through.

3 ASSEMBLE THE SANDWICHES: Fill each sandwich or wrap with equal amounts of the seitan, cabbage salad, basil, cilantro, and additional sauce, plus a squeeze of lime, if desired.

FOR 1 SANDWICH:
CALORIES: 455
PROTEIN: 32 GRAMS (1.5 BLOCKS)
CARBOHYDRATES: 58 GRAMS (3 BLOCKS)
FAT: 13 GRAMS (1.5 BLOCKS)

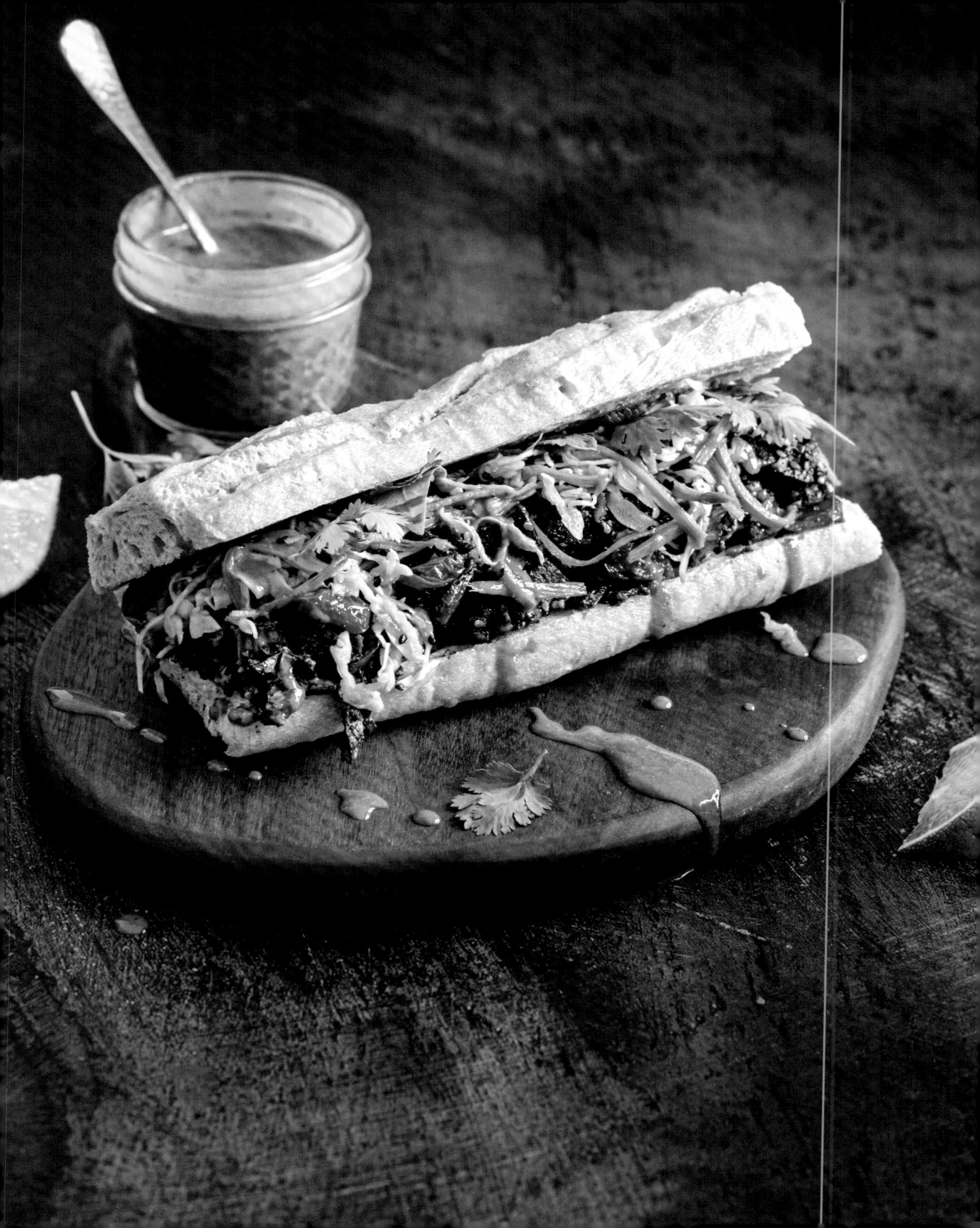

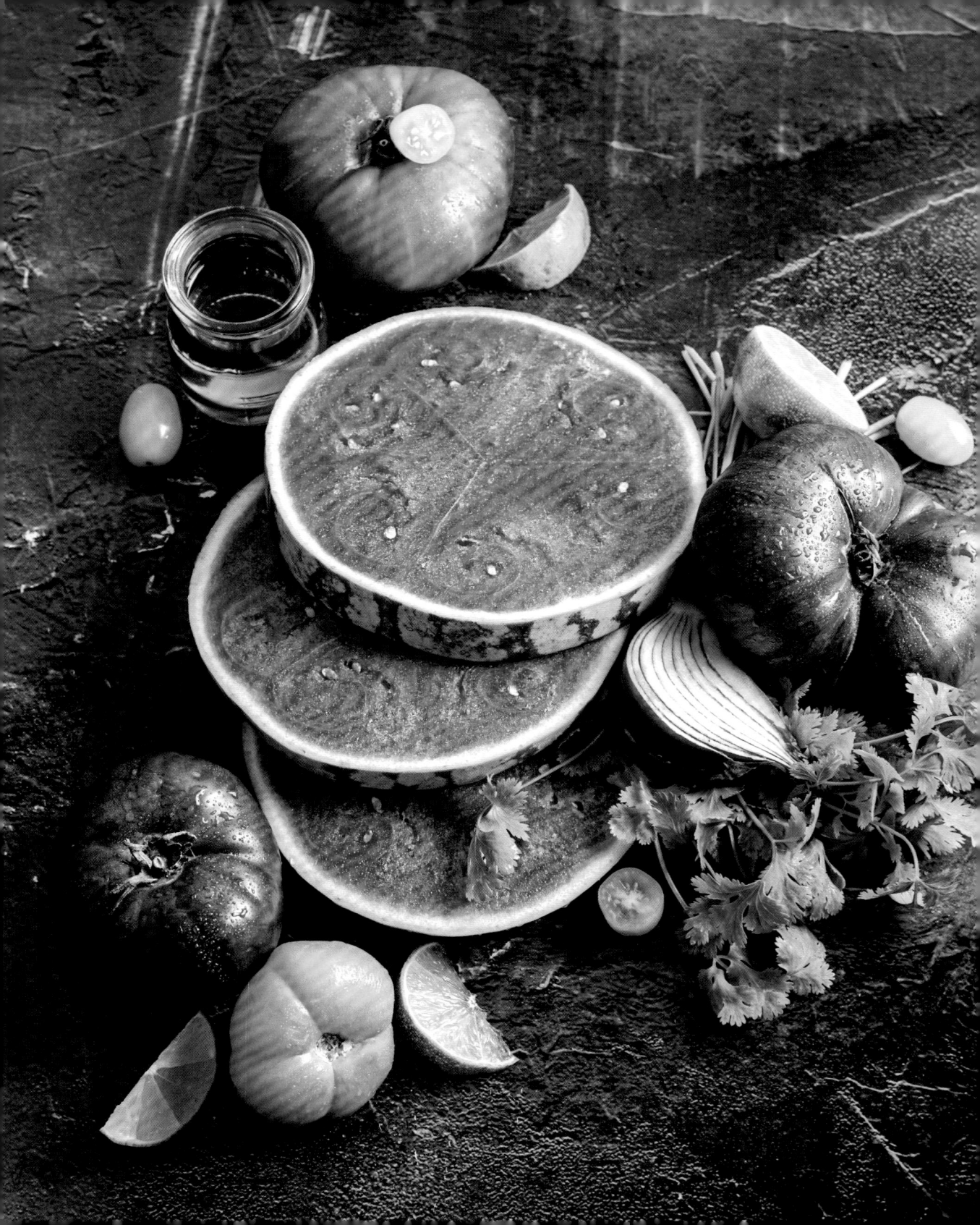

WATERMELON GAZPACHO

Fresh was the mission of this recipe, so I have to say that this dish is definitely Mission Accomplished. It's a raw soup, which means there's no need to cook anything, and you can eat it room temperature or chilled, which makes it perfect for when it's too hot to mess with the stove. **SERVES 4.**

3¼ cups diced seedless watermelon

¾ cup diced tomato, such as Roma or an heirloom variety

2 tablespoons minced red onion

2 tablespoons fresh lime juice

1 tablespoon minced shallot

1 tablespoon apple cider vinegar

1 tablespoon extra-virgin olive oil

½ cup finely chopped fresh cilantro

1 teaspoon sea salt, plus more to taste

1 In a high-speed blender, add 2¼ cups of the watermelon, plus the tomato, onion, lime juice, shallot, vinegar, and oil. Pulse until mostly smooth, being careful not to overblend.

2 Transfer the mixture to a serving bowl and add the remaining 1 cup of watermelon, the cilantro, and salt. Stir gently to combine and adjust the seasoning as desired. Divide between bowls and serve.

FOR 1 SERVING:
CALORIES: 80
PROTEIN: 1 GRAM (0 BLOCKS)
CARBOHYDRATES: 11 GRAMS (0.5 BLOCK)
FAT: 3.5 GRAMS (0.5 BLOCK)

AVOXO SALAD

Remember when you weren't vegan and you had that steak with the grill lines, and for some reason those lines made it taste better? Now imagine that on an avocado. Just think about that for a minute. Grilling makes just about *everything* taste better, including asparagus and broccoli. Toss it all together with a little dressing. *That's* a salad. **SERVES 1**

½ Hass avocado, pitted, peeled, and sliced

4 stalks asparagus, woody ends trimmed

½ cup large broccoli florets

1 teaspoon extra-virgin olive oil

Sea salt and ground black pepper, to taste

2 tablespoons Red Wine Vinaigrette (page 268)

¼ cup canned chickpeas, drained and rinsed

¼ cup pea sprouts

1 Preheat your grill or grill pan to high heat.

2 In a bowl, combine the avocado, asparagus, and broccoli. Toss with the olive oil to coat and season with salt and pepper.

3 Carefully lay everything on the grill. Cook, flipping occasionally, until the avocado and vegetables are nice and charred on all sides, 8 to 10 minutes.

4 Transfer everything to a bowl, drizzle with the vinaigrette, top with the chickpeas and sprouts, and enjoy.

FOR 1 SERVING:
CALORIES: 430
PROTEIN: 17 GRAMS (1 BLOCK)
CARBOHYDRATES: 43 GRAMS (2 BLOCKS)
FAT: 27 GRAMS (2.5 BLOCKS)

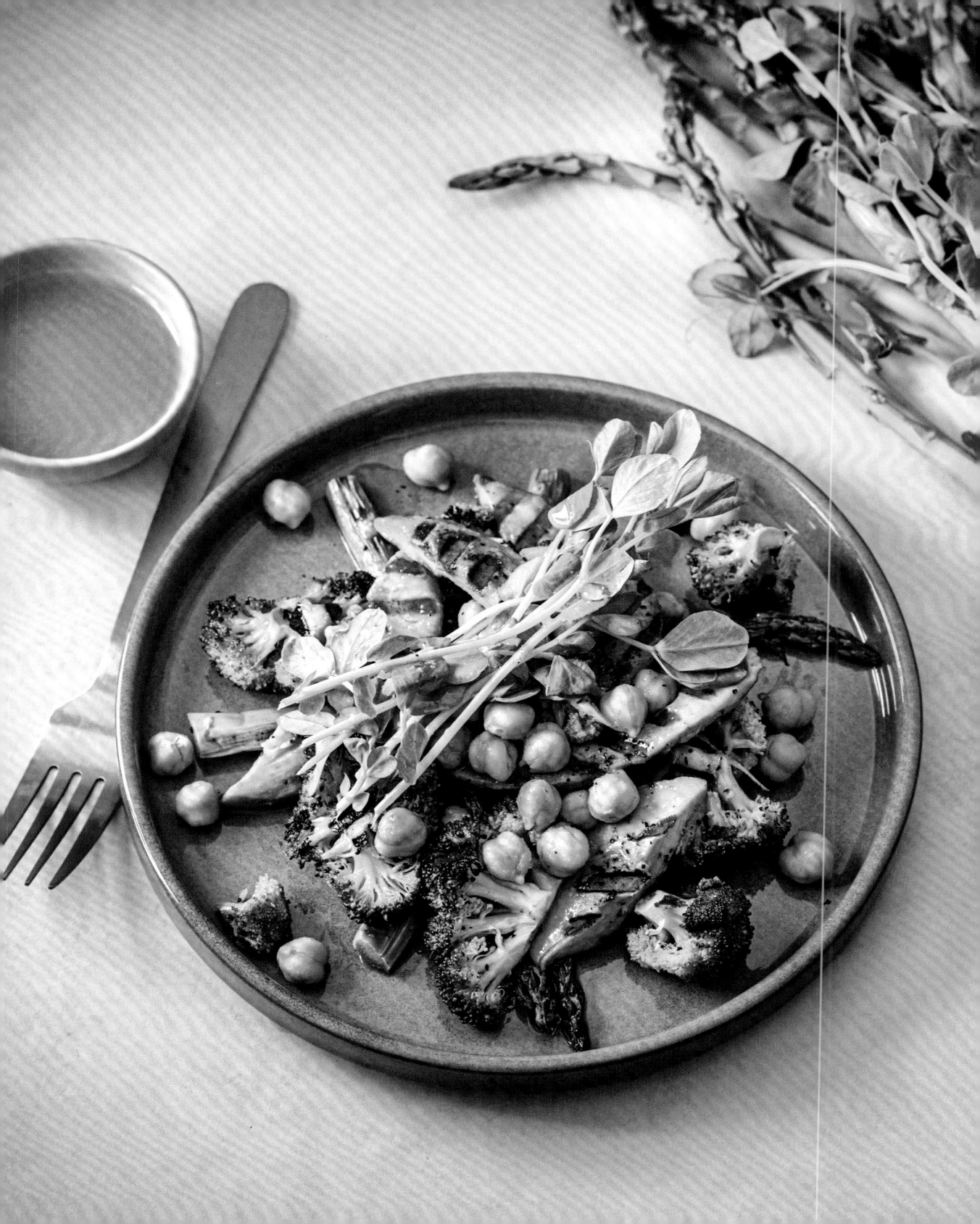

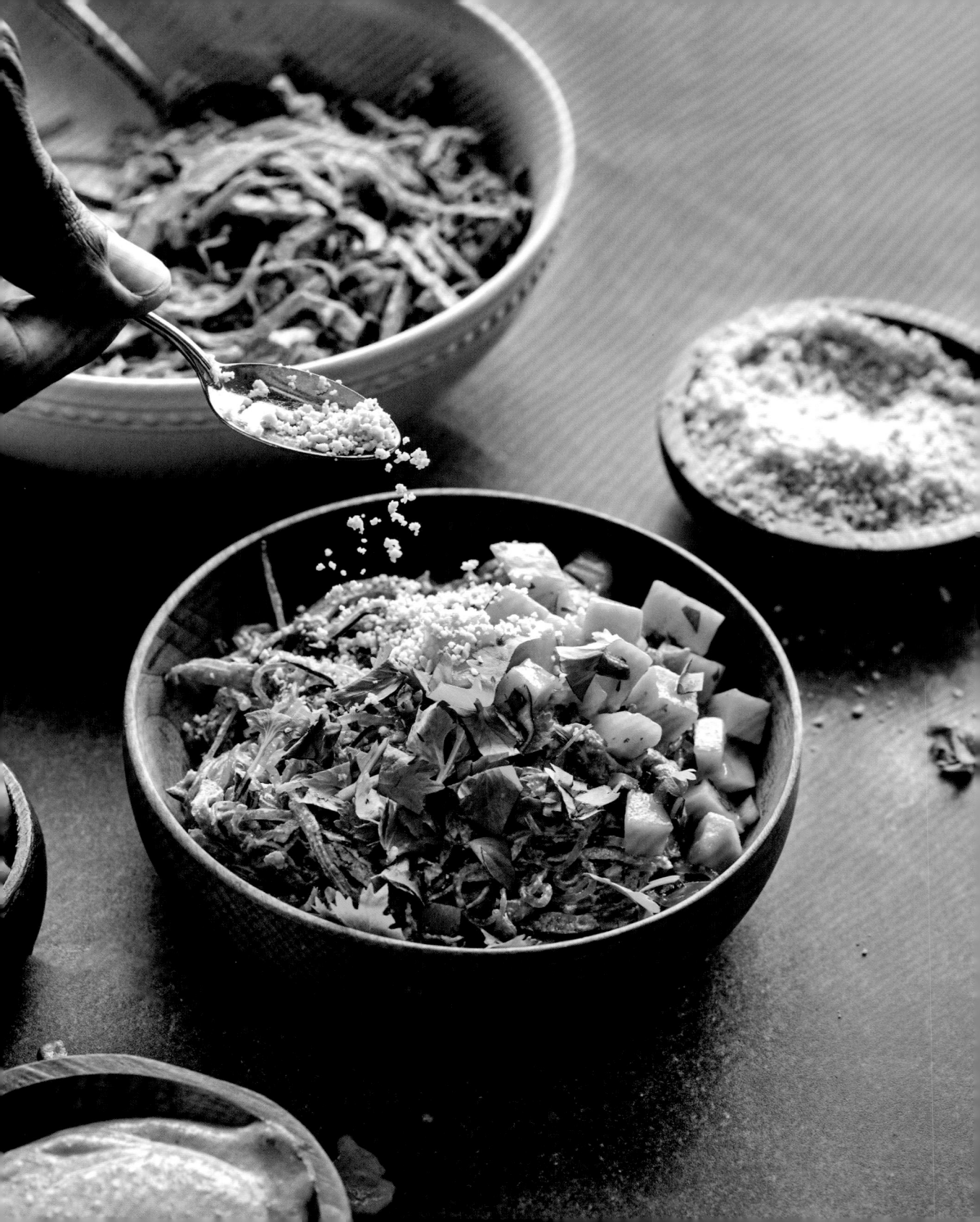

READING RAINBOW
BOWL

This baby just brings color to your life. The kelp noodles might sound funky, but they have a texture just like traditional noodles and are gluten-free and rich in nutrients like calcium, iron, vitamin K, and iodine. They are not as hard to find as you might think (even Walmart carries them now). **SERVES 2**

FOR THE KELP NOODLES

1 cup cold water

1 tablespoon fresh lemon juice

1 (12-ounce) bag kelp noodles (I like Sea Tangle), drained and rinsed

FOR THE RAINBOW VEGETABLES

1 cup shredded carrots

1 cup shredded purple cabbage

1 cup thinly sliced red bell pepper

FOR SERVING

½ cup Almond Ginger Dressing (page 276)

½ cup Mango Salsa (page 272)

¼ cup Cashew Crumble (page 271)

2 tablespoons chopped fresh cilantro

1 MAKE THE KELP NOODLES: In a medium bowl, stir together the cold water and lemon juice. Add the drained kelp noodles and soak until they're tender enough to chew, 1 to 2 hours. (Go ahead and take a nibble to test it out.) The lemon will help break down the noodles for a nice texture. Drain well.

2 ASSEMBLE THE BOWLS: In a large bowl, toss the drained kelp noodles with the carrots, cabbage, and bell pepper. Add the almond ginger dressing and toss to coat. Divide the mixture between two bowls and top with the mango salsa, cashew crumble, and cilantro.

FOR 1 SERVING:
CALORIES: 330
PROTEIN: 10 GRAMS (0.5 BLOCK)
CARBOHYDRATES: 34 GRAMS (1.5 BLOCKS)
FAT: 22 GRAMS (2 BLOCKS)

BIG PAPA-YA SALAD

I love big papayas and I cannot lie. Especially when they're still green and haven't gotten sweet yet. They're juicy, crunchy, and the perfect element to bring a salad to the next level. This one gets a Thai-style kick from a spicy chili and lime dressing. **SERVES 4**

2 cups peeled and shredded green (unripe) papaya (Do not use ripe papaya!)

½ cup shredded carrots

½ cup halved grape tomatoes

½ cup green beans, trimmed and cut into 1-inch pieces

½ cup Spicy Chili Lime Dressing (page 275)

¼ cup chopped fresh cilantro

1 tablespoon thinly sliced scallions

2 tablespoons Cashew Crumble (page 271)

6 fresh Thai basil leaves

In a large bowl, toss the green papaya, carrots, tomatoes, and green beans with the dressing until well coated. Top with the cilantro, scallions, cashew crumble, and Thai basil.

FOR 1 SERVING:
CALORIES: 150
PROTEIN: 3 GRAMS (0 BLOCKS)
CARBOHYDRATES: 14 GRAMS (0.5 BLOCK)
FAT: 11 GRAMS (1 BLOCK)

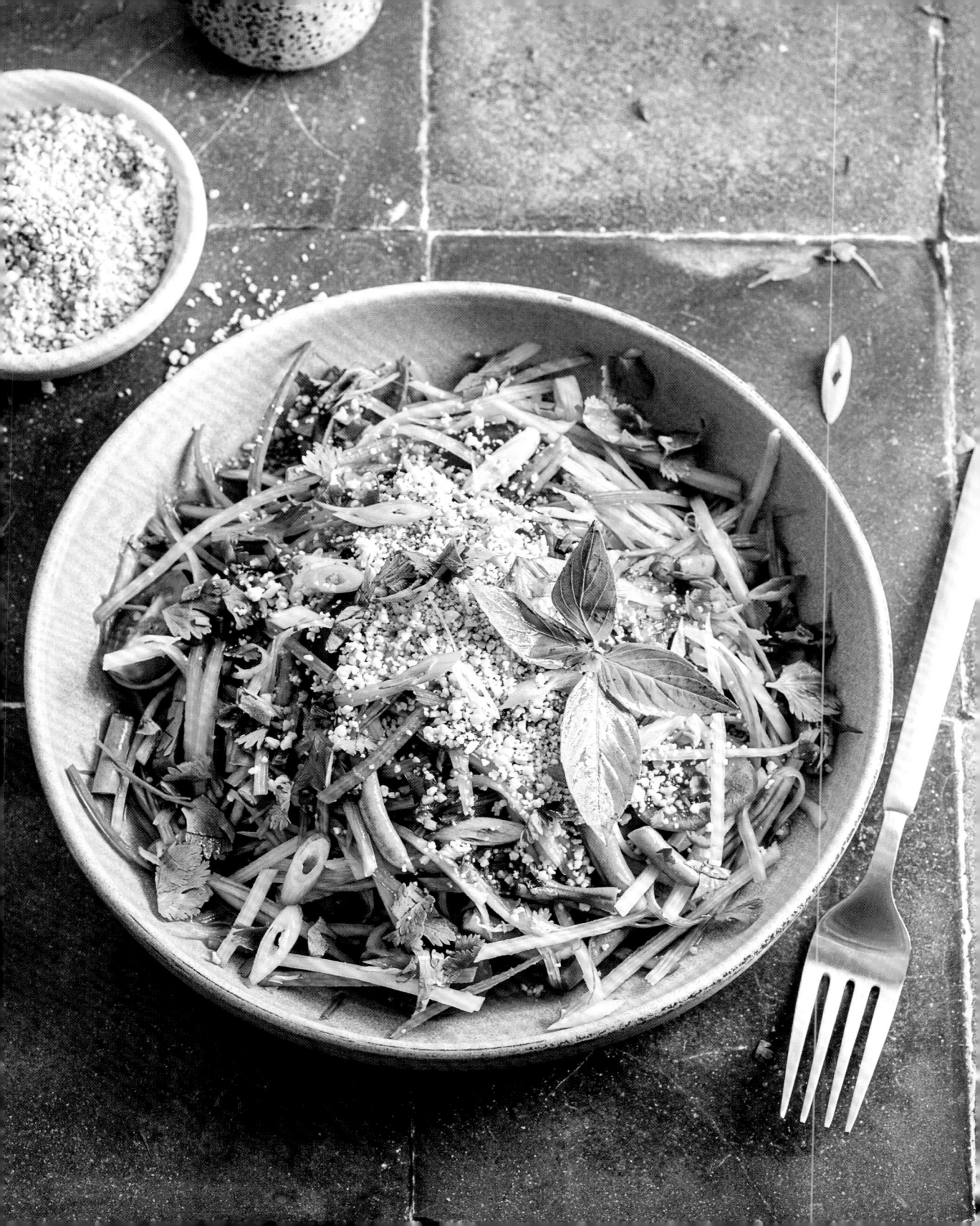

SOUTH BY SOUTHWEST
SALAD

I gave this salad the name I did because if you've ever been to that festival, then you know it's a complete party—and that's exactly what this salad is, a whole damn party in your mouth. What I also love about it is that you can prep a big batch of black beans, slaw, and pico de gallo in advance so that you can make this salad throughout the week. **SERVES 4**

FOR THE SEASONED BLACK BEANS

1 pound dried black beans, soaked overnight, or 2 (15-ounce) cans black beans, drained and rinsed

8 cups filtered water (if using dried beans)

¼ cup extra-virgin olive oil

½ cup diced yellow onion

2 garlic cloves, minced

2 teaspoons ground coriander

2 teaspoons ground cumin

2 teaspoons dried thyme

2 teaspoons dried oregano leaves

1 bay leaf

2 teaspoons sea salt, plus more to taste

FOR THE JICAMA SLAW

1 tablespoon fresh lime juice

1 tablespoon agave nectar

1 teaspoon apple cider vinegar

1 teaspoon sea salt

1 teaspoon chili powder

½ teaspoon ground black pepper

2 cups shredded jicama

½ cup shredded carrots

¼ cup finely chopped fresh cilantro

¼ cup diced red onion

FOR THE PICO DE GALLO

½ cup diced yellow onion

1 small jalapeño, seeded and diced

2 tablespoons fresh lime juice

2 teaspoons sea salt, plus more to taste

1 pound Roma tomatoes, diced (about 6 tomatoes)

¼ cup finely chopped fresh cilantro

FOR THE SALAD

4 cups chopped romaine lettuce

¼ cup Cilantro Lime Dressing (page 274)

2 tablespoons Holy Moly Guacamole (page 262) or store-bought

½ cup Cashew Sour Cream (page 277)

Tortilla chips, for serving

1 **MAKE THE SEASONED BLACK BEANS:** If using dried beans, in a slow cooker, combine the soaked beans with the water, olive oil, onion, garlic, coriander, cumin, thyme, oregano, and bay leaf. Cover the pot and cook on the low setting until the beans are fully cooked, 6 to 8 hours. Stir in the salt and adjust the seasoning as needed. If you can, let the cooked beans sit for a while before serving. The longer they sit, the better the flavor.

If using canned beans, cook on the stovetop instead: In a medium saucepan or pot over medium heat, warm the olive oil. Add the onion and cook until softened, then add the garlic and cook for another minute. Add the beans with their liquid, the seasonings, and the salt and mix well. Simmer for 3 to 5 minutes, until heated through. Adjust the seasoning as needed.

2 **MAKE THE JICAMA SLAW:** In a medium bowl, whisk together the lime juice, agave, vinegar, salt, chili powder, and black pepper. Add the jicama, carrot, cilantro, and onion and toss to coat.

3 **MAKE THE PICO DE GALLO:** In a medium bowl, toss the onion and jalapeño with the lime juice and salt and let sit for 5 minutes. Add the tomatoes and cilantro and stir to combine. Taste and adjust the seasoning and let sit another 15 minutes before serving.

4 **ASSEMBLE THE SALAD:** In a large bowl, toss the romaine with the dressing. Divide the salad between bowls and top with ½ cup each of the black beans, jicama slaw, and pico de gallo. Finish with the guacamole and drizzle with the cashew sour cream. Serve with tortilla chips.

FOR 1 SERVING:
CALORIES: 500
PROTEIN: 16 GRAMS (1 BLOCK)
CARBOHYDRATES: 57 GRAMS (3 BLOCKS)
FAT: 30 GRAMS (3 BLOCKS)

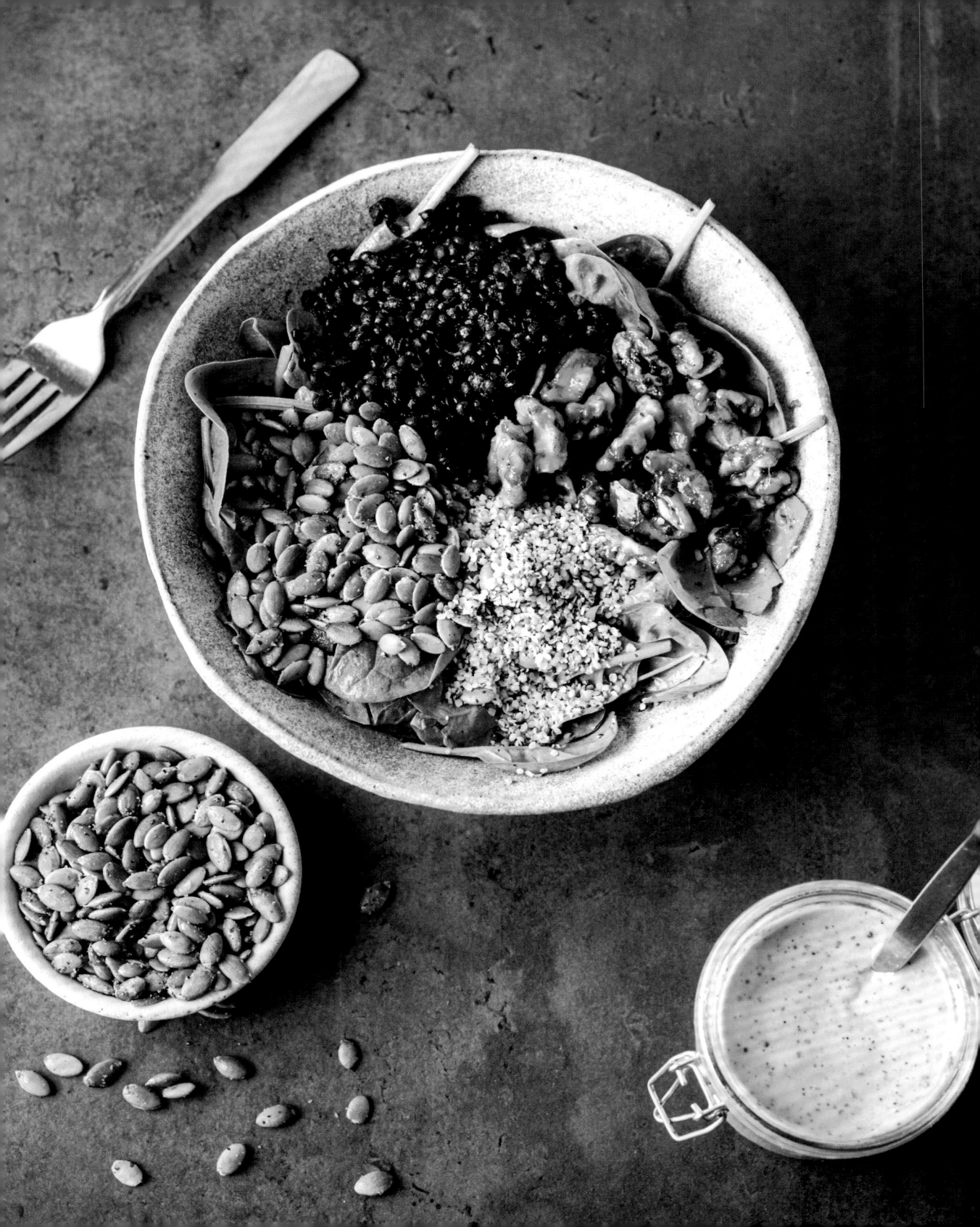

PROTEIN POWER SALAD

This salad dispels the myth that vegans don't get enough protein. Between the lentils, candied walnuts, toasted hull-less pumpkin seeds (or pepitas, if you're fancy), and hempseeds, you've got some serious horsepower. You'll be left with extra lentils, candied walnuts, and toasted pepitas, which you can store in the fridge for up to a week and use to dress up your next few lunches and dinners. **SERVES 4**

FOR THE SMOKY BLACK LENTILS

2 cups vegetable broth (I like Imagine's No-Chicken Broth)

1 cup dried black lentils, sorted, rinsed, and any small stones discarded

2 teaspoons smoked paprika

1 teaspoon dried thyme

1 teaspoon sea salt, plus more to taste

FOR THE CANDIED WALNUTS

1 cup walnuts

¼ cup maple syrup

1 teaspoon extra-virgin olive oil

½ teaspoon sea salt

1 teaspoon ground black pepper

FOR THE TOASTED PEPITAS

1 cup raw pepitas

1 teaspoon maple syrup

½ teaspoon sea salt

1 teaspoon ground black pepper

FOR THE SALAD

8 cups baby spinach

1 cup Walnut Vinaigrette (page 265)

¼ cup hempseeds

RECIPE CONTINUES >>

1 MAKE THE LENTILS: In a large saucepan over medium-high heat, combine the broth, lentils, smoked paprika, thyme, salt, and 1 cup of water. Bring to a boil, stirring occasionally, and reduce the heat to low. Cover and simmer until tender, 15 to 20 minutes. Remove the pan from the heat and drain any excess liquid. Taste and adjust the seasoning as desired. Cover and set aside to keep warm.

2 MAKE THE CANDIED WALNUTS AND TOASTED PEPITAS: Preheat the oven to 350°F. Line two baking sheets with parchment paper.

3 In a medium bowl, toss together the walnuts, maple syrup, olive oil, salt, and pepper. Spread the walnuts on the first prepared baking sheet. In the same medium bowl, toss together the pepitas, maple syrup, salt, and pepper. Spread the pepitas onto the second prepared baking sheet. Bake until the walnuts and pepitas are golden brown, about 10 minutes. Set aside to cool.

4 MAKE THE SALAD: In a large bowl, toss the baby spinach with the walnut vinaigrette. Divide the dressed greens between bowls and top each salad with ½ cup of the warm lentils, 1 tablespoon of the candied walnuts, 1 tablespoon of the toasted pepitas, and 1 tablespoon of the hempseeds.

FOR 1 SERVING:
CALORIES: 860
PROTEIN: 40 GRAMS (2 BLOCKS)
CARBOHYDRATES: 73 GRAMS (3.5 BLOCKS)
FAT: 53 GRAMS (5.5 BLOCKS)

BADASS VEGAN

JAPANESE COLD SOBA

Oodles of noodles here. This dish has been a staple of mine for so long because it's quick, easy, and just tastes so damn good. Plus, soba noodles are made from buckwheat, which can help regulate blood sugar, improve heart health, alleviate inflammation, and potentially prevent cancer.
SERVES 8

FOR THE SOBA NOODLES

Sea salt, to taste

1 (10-ounce) package soba noodles (my favorite is Hakubaku)

½ teaspoon sesame oil

FOR THE PEANUT SAUCE

½ cup unsweetened peanut butter

½ cup filtered water

2 tablespoons maple syrup

2 tablespoons brown rice syrup

1 teaspoon fresh lime juice

1 tablespoon minced fresh ginger

1 teaspoon minced garlic

½ teaspoon sea salt

Pinch of cayenne pepper

2 tablespoons finely chopped fresh cilantro

FOR SERVING

1 tablespoon roasted, salted peanuts

2 teaspoons black sesame seeds

2 teaspoons thinly sliced scallions

1 lime, cut into wedges

2 cups Miso-Glazed Tempeh (page 235; optional)

LUNCH

RECIPE CONTINUES >>

1 MAKE THE NOODLES: Bring a medium pot of salted water to a boil. Cook the soba noodles according to the package instructions. Drain the noodles, toss with the sesame oil, and chill in the refrigerator while you make the peanut sauce.

2 MAKE THE PEANUT SAUCE: In a high-speed blender, add the peanut butter, water, maple syrup, brown rice syrup, lime juice, ginger, garlic, salt, and cayenne and blend until very smooth. Add the cilantro and blend again until just incorporated. Store extra dressing in an airtight container in the refrigerator for 5 to 6 days.

3 SERVE: In a large bowl, toss the cold soba noodles with enough sauce to coat. Divide the noodles between bowls and top with the peanuts, sesame seeds, and scallions. Serve with the lime wedges and miso-glazed grilled tempeh for added protein, if desired.

FOR 1 SERVING:
CALORIES: 531 (5 BLOCKS)
PROTEIN: 29 GRAMS (2.5 BLOCKS)
CARBOHYDRATES: 53 GRAMS (5 BLOCKS)
FAT: 21.5 GRAMS (2 BLOCKS)

BADASS VEGAN

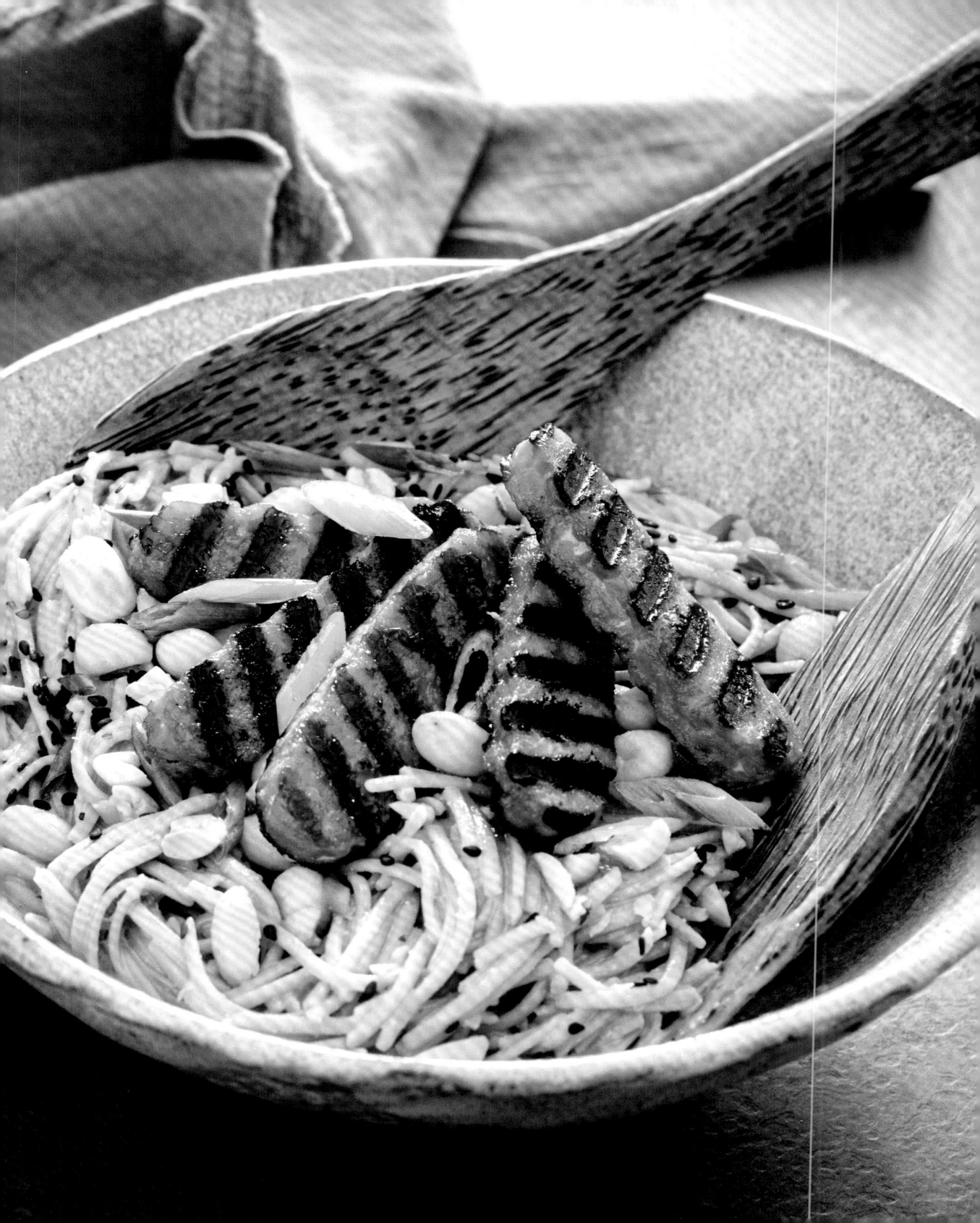

MUSHROOM 'VICHE

Unlike a traditional ceviche that's made with fish, I got inspired by my brothers over at Wicked Healthy and tried a version using mushrooms. By leaving the oceans alone and going with fantastic fungi instead, you're not only pleasing your taste buds with this salad; you're making the planet pretty happy too. **SERVES 8**

FOR THE CITRUS DRESSING

½ cup chopped fresh cilantro

½ cup fresh lemon juice

½ cup fresh lime juice

¼ cup fresh orange juice

2 tablespoons minced shallot

1 tablespoon sea salt, plus more to taste

2 teaspoons minced garlic

1 cup extra-virgin olive oil

FOR THE CEVICHE

1 cup thinly sliced king oyster mushrooms, cut into 1-inch strips

1 cup thinly sliced coconut meat

1 cup halved cherry or grape tomatoes

½ cup diced orange or red bell pepper

¼ cup finely chopped fresh cilantro

¼ cup finely diced red onion

½ to 1 jalapeño, seeded and minced (depending on your heat preference)

1 Hass avocado, peeled, pitted, and diced

FOR SERVING

8 cups organic blue corn tortilla chips

1 **MAKE THE DRESSING:** In a blender, add the cilantro, lemon juice, lime juice, orange juice, shallot, salt, and garlic and blend until smooth. With the blender running, stream in the olive oil and continue blending until the dressing is emulsified. Taste to check for seasoning and adjust if needed.

2 **MAKE THE CEVICHE:** In a large bowl, toss the mushrooms, coconut, tomatoes, bell pepper, cilantro, onion, and jalapeño with almost all of the citrus dressing. Check the seasoning and add more salt or dressing to taste. Let the mixture marinate until the mushrooms have absorbed the flavor of the dressing, 20 to 30 minutes. Add the avocado and gently toss once more. Serve with about 1 cup of tortilla chips per person, but you know how it is with chips.

FOR 1 SERVING:
CALORIES: 410
PROTEIN: 2.5 GRAMS (0 BLOCKS)
CARBOHYDRATES: 14 GRAMS (1 BLOCK)
FAT: 40 GRAMS (4 BLOCKS)

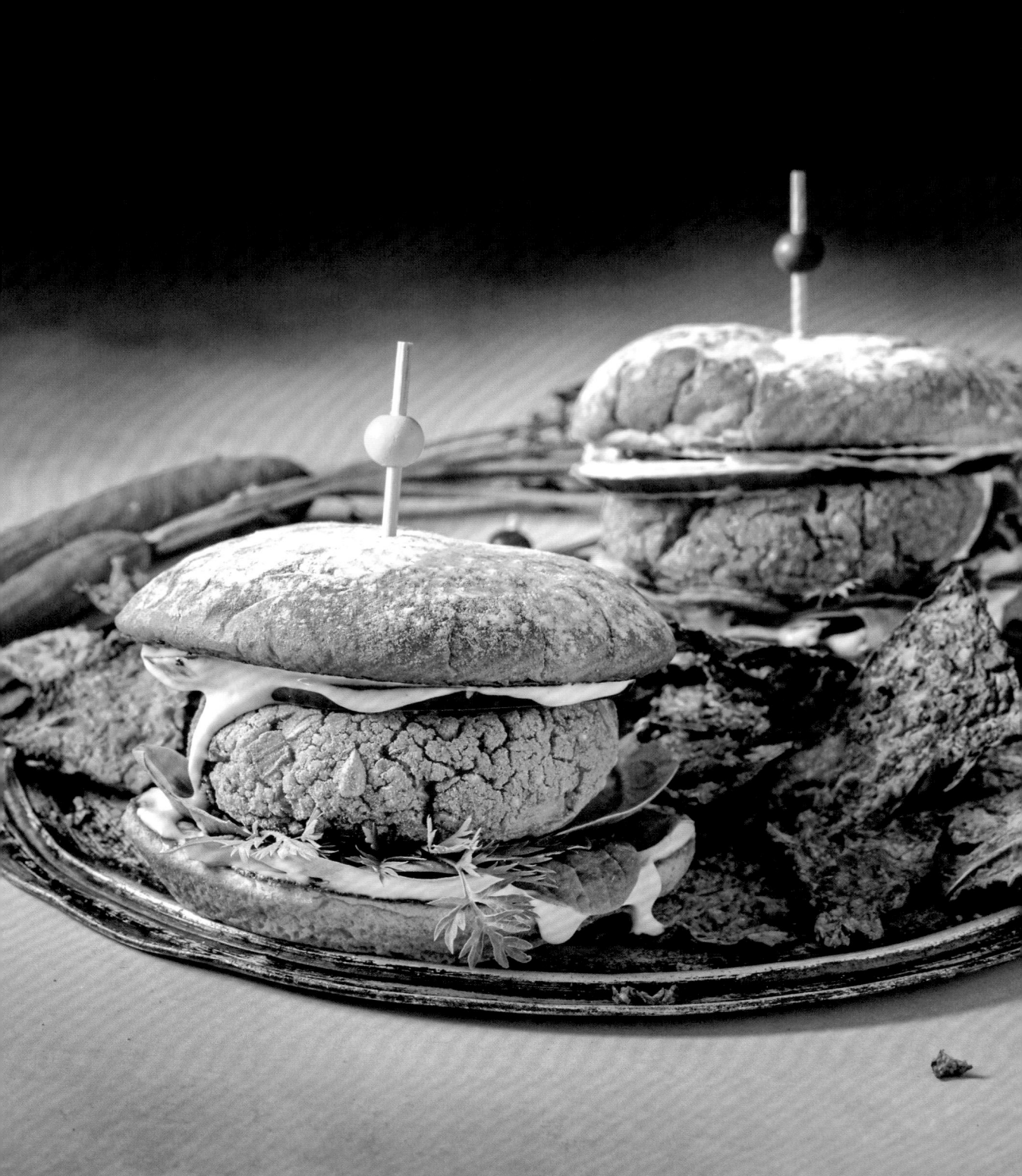

BUNNY BURGERS
WITH COLLARD CHIPS

Sorry, but I can't think about these burgers without giving a shout-out to my favorite carrot-loving bunny, Bugs. *What's up, Doc?* This isn't the kind of burger you'll find at your local grill, but it is the kind of burger you can serve to your friends and they'll love you for the rest of their lives. Toasted and cooked millet gives the patties structure, and all the spices like cumin and chili powder bring the mouthgasm. You could also just keep these all for yourself—that's totally fine too. **SERVES 6**

FOR THE COLLARD CHIPS

½ cup fresh lemon juice

½ cup sunflower seeds

¼ cup macadamia nuts

¾ cup chopped red bell pepper

1½ tablespoons nutritional yeast

1 teaspoon chili powder

1 teaspoon garlic powder

1 teaspoon onion powder

1 teaspoon sea salt

1 teaspoon ground black pepper

¼ teaspoon chipotle powder

1 pound collard greens, stems removed and leaves cut into triangles

FOR THE BUNNY BURGERS

½ cup uncooked millet

Sea salt, to taste

3 medium carrots, plus greens

1½ teaspoons extra-virgin olive oil

1 medium onion, chopped

⅓ cup sunflower seeds

1 cup cooked or canned peas, drained and rinsed

3 tablespoons ground flaxseeds

1 tablespoon tamari soy sauce

1 teaspoon ground cumin

½ teaspoon chili powder

3 tablespoons buckwheat flour

Ground black pepper, to taste

RECIPE CONTINUES >>

1 **MAKE THE COLLARD CHIPS:** Preheat the oven to 325°F.

2 In a high-speed blender, add the lemon juice, sunflower seeds, macadamia nuts, bell pepper, nutritional yeast, chili powder, garlic powder, onion powder, salt, black pepper, and chipotle powder and blend until completely smooth.

3 In a large bowl, toss together the collard greens and dressing, making sure each leaf is well coated. Spread the dressed greens onto a baking sheet in an even layer, dividing the greens between two baking sheets if needed.

4 Bake the chips until dried and crispy, flipping them halfway through, 10 to 15 minutes. Store in a zip-top bag at room temperature for up to 1 week.

5 **MAKE THE BURGERS:** In a medium pot over medium heat, toast the millet until fragrant and golden brown, 4 to 5 minutes. Add 2 cups of water and a pinch of salt to the pot and bring to a boil. Reduce the heat to a simmer, cover, and cook until the millet has absorbed all the water, about 15 minutes. Remove the pot from the heat and set aside to cool.

6 While the millet cooks, peel and dice the carrots into small cubes. Reserve the greens. Add the carrots to a small pot with just enough cold water to cover. Bring to a boil and cook until the carrots can easily be pierced with a knife, 4 to 5 minutes. Drain, rinse with cold water, and set aside to cool.

7 In a large pan over medium heat, heat the oil. Add the onion and cook until golden brown, about 7 minutes. Transfer the onion to a bowl, reduce the heat to low, and add the sunflower seeds to the pan. Toast the seeds until they're fragrant and just beginning to brown, about 1 minute. Remove the pan from the heat.

8 Preheat the oven to 375°F. Line a baking sheet with parchment paper.

9 In a blender or food processor, combine the millet, peas, carrots, flaxseeds, tamari, cumin, chili powder, 1 tablespoon of the buckwheat flour, and a pinch of black pepper. Blend until the mixture combines and thickens. Pause to add the onion, sunflower seeds, and two sprigs of the carrot greens. Blend again until the mixture is fully combined, moist, and sticky.

10 Form the mixture into 6 equal patties. Lightly coat them with the remaining 2 tablespoons buckwheat flour and lay them on the prepared baking sheet. Bake for 25 minutes, flip, and bake for another 15 to 20 minutes, until the patties are crisped on the outside and warmed through. Serve hot with the collard chips and your favorite vegan fixin's.

FOR 1 SERVING:
CALORIES: 430
PROTEIN: 18 GRAMS (1 BLOCK)
CARBOHYDRATES: 59 GRAMS (3 BLOCKS)
FAT: 20 GRAMS (2 BLOCKS)

BIG-ASS SALAD

Eat your damn vegetables. And make this spiced tempeh because it yields a batch big enough to throw into salads, soups, sandwiches, and wraps all week long. Just remember to plan for this meal in advance; marinating the tempeh overnight makes all the difference. **SERVES 4**

FOR THE BLACKENED TEMPEH

1 (8-ounce) package tempeh, cut into ½-inch squares

½ cup safflower or other neutral oil

¼ cup brown rice syrup

¼ cup tamari soy sauce

¼ cup stone-ground mustard

¼ cup fresh lemon juice

2 tablespoons gluten-free flour mix (such as Bob's Red Mill)

2 teaspoons paprika

2 teaspoons ground cumin

2 teaspoons chili powder

2 teaspoons dried oregano

2 teaspoons garlic powder

2 teaspoons onion powder

2 teaspoons dried thyme leaves

1½ teaspoons sea salt

1 teaspoon ground black pepper

Pinch of cayenne pepper

FOR THE SALAD

4 cups mixed greens

½ cup cooked chickpeas, drained and rinsed

½ cup chopped apple

½ cup halved cherry tomatoes

½ cup shredded or julienned carrots

½ cup diced cucumber

¼ cup diced red bell pepper

2 tablespoons finely diced red onion

2 tablespoons sunflower seeds

¼ cup Balsamic Vinaigrette (page 280), plus more if needed

1 **MAKE THE TEMPEH:** Place the tempeh pieces in a large zip-top plastic bag.

2 In a medium bowl, whisk together the oil, brown rice syrup, tamari, mustard, and lemon juice. Pour the marinade over the tempeh in the bag. Carefully push out the excess air and seal the bag. Marinate the tempeh in the refrigerator for at least 6 hours, ideally overnight.

3 Preheat the oven to 350°F. Line a baking sheet with parchment paper.

4 In a medium bowl, whisk together the gluten-free flour, paprika, cumin, chili powder, oregano, garlic powder, onion powder, thyme, salt, black pepper, and cayenne. Remove the tempeh pieces from the marinade, shaking off any excess liquid. Dredge the marinated tempeh in the spice mixture and place on the prepared baking sheet.

5 Bake the tempeh for 15 minutes, flip the tempeh over, and bake for another 15 minutes, until it is browned and crispy.

6 **ASSEMBLE THE SALAD:** In a large bowl, toss the greens, chickpeas, apple, tomatoes, carrots, cucumber, bell pepper, onion, and sunflower seeds with the balsamic vinaigrette until the salad is thoroughly coated. Taste and add more dressing if desired. Top with 1 cup of the blackened tempeh.

FOR 1 SERVING:
CALORIES: 710
PROTEIN: 27 GRAMS (1.5 BLOCKS)
CARBOHYDRATES: 67 GRAMS (3.5 BLOCKS)
FAT: 43 GRAMS (4.5 BLOCKS)

CARIBBEAN TOFU SALAD SANDWICHES

Nah, this ain't some bullshit mock chicken salad. Here cubed tofu is tossed with some creamy dressing with a taste of the islands like nothing you've experienced before. Honestly, until you taste this, you haven't been living. **SERVES 4**

FOR THE DRESSING

8 ounces organic silken tofu (I prefer Wildwood brand)

2 tablespoons apple cider vinegar

2 tablespoons fresh lime juice

2 tablespoons coconut oil

1 tablespoon unsweetened shredded coconut

2 teaspoons minced garlic

1 Medjool date, pitted

2 teaspoons ground turmeric

2 teaspoons ground coriander

1 teaspoon sea salt

½ teaspoon onion powder

½ teaspoon garlic powder

½ teaspoon ground ginger

½ teaspoon garam masala

½ teaspoon ground yellow mustard

½ teaspoon ground black pepper

½ teaspoon ground cumin

FOR THE TOFU SALAD

8 ounces firm tofu, cut into ¼-inch to ½-inch cubes (I prefer Wildwood brand)

½ cup diced red apple, any variety

¼ cup diced celery

¼ cup finely diced onion

1 tablespoon chopped fresh parsley

2 teaspoons chopped fresh dill

FOR THE SANDWICHES

8 slices bread (I like Dave's Killer Good Seed Bread) or 4 large whole wheat wraps (I like La Tortilla Factory)

1 cup baby spinach

¼ cup shredded carrots

1 **MAKE THE DRESSING:** In a high-speed blender, add the silken tofu, vinegar, lime juice, coconut oil, coconut, garlic, date, turmeric, coriander, salt, onion powder, garlic powder, ground ginger, garam masala, ground mustard, pepper, and cumin and blend until completely smooth.

2 **MAKE THE TOFU SALAD:** In a medium bowl, add the cubed tofu, apple, celery, onion, parsley, and dill. Add 1 cup of the dressing and toss to combine. You can add more dressing here, if desired, or save any extra to spread on the sandwiches.

3 **MAKE THE SANDWICHES:** For each sandwich, scoop about ½ cup of the tofu salad onto a slice of bread. Top with a small handful of the baby spinach and about a tablespoon of the shredded carrots. Spread the other piece of bread with any extra dressing, if desired, and top the sandwich.

FOR 1 SANDWICH:
CALORIES: 420
PROTEIN: 23 GRAMS (1 BLOCK)
CARBOHYDRATES: 54 GRAMS (2.5 BLOCKS)
FAT: 18 GRAMS (2 BLOCKS)

COUNTRY-STYLE
MISO SOUP

I love me some miso soup. But this ain't the shit you get from some restaurants that serve you watered-down tofu. This here is country style, or *butajiru*, as it's called in parts of Japan. It's loaded with veggies like radish, carrots, cabbage, and mushrooms and has all that miso umami flavor.

MAKES ABOUT 5 CUPS

4 cups filtered water

½ cup sliced daikon radish, cut into ¼-inch half-moons

½ cup sliced carrots, cut into ¼-inch half-moons

½ cup sliced celery, cut into ¼-inch half-moons

½ cup sliced yellow onion, cut into ¼-inch half-moons

3 shiitake mushrooms, stems trimmed and caps sliced into ⅛-inch strips

1 cup sliced napa cabbage, cut into ¼-inch strips

¼ cup white miso

1 tablespoon dried wakame

Thinly sliced scallions, for serving

1 In a large pot over medium-high heat, add the water, daikon, carrots, celery, onion, and mushrooms and bring to a boil. Reduce the heat to medium-low and simmer until the celery is fully cooked, about 12 minutes.

2 Remove the soup from the heat and stir in the cabbage, miso, and wakame. Stir until the miso is fully dissolved and the cabbage is wilted. Divide between bowls and top with the sliced scallions.

FOR 1 CUP:
CALORIES: 110
PROTEIN: 6 GRAMS (0.5 BLOCK)
CARBOHYDRATES: 20 GRAMS (1 BLOCK)
FAT: 2.5 GRAMS (0.5 BLOCK)

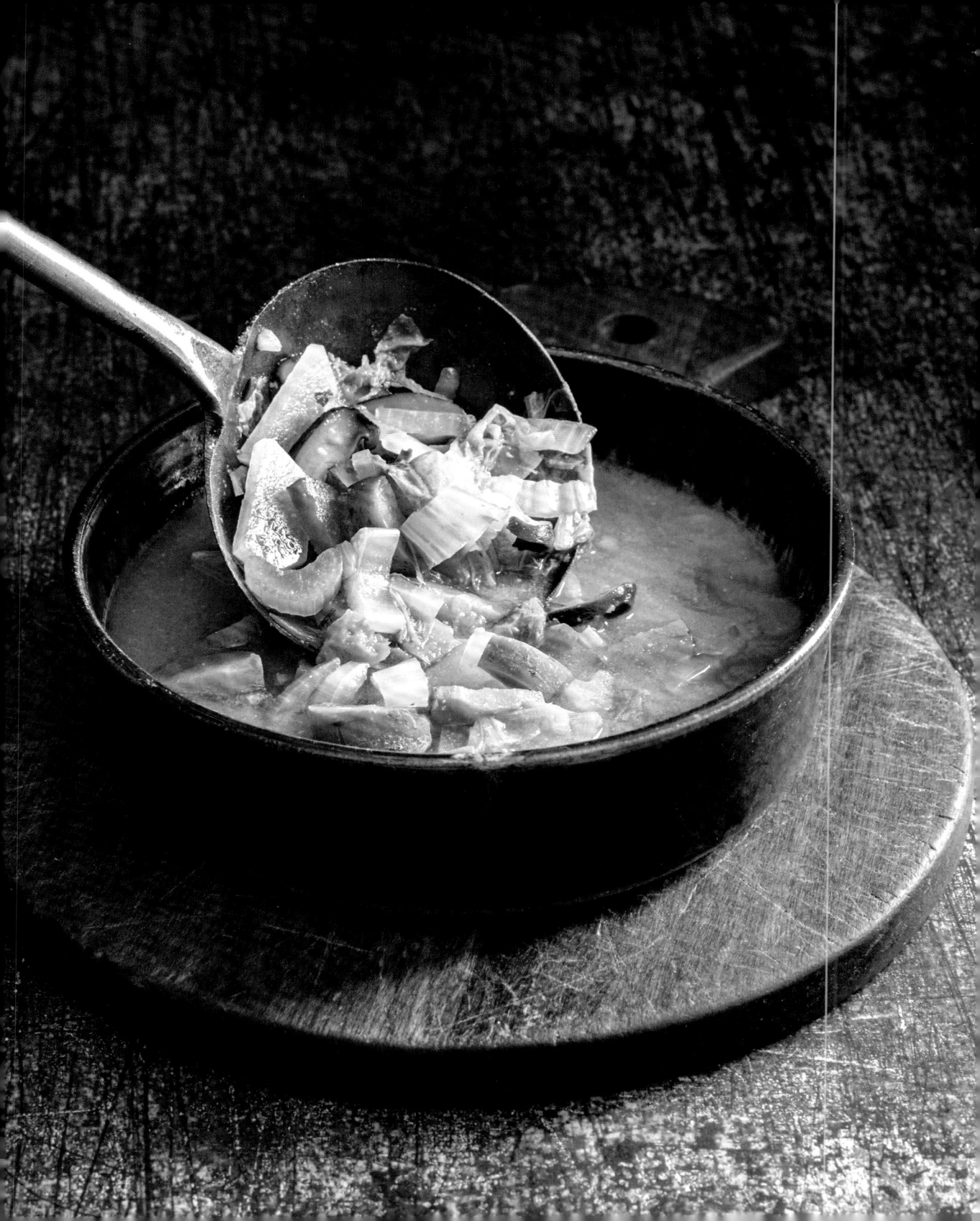

CHAPTER 19

DINNER

SMASHED POTATOES
AND BROWN GRAVY
WITH COLLARD GREENS

Some people think that just because they've gone vegan they need to leave behind heart-warming, stick-to-your-ribs, cry-for-your-mama soul food. But this dish is proof that (1) it's just not true, and (2) you'll never look back. Just be sure to wash your collards well, because you don't want to bite into any grit. **SERVES 6**

FOR THE GRAVY

⅓ cup nutritional yeast

⅓ cup gluten-free flour mix (such as Bob's Red Mill)

⅓ cup safflower oil

¼ cup diced yellow onion

1 teaspoon minced garlic

1 teaspoon fresh thyme leaves

1 teaspoon dried sage

½ teaspoon ground black pepper

3 tablespoons tamari soy sauce

½ teaspoon sea salt, plus more to taste

FOR THE SMASHED POTATOES

3 large Yukon Gold potatoes, peeled and cut into 1-inch pieces

1 teaspoon sea salt, plus more for cooking the potatoes

¼ cup extra-virgin olive oil

½ teaspoon ground black pepper

FOR THE COLLARD GREENS

¼ cup extra-virgin olive oil

2 tablespoons diced yellow onion

1 tablespoon minced garlic

2 teaspoons smoked paprika

1 teaspoon sea salt, plus more to taste

1 teaspoon ground black pepper

1 bunch collard greens (1½–2 pounds), stems removed and leaves cut into 1-inch strips

RECIPE CONTINUES >>

1 MAKE THE GRAVY: In a large, dry pot over medium heat, toast the nutritional yeast and flour, stirring frequently, until lightly browned and fragrant, 3 minutes. Set aside.

2 In a large nonstick pan over medium-high heat, heat the oil. Add the onion and cook, stirring, until softened, about 5 minutes. Add the garlic, thyme, sage, and pepper and reduce the heat to low. Cook, stirring occasionally, for about 5 more minutes. Add the toasted yeast and flour mixture, increase the heat to medium-high, and whisk rapidly until the mixture is golden brown, 3 minutes. Add 4½ cups of water and whisk continuously until the texture becomes very creamy and smooth, about 15 minutes. Whisk in the tamari and salt. Taste and adjust the seasoning if needed. Remove the pan from the heat. If desired, strain the gravy through a fine-mesh strainer for a perfectly smooth texture. Return the gravy to the pan and cover to keep warm.

3 MAKE THE SMASHED POTATOES: Add the potatoes to a large pot of salted water. Set the pot over medium-high heat, bring to a boil, and cook the potatoes until very tender when pierced with a knife or fork, 12 to 15 minutes.

4 Drain the potatoes and reserve about 1 cup of the cooking water. (You'll use part of this for the potatoes and part for the collards.) Return the potatoes to the pot and add the olive oil, the 1 teaspoon of salt, and the pepper. Use a potato masher or fork to smash the potatoes into a rustic texture, adding cooking water to thin them out as needed. Cover to keep warm.

5 MAKE THE COLLARD GREENS: In a large nonstick pan over medium heat, heat the olive oil. Add the onion, garlic, smoked paprika, salt, and pepper and cook until the onion is translucent, about 10 minutes. Reduce the heat to low and add the collard greens. Cook, stirring occasionally and adding a splash of potato cooking water as needed to prevent browning, until the collards are very tender, 8 to 10 minutes. Taste and adjust the seasoning if desired.

6 Serve the smashed potatoes smothered in the gravy with the collard greens on the side.

FOR 1 SERVING:
CALORIES: 670
PROTEIN: 20 GRAMS (1 BLOCK)
CARBOHYDRATES: 63 GRAMS (3 BLOCKS)
FAT: 44 GRAMS (4.5 BLOCKS)

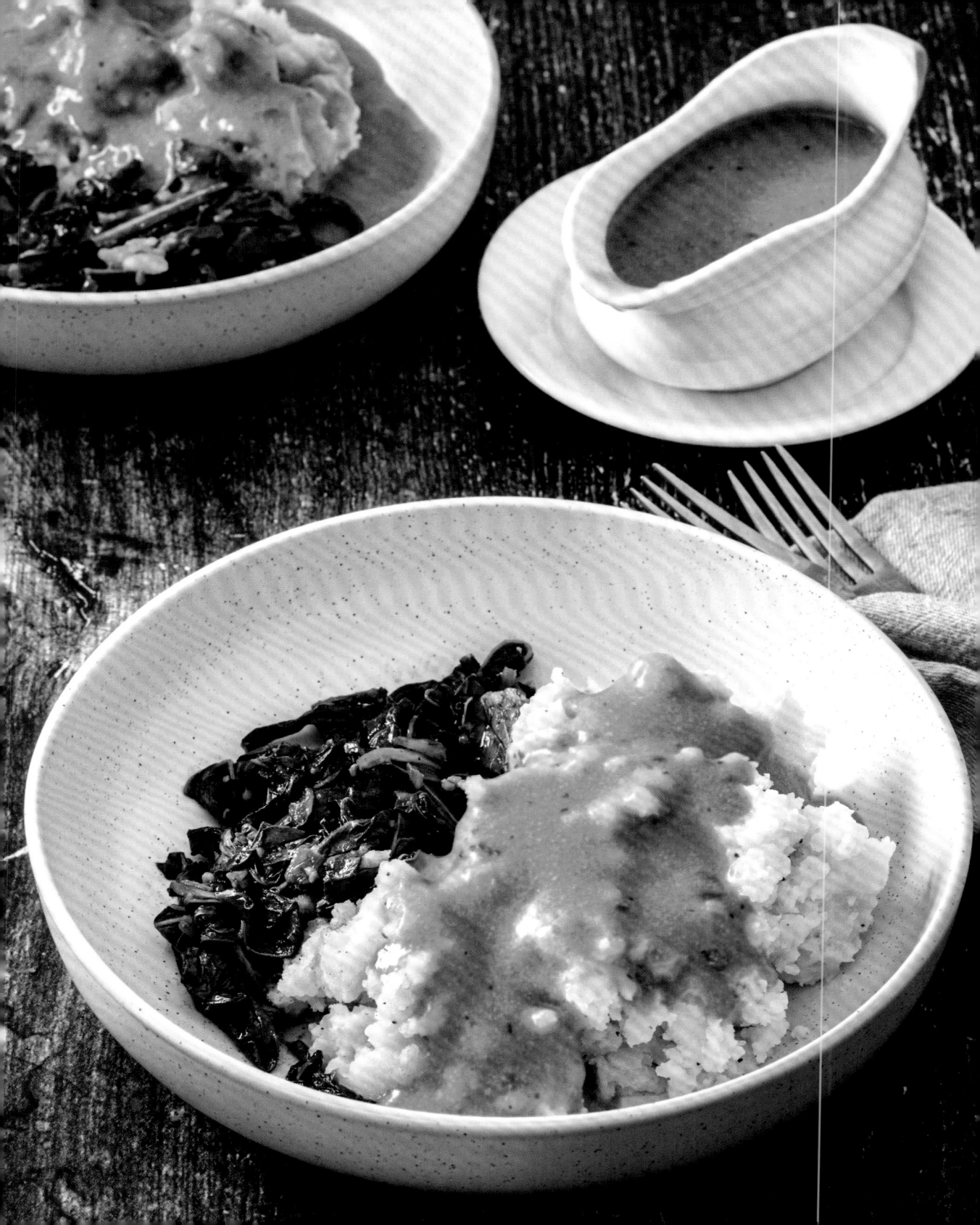

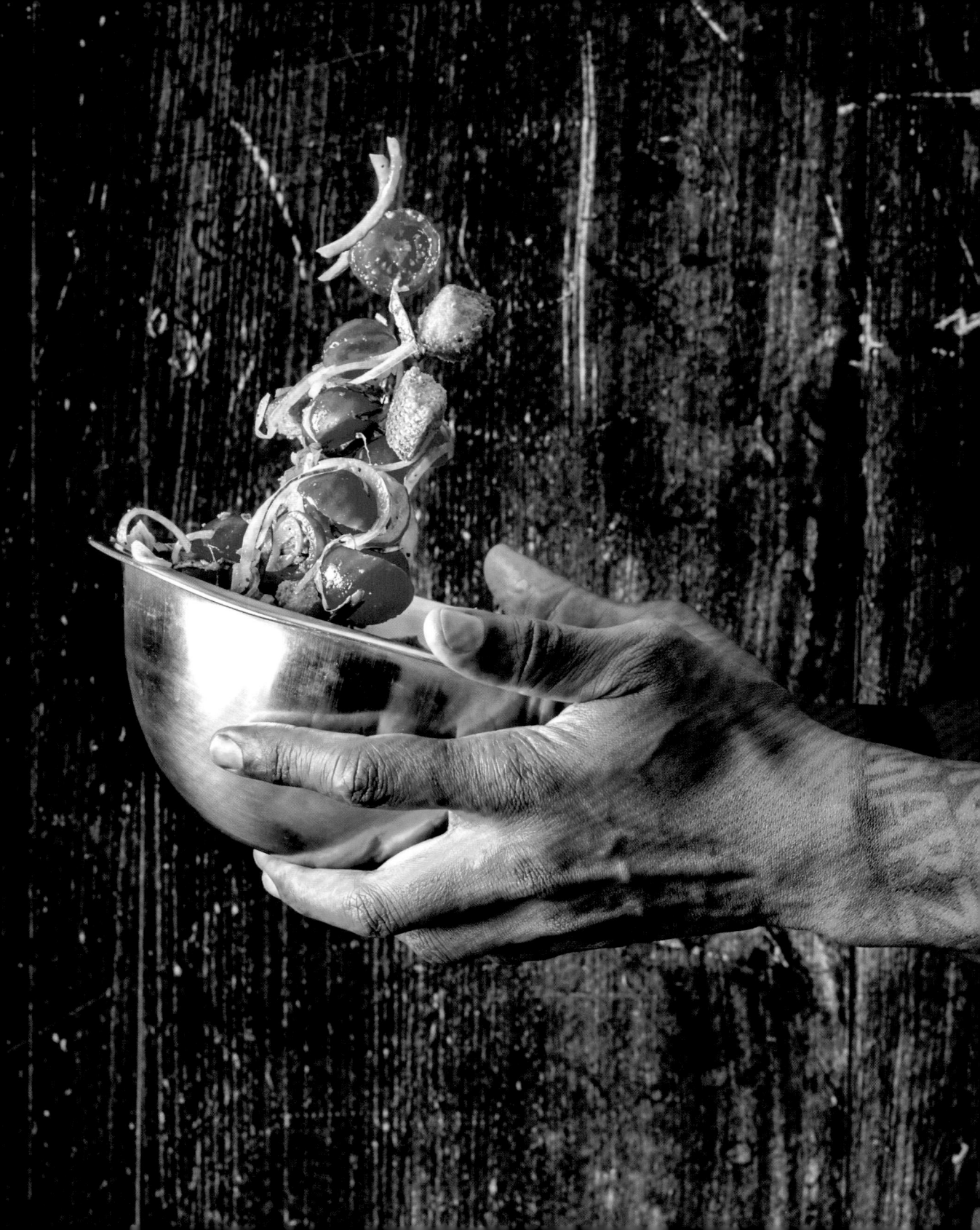

PANZANELLA SALAD

Have you ever had a salad made out of fresh-ass bread? Yeah, I bet just the thought makes your brain light up . . . wait until you actually eat it. **SERVES 4.**

4 cups (1-inch) cubed baguette or ciabatta bread

¼ cup extra-virgin olive oil

Sea salt and ground black pepper, to taste

4 cups halved cherry or grape tomatoes

½ cup Red Wine Vinaigrette (page 268)

½ cup fresh chiffonade-cut basil leaves

½ cup very thinly sliced red onion (a mandoline works great here)

1 Preheat the oven to 350°F.

2 In a large bowl, toss the bread cubes with the olive oil, salt, and pepper. Arrange the bread in a single layer on a baking sheet and bake until golden brown, about 10 minutes.

3 Transfer the toasted bread cubes to a large bowl and toss with the tomatoes, vinaigrette, basil, and onion. Set the salad aside for at least 15 minutes before serving to let the bread soak up the dressing.

FOR 1 SERVING:
CALORIES: 270
PROTEIN: 5 GRAMS (0.5 BLOCK)
CARBOHYDRATES: 26 GRAMS (1.5 BLOCKS)
FAT: 17 GRAMS (1.5 BLOCKS)

PASTA AL PESTO

The beauty of this pasta is that you'd never guess it skips the dairy. Even though traditional pesto gets its creamy texture and salty bite from Parmesan, you can get the same flavor and texture with pine nuts, olive oil, garlic, and nutritional yeast.

Use any type of pasta, regular or gluten-free, for this recipe. For a higher-protein dish, try red lentil pasta. Pasta with pesto is also very delicious served cold. So if you have leftovers, you will have an easy snack for later. The pasta water from the cooked pasta helps the sauce to stick! **SERVES 4**

2 cups packed fresh basil, stems removed

½ cup extra-virgin olive oil

¼ cup pine nuts or blanched, sliced almonds

2 garlic cloves

2 teaspoons nutritional yeast

2 teaspoons fresh lemon juice

1 teaspoon sea salt, plus more for the pasta water

½ teaspoon ground black pepper

¼ teaspoon crushed red pepper (optional)

1 (16-ounce) box of pasta of your choice

1 In a high-speed blender or food processor, add the basil, olive oil, pine nuts, garlic, nutritional yeast, lemon juice, salt, black pepper, and crushed red pepper, if using. Blend until smooth and set aside.

2 Fill a large pot with generously salted water and bring it to a boil over medium-high heat. Add the pasta and cook according to the package instructions.

3 Transfer the pesto to a large pan over low heat. Gently warm the pesto, stirring occasionally, while the pasta finishes cooking. Add about 2 tablespoons of the pasta cooking water to the pesto. Drain the pasta, add it to the pesto, and toss gently to coat completely.

FOR 1 SERVING:
CALORIES: 750
PROTEIN: 19 GRAMS (1 BLOCK)
CARBOHYDRATES: 90 GRAMS (4.5 BLOCKS)
FAT: 38 GRAMS (4 BLOCKS)

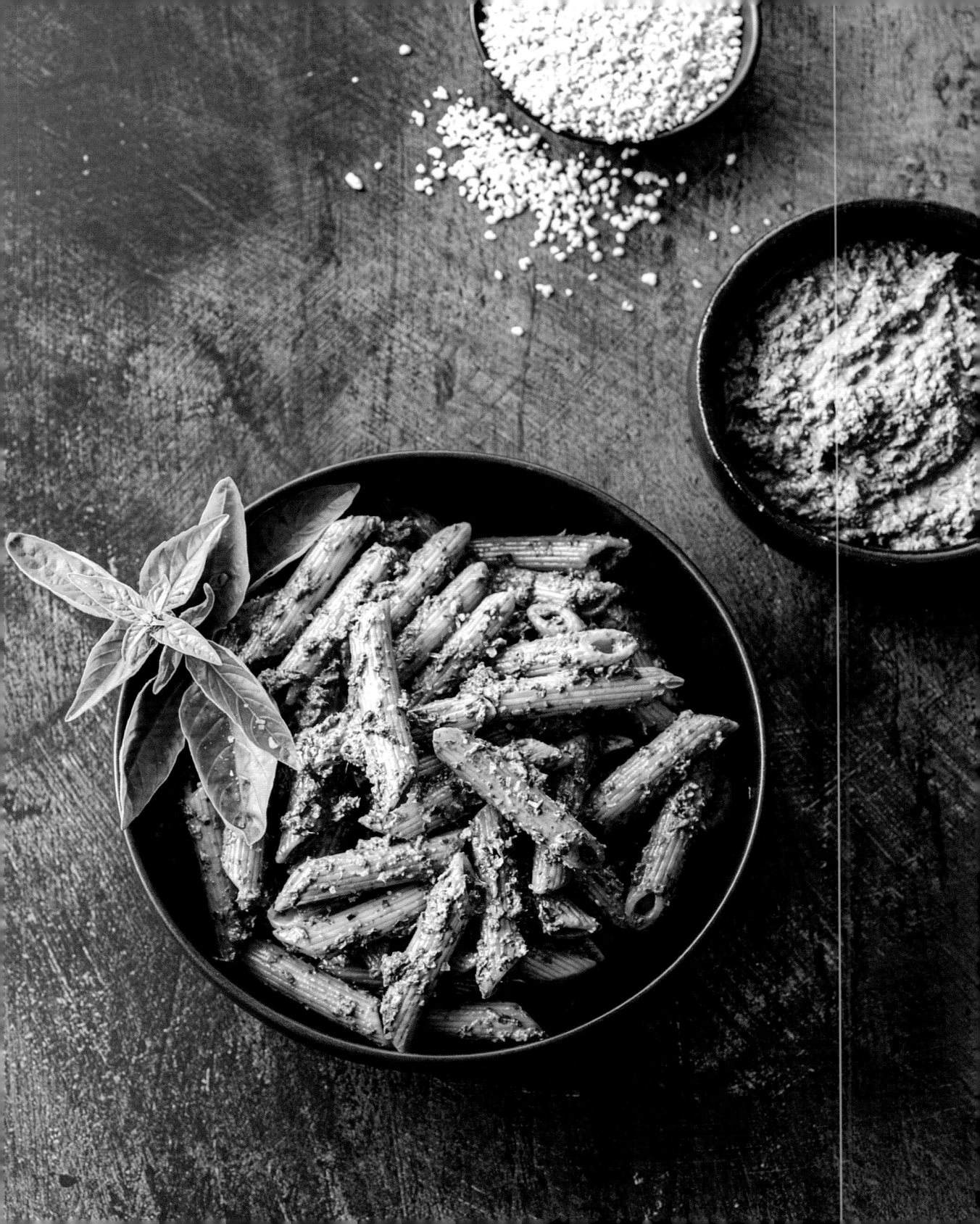

SMOKY SPICY MOUNTAIN CHILI

This chili is named after the first time I ever made it—when I was in the mountains of North Carolina. I was staying in a cabin with most of my extended family, and I served them this dish without telling them it was vegan. Needless to say, everybody loved it. To anyone who ever said that vegan food can't be flavorful, grab a spoon. And a glass of water. Because this chili is about to kick your ass.

Note: While this recipe is tasty when served the same day it's cooked, preparing the tempeh and corn the day before you put the chili together saves time. **SERVES 6**

FOR THE BEANS

½ cup dried pinto beans

½ cup dried black beans

¼ cup dried red kidney beans

1 piece kombu seaweed
(5–10 feet/
1.5–3 m long,
and 8–12 inches/
20–30 cm wide)

FOR THE SEASONED TEMPEH

1 (8-ounce) package tempeh

1 tablespoon extra-virgin olive oil

2 teaspoons dried oregano

2 teaspoons smoked paprika

2 teaspoons paprika

2 teaspoons chili powder

2 teaspoons ground cumin

2 teaspoons sea salt

2 teaspoons ground black pepper

1 teaspoon crushed red pepper

½ teaspoon ground cayenne pepper

FOR THE ROASTED CORN

Kernels from 2 ears of corn

2 tablespoons extra-virgin olive oil

1 teaspoon sea salt

1 teaspoon ground black pepper

FOR THE CHILI

3 dried bay leaves

¼ cup safflower oil

1 cup diced yellow onion

½ cup diced celery

½ cup diced red bell pepper

½ cup diced green bell pepper

½ jalapeño, minced (seeds removed if desired)

1 tablespoon minced garlic

1 tablespoon chili powder

2 teaspoons ground cumin

2 teaspoons ground coriander

2 teaspoons smoked paprika

Pinch of cayenne pepper (optional)

2 tablespoons tomato paste

1 cup canned diced tomatoes (preferably a fire-roasted variety such as Muir Glen)

½ cup chopped Tuscan kale (also sold as black or lacinato kale)

1 tablespoon tamari soy sauce

2 teaspoons sea salt, plus more to taste

1 teaspoon ground black pepper

½ cup chopped fresh cilantro

FOR SERVING

Chopped fresh cilantro

Lime wedges

Cashew Sour Cream (page 277)

1 **PREPARE THE BEANS:** In a large pot, combine the pinto beans, black beans, kidney beans, kombu, and enough water to cover by about 3 inches. Cover the pot and let the beans soak at room temperature overnight.

2 **MAKE THE SEASONED TEMPEH:** In a large bowl, add the tempeh, oil, oregano, smoked paprika, paprika, chili powder, cumin, salt, black pepper, crushed red pepper, and cayenne. Use your hands to mix, massage, and break down the tempeh into the seasonings. Let sit for 30 minutes.

3 **MAKE THE ROASTED CORN:** Preheat the oven to 350°F.

4 In a medium bowl, toss the corn with the oil, salt, and black pepper. Spread the corn in a single layer on a baking sheet and roast until tender and slightly browned, 15 to 20 minutes. Set aside.

RECIPE CONTINUES >>

5 MAKE THE CHILI: Drain and rinse the soaked beans, reserving the kombu. Add the beans and kombu back into the pot and add the bay leaves and fresh water to cover by 2 inches. Set the pot over high heat, cover, and bring to a boil. Reduce the heat to medium and let the beans simmer, covered, until softened but not yet fully tender, 40 to 45 minutes.

6 In another large pot over medium heat, heat the safflower oil. Add the onion and cook, stirring, for 5 minutes. Add the celery, red bell pepper, green bell pepper, jalapeño, garlic, chili powder, cumin, coriander, smoked paprika, and cayenne, if using, and continue to cook, stirring frequently, until tender, about 10 minutes.

7 Add ½ cup of the seasoned tempeh and the tomato paste and cook for 5 minutes. (Reserve the remaining tempeh as a tasty addition for other recipes.) Remove the kombu and bay leaves and transfer the beans and their cooking liquid to the tempeh and vegetables. Add the diced tomatoes and bring the mixture to a boil. Reduce the heat to low, cover, and simmer, stirring occasionally, until the beans are tender, about 20 minutes. Remove the lid and continue simmering, stirring occasionally, until the mixture thickens slightly and the flavors blend, about 15 more minutes. Add ½ cup of water to thin the chili if desired.

8 Stir in the roasted corn, plus the kale, tamari, salt, and black pepper. Taste and adjust the seasoning if desired. Remove the pot from the heat and stir in the cilantro.

9 SERVE: Divide the chili between bowls and serve with additional chopped cilantro, lime wedges, and cashew sour cream.

FOR 1 SERVING:
CALORIES: 380
PROTEIN: 22 GRAMS (1 BLOCK)
CARBOHYDRATES: 44 GRAMS (2 BLOCKS)
FAT: 19 GRAMS (2 BLOCKS)

YAKISOBA
(OODLES OF SOBA NOODLES)

This ain't that old dollar-store package of dried-up sodium sticks. This is a "feel it in your soul" kind of noodle dish that'll make you feel like the Asian mama you never had just had you home for dinner. You'll end up with more sauce than you'll need for this recipe, but it'll last about a week in the fridge. Toss it into your grain bowls or onto roasted vegetables anytime you want a little extra flavor. **SERVES 4.**

FOR THE GINGER TAMARI SAUCE

⅓ cup tamari soy sauce

⅓ cup brown rice syrup

2 tablespoons grated fresh ginger

2 tablespoons brown rice vinegar

2 teaspoons tahini

1 teaspoon minced garlic

2 teaspoons minced shallot

1 teaspoon paprika

Pinch of cayenne pepper

¼ cup sesame oil

FOR THE MISO-GLAZED TEMPEH

½ cup brown rice syrup

¼ cup white miso

1 tablespoon tamari soy sauce

1 tablespoon fresh lemon juice

1 tablespoon minced fresh ginger

2 tablespoons sesame oil

1 (8-ounce) package tempeh, cut into ¼-inch strips

FOR THE YAKISOBA BOWLS

1 tablespoon Caramelized Onions (page 257; optional)

½ cup shredded green or purple cabbage

½ cup shredded carrots

½ cup thinly sliced red bell pepper

¼ cup snap peas, strings removed

¼ cup broccoli florets, cut into bite-size pieces

1 (10-ounce) package soba noodles, cooked according to package instructions, ¼ cup cooking water reserved

FOR SERVING

Pickled Purple Cabbage (page 255)

Thinly sliced scallions, white and light green parts only

Black sesame seeds

RECIPE CONTINUES >>

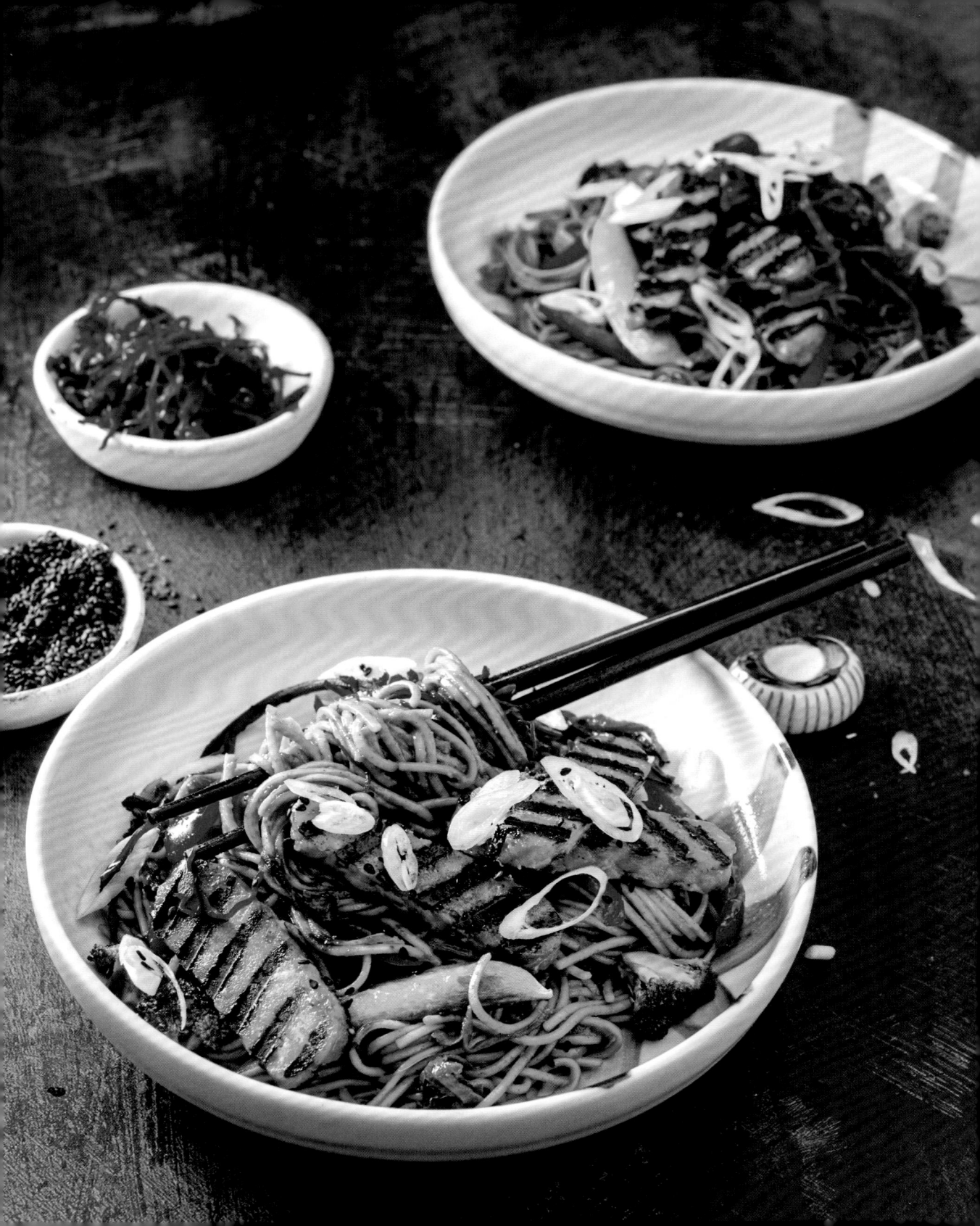

1. **MAKE THE GINGER TAMARI SAUCE:** In a high-speed blender, add the tamari, rice syrup, ginger, vinegar, tahini, garlic, shallot, paprika, and cayenne and blend on medium speed until very smooth. Reduce the blender speed to medium-low and slowly stream in the oil, blending until emulsified.

2. **MAKE THE MISO-GLAZED TEMPEH:** In a high-speed blender, add the rice syrup, miso, tamari, lemon juice, ginger, and 2 tablespoons of water and blend on medium speed until completely smooth. Reduce the blender speed to medium-low and slowly stream in the oil, blending until emulsified.

3. In a medium bowl, add the tempeh strips and the glaze. Gently toss to coat the tempeh, being careful not to break the pieces. Marinate the tempeh in the refrigerator for at least 30 minutes and up to overnight.

4. Heat a grill or grill pan to medium-high. Grill the tempeh strips for 2 minutes per side. Transfer the grilled tempeh to a plate and set aside.

5. **MAKE THE YAKISOBA BOWLS:** In a large nonstick pan over medium-high heat, heat ½ cup of the ginger tamari sauce with the caramelized onions, if using. Add the cabbage, carrots, bell pepper, snap peas, and broccoli and toss in the sauce. Cook, stirring, until the vegetables begin to soften, about 5 minutes. Add the cooked soba noodles and a splash of the noodle cooking water. Cook until the vegetables are tender and the noodles are coated in the sauce, another 2 to 3 minutes.

6. **SERVE:** Transfer the noodle mixture to a serving bowl and top with the tempeh. Serve with the pickled purple cabbage, scallions, and sesame seeds.

FOR 1 SERVING:
CALORIES: 260
PROTEIN: 7 GRAMS (0.5 BLOCK)
CARBOHYDRATES: 42 GRAMS (4 BLOCKS)
FAT: 8 GRAMS (1 BLOCK)

SPICY ASIAN RICE PAPER ROLLS

Sandwich wraps are nice and all, but sometimes you want something a little lighter. That's when I reach for the rice paper wraps, which are made from rice, water, tapioca flour, and salt and have a soft texture that you can use to bundle up just about anything. **SERVES 4.**

BADASS VEGAN

4 (9-inch/22 cm) sheets rice paper

16 (¼-inch-thick) strips Marinated and Grilled Tofu (page 247)

1 fresh mango, sliced into long, thin pieces

1 red bell pepper, seeded and sliced thin

1 bunch fresh cilantro, stems removed and leaves chopped

1 bunch fresh mint, leaves removed from the stems

1 bunch fresh basil, leaves removed from the stems

¼ cup shredded carrots

¼ cup shredded daikon radish

½ cup sunflower sprouts, pea shoots, or other sprouts of choice

¼ cup Peanut Jalapeño Crumble (page 266)

½ cup Tahini Ginger Dressing (page 269)

Dip the rice paper briefly in cold water and set it on a flat surface. Leaving a border along the top and bottom edges, layer four strips of tofu and one-fourth of the mango, bell pepper, cilantro, mint, basil, carrots, and daikon. Arrange a fourth of the sunflower sprouts with the green sprouts facing out so they stick out of the ends of the roll. Sprinkle the peanut jalapeño crumble on top and roll the rice paper up, sushi style. Repeat with the remaining rolls. Cut the rolls in half and serve with the dressing.

FOR 1 ROLL:
CALORIES: 380
PROTEIN: 17 GRAMS (1 BLOCK)
CARBOHYDRATES: 30 GRAMS (1.5 BLOCKS)
FAT: 25 GRAMS (2.5 BLOCKS)

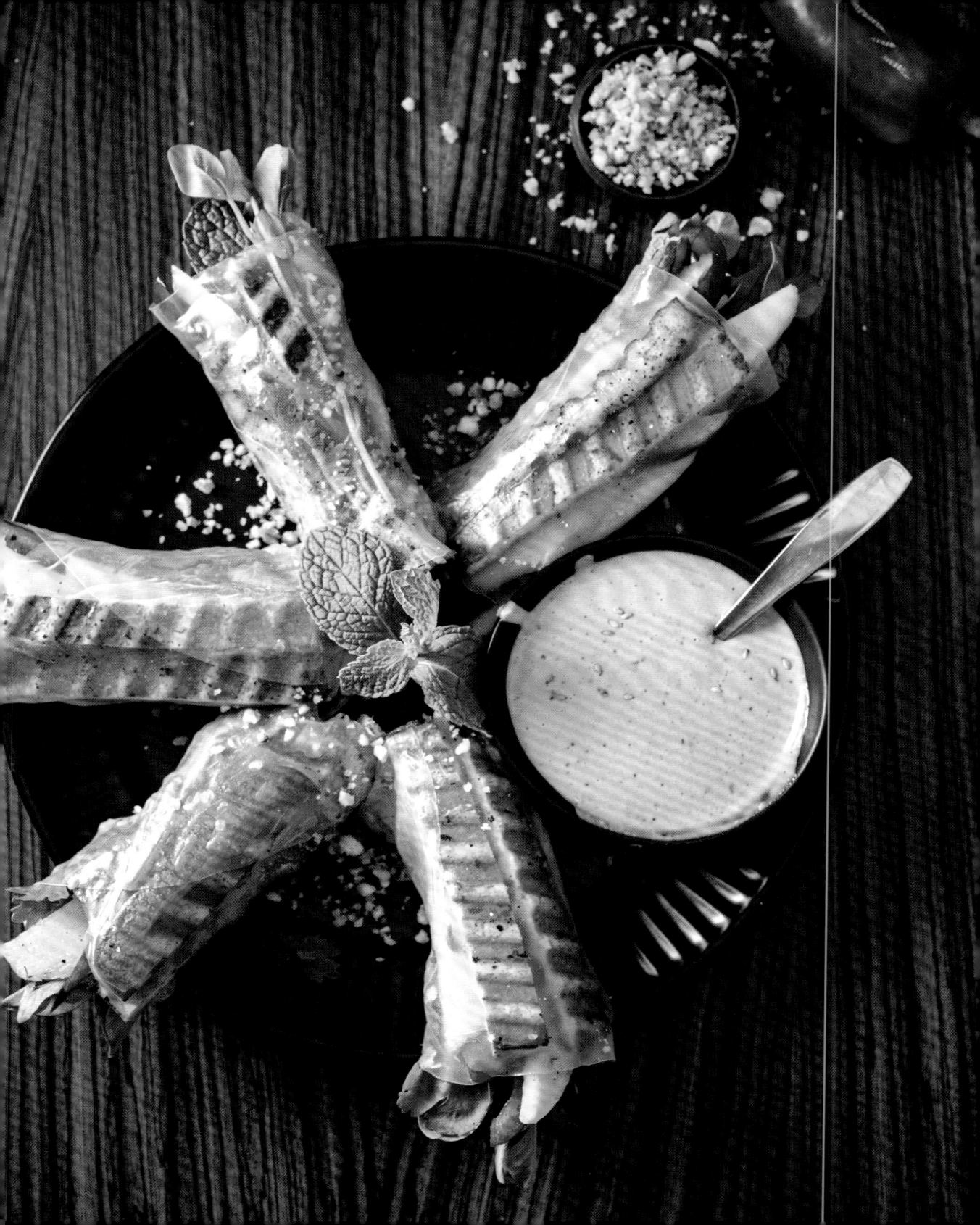

SAINT LOUIS BBQ

When I was growing up in the STL, there was nothing like a BBQ cookout because of how it brings people together, except it usually featured things like ribs and brisket. I wanted to keep the tasty tradition of love and family but drop the cruelty, so I came up with a version that still gets the family to come through and ask the age-old question of "Is this really vegan?" **SERVES 4**

FOR THE BBQ SAUCE

2 Roma tomatoes, halved

1 teaspoon extra-virgin olive oil

1½ teaspoons sea salt, plus more for the tomatoes

½ teaspoon ground black pepper, plus more for the tomatoes

¼ cup safflower oil

½ cup chopped yellow onion

2 teaspoons minced garlic

½ cup cubed mango, fresh or frozen and thawed

1 cup canned diced fire-roasted tomatoes (such as Muir Glen)

¼ cup maple syrup

2 tablespoons tomato paste

2 tablespoons apple cider vinegar

2 teaspoons fresh lemon juice

2 teaspoons molasses

2 teaspoons tamari soy sauce

2 teaspoons smoked paprika

2 teaspoons ground mustard

½ teaspoon onion powder

½ teaspoon garlic powder

Pinch of cayenne pepper

FOR THE RED POTATO SALAD

4 cups well-scrubbed, cubed or diced red potatoes

1 teaspoon sea salt, plus more for cooking the potatoes

¾ cup Cashew Aioli (page 278)

¼ cup finely diced celery

2 tablespoons thinly sliced scallions, white and light green parts only

1 tablespoon chopped fresh dill

½ teaspoon ground black pepper

FOR THE JACKFRUIT PULLED PORK

2 tablespoons safflower oil

½ cup diced yellow onion

2 teaspoons minced garlic

1 teaspoon paprika

1 teaspoon smoked paprika

1 teaspoon chili powder

1 teaspoon ground cumin

1 teaspoon sea salt

½ teaspoon ground black pepper

1 (10.6-ounce) box Upton's Naturals Original Jackfruit or 1 (14-ounce) can young jackfruit in brine, drained and rinsed

FOR SERVING

4 vegan brioche or ciabatta buns (or regular ol' hamburger buns), sliced

Cashew Aioli (page 278)

Pickled Purple Cabbage (page 255)

1 **MAKE THE BBQ SAUCE:** Preheat the oven to 375°F.

2 Brush the tomato halves with the olive oil and season with salt and pepper. Place the tomatoes cut side up on a baking sheet and roast until dried slightly and browned at the edges, 25 minutes. Set aside to cool.

3 In a large saucepan over medium heat, heat the safflower oil. Add the onion and garlic and cook, stirring, until the onion is translucent, about 10 minutes. Reduce the heat to low, add the mango, and cook for 10 more minutes. Add the oven-roasted tomatoes, canned tomatoes, maple syrup, tomato paste, vinegar, lemon juice, molasses, tamari, smoked paprika, ground mustard, the 1½ teaspoons of salt, the ½ teaspoon of black pepper, the onion powder, garlic powder, cayenne, and ½ cup of water. Stir to combine. Increase the heat to medium-high and bring the mixture to a boil. Reduce the heat to low and simmer the sauce for 1 hour, stirring occasionally.

RECIPE CONTINUES >>

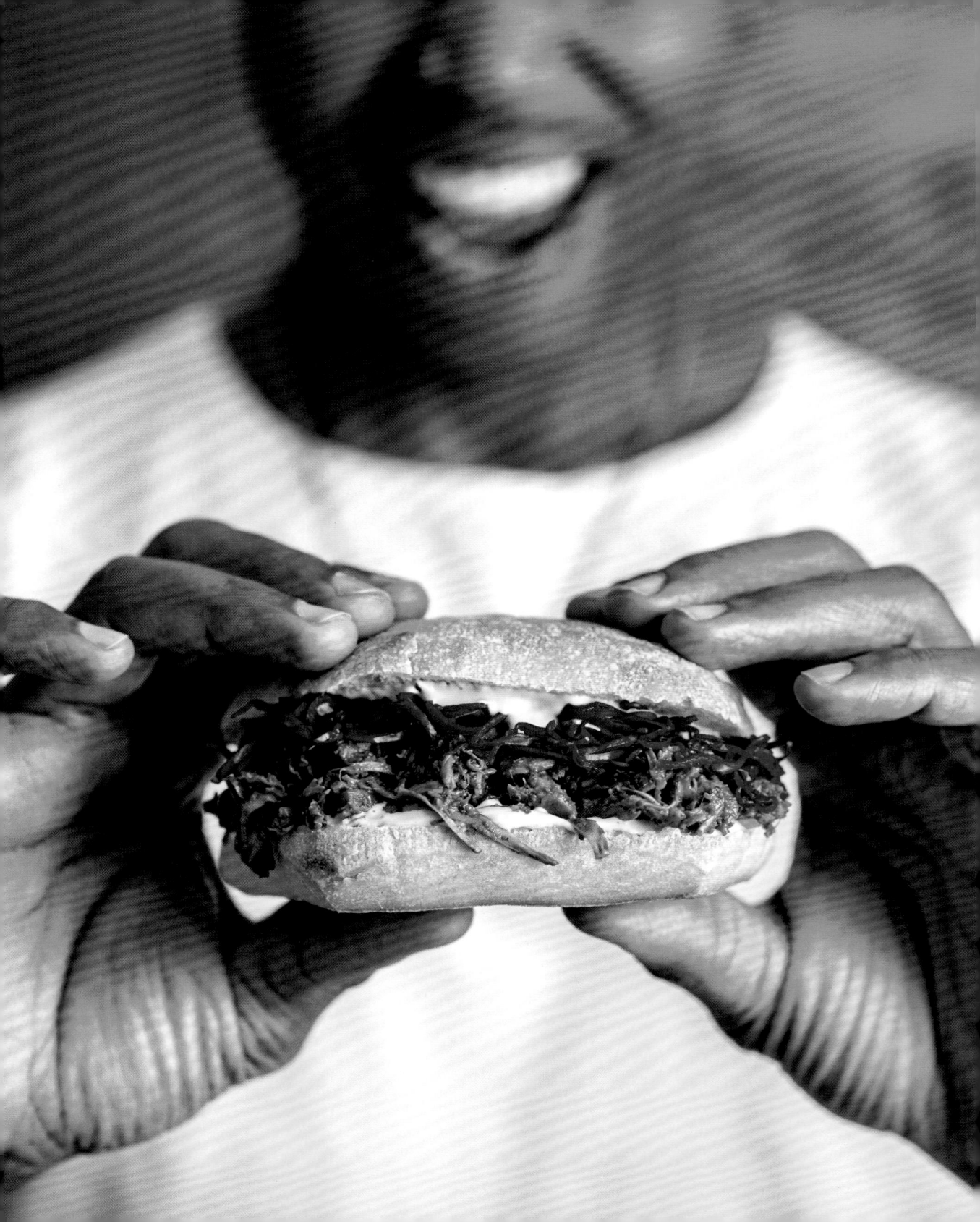

4 Remove the saucepan from the heat and use an immersion blender to puree the sauce until completely smooth. Set aside.

5 **MAKE THE RED POTATO SALAD:** In a large pot, add the potatoes and enough cold water to cover. Generously salt the water. Set the pot over high heat and bring to a boil. Reduce the heat to medium to keep the water boiling lightly and cook until the potatoes are soft enough to be pierced easily with a knife, about 12 minutes. Drain the potatoes and set aside to cool.

6 In a large bowl, whisk together the cashew aioli, celery, scallions, dill, the 1 teaspoon of salt, and the pepper. Add the potatoes and carefully toss to coat. Set aside to let the flavors mingle.

7 **MAKE THE JACKFRUIT PULLED PORK:** In a large nonstick pan over medium-high heat, heat the oil. Add the onion, garlic, paprika, smoked paprika, chili powder, cumin, salt, and pepper and cook, stirring, for 5 minutes. Add the jackfruit and a splash of water and cook for another 15 minutes, breaking down the jackfruit gently as you stir. Add ½ cup of the BBQ sauce and reduce the heat to medium-low. Continue stirring and cooking until the sauce has thickened slightly, 10 to 15 minutes.

8 **SERVE:** Top the buns with a generous scoop of the jackfruit pulled pork, additional BBQ sauce, the cashew aioli, and the pickled purple cabbage. Serve with the potato salad.

FOR 1 SERVING:
CALORIES: 780
PROTEIN: 15 GRAMS (1 BLOCK)
CARBOHYDRATES: 117 GRAMS (6 BLOCKS)
FAT: 32 GRAMS (3 BLOCKS)

C.R.E.A.M. PASTA
(CREAM RULES EVERYTHING AROUND MUSHROOMS)

Sure, you've had pasta with some mushrooms on top before, but have you ever witnessed a party with pasta, mushrooms, *and* a garlicky, cheesy, vegan cream sauce all together? That's what this is—a party that pasta invited the mushrooms and sauce to come out to, and now they're taking that party to your mouth. Boom. **SERVES 3**

8 ounces penne pasta

5 ounces button mushrooms, sliced

½ large red onion, diced

3 garlic cloves, minced

½ cup low-sodium vegetable broth or water

½ cup tahini

¼ cup unsweetened almond milk (see page 179), cashew milk, or water, plus more if needed

2 tablespoons apple cider vinegar

1 tablespoon fresh lemon juice

2 tablespoons nutritional yeast

½ teaspoon sea salt, plus more to taste

1 teaspoon maple syrup (optional)

Handful of chopped fresh parsley, for serving

1 Cook the pasta according to the package instructions. Drain and set aside.

2 Meanwhile, in a large nonstick pan over medium-low heat, cook the mushrooms until tender, about 10 minutes. Transfer the mushrooms to a bowl or plate, leaving their juice in the pan.

3 In the same pan, cook the onion and garlic in the leftover mushroom juice until the onion is translucent, about 5 minutes. Add the vegetable broth and cook until all the liquid is absorbed, 6 to 7 minutes. Remove the pan from the heat and set aside.

4 In a bowl, combine the tahini, almond milk, vinegar, lemon juice, nutritional

RECIPE CONTINUES >>

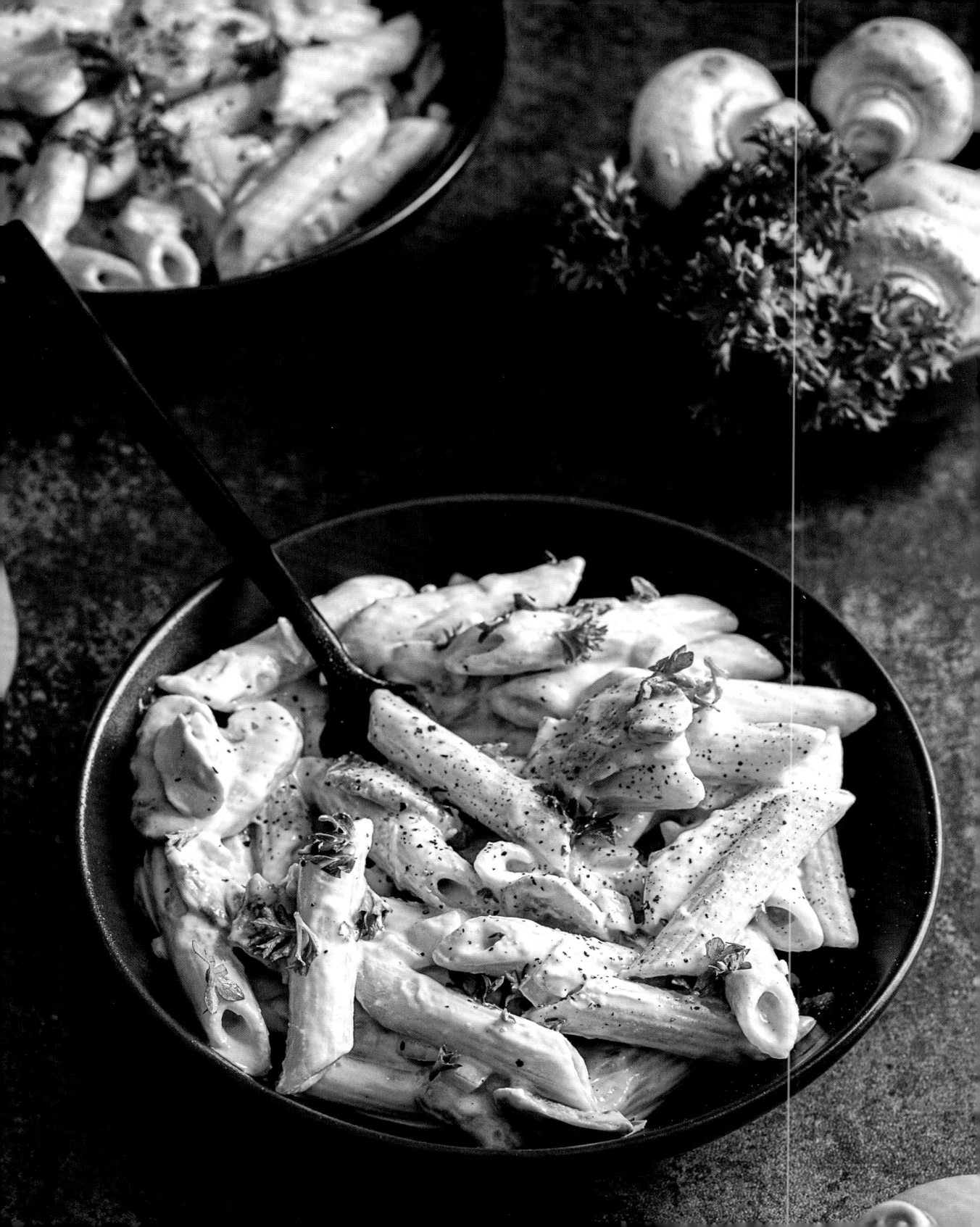

yeast, salt, and maple syrup, if using. Whisk together until smooth. Season with more salt to taste, if needed.

5 Pour the tahini sauce into the pan with the onion mixture and heat over medium-low. Whisk until the mixture warms through, then remove the pan from the heat. Immediately add the pasta and mushrooms to the sauce and stir to combine. If the sauce is too thick, add more almond milk or water until it reaches your desired consistency. Top with the parsley and serve hot.

FOR 1 SERVING:
CALORIES: 580
PROTEIN: 22 GRAMS (1 BLOCK)
CARBOHYDRATES: 65 GRAMS (3.5 BLOCKS)
FAT: 30 GRAMS (3.5 BLOCKS)

MARINATED AND GRILLED
TOFU

Next time someone tells you tofu doesn't have any flavor, instead of telling them just how stupid they sound, let them try this recipe. **SERVES 5**

½ cup extra-virgin olive oil

½ cup fresh lemon juice

½ cup tamari soy sauce

2 tablespoons minced garlic

1 tablespoon chopped fresh basil

1 tablespoon chopped fresh dill

1 tablespoon chopped fresh parsley

1 tablespoon ground black pepper

1 (16-ounce) package superfirm high-protein tofu (such as Wildwood)

1 In a high-speed blender, add the olive oil, lemon juice, tamari, garlic, basil, dill, parsley, and pepper and blend until emulsified.

2 Cut the tofu into ¼-inch-thick slices and arrange them in an even layer in a glass dish or nonreactive pan. Pour the marinade over the tofu and flip to coat both sides. Marinate, refrigerated, for at least 4 hours, turning the tofu halfway through.

3 Preheat a grill to medium-high heat.

4 Grill the tofu on each side until black grill marks form; this indicates perfect grill flavor. Be careful when flipping the tofu as it will be delicate. Serve immediately with your favorite salad or grains, or store in an airtight container in the refrigerator for up to 1 week.

FOR 1 SERVING:
CALORIES: 340
PROTEIN: 17 GRAMS (1 BLOCK)
CARBOHYDRATES: 7 GRAMS (0.5 BLOCK)
FAT: 28 GRAMS (3 BLOCKS)

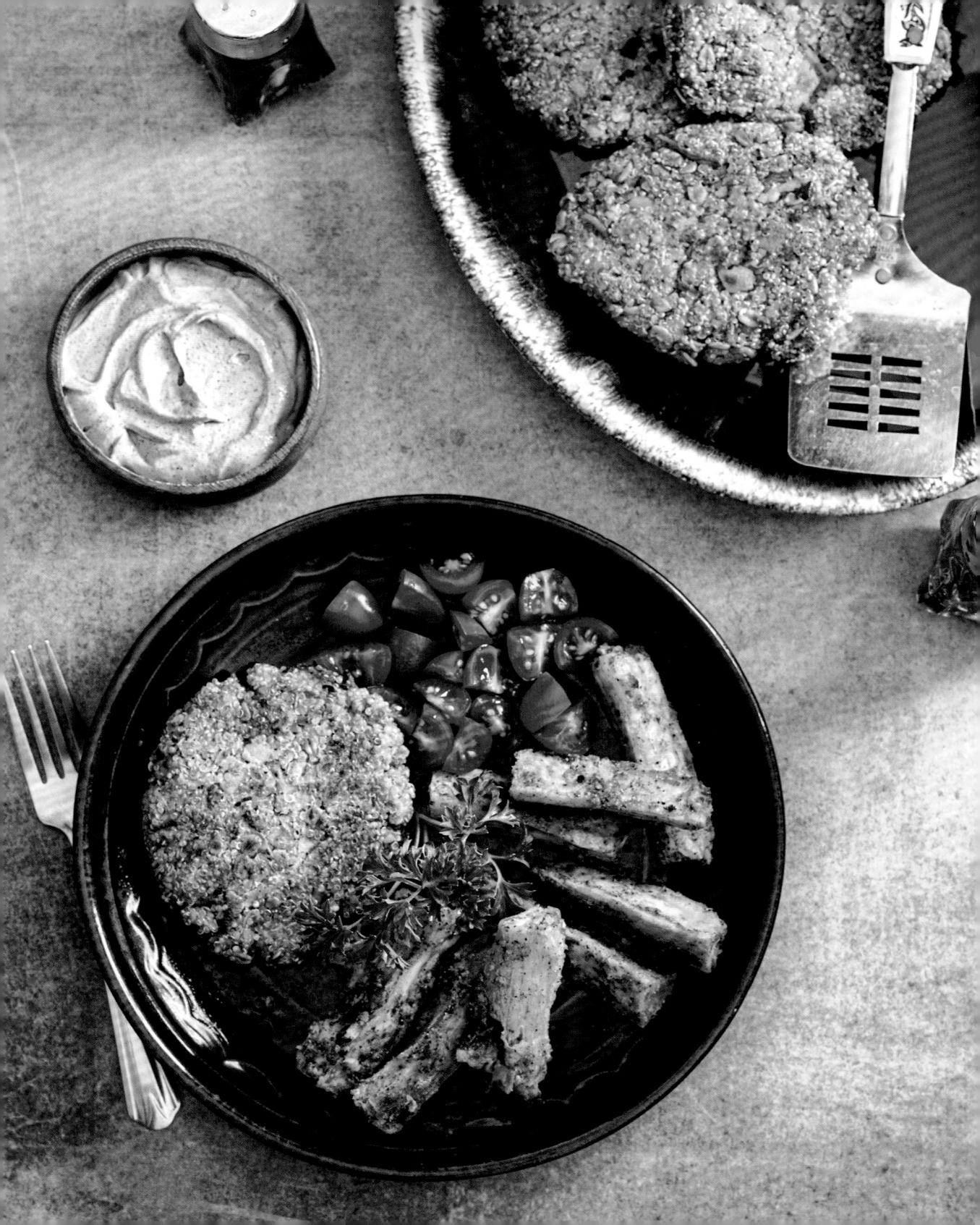

OINKLESS CUTLETS
WITH YUCA FRIES

If you're like me, then you remember when your mom used to make pork chops and all you could think about was eating that fried goodness, including the extra ring of fat we knew wasn't good for us but we'd eat anyway. Well you can still have that—flavor and all—just without the guilt and heart disease. Cooked grains flavored with ginger, chili paste, and garam masala make for a hearty, meaty, crispy cutlet that no one would guess is plant-based if you didn't tell 'em. To mix it up from the yuca fries, I suggest serving these with a side of grains (like more quinoa, which you could make at the same time you cook the quinoa for the cutlets) and fresh veggies like chopped tomato. **SERVES 4**

1 cup uncooked quinoa, rinsed

Sea salt, to taste

1 large Yukon Gold potato

1 cup rolled oats, toasted in a pan until fragrant

½ medium carrot, grated

1 teaspoon fresh ginger paste or grated fresh ginger

¼ green chili, seeded, chopped, and crushed into a paste

½ teaspoon garam masala

Ground black pepper, to taste

Vegetable oil, as needed

Yuca Fries with Chipotle Cashew Aioli, for serving (recipe follows)

1 In a medium pot over medium-low heat, combine the quinoa with 2 cups of water and a pinch of salt. Cook until the quinoa absorbs all the water, about 15 minutes. Set aside.

2 In a small or medium pot, add the potato and enough cold water to cover it by an inch. Bring to a boil, reduce to a simmer, and cook until the potato can easily be pierced with a fork or knife, 8 to 12 minutes. Drain the pot, and when the potato is cool enough to handle, remove and discard the skin, mash it with a fork, and set it aside.

RECIPE CONTINUES >>

3 In a large bowl, combine the quinoa and mashed potato with the oats, carrot, ginger, chili, and garam masala. Season to taste with salt and pepper. Shape the mixture into four equal patties. Flatten the patties with your palm so they're about ½ inch thick.

4 In a large pan over medium-high heat, add enough oil to just coat the bottom of the pan. When the oil begins to shimmer, add the cutlets and fry until golden brown, about 2 minutes per side. Serve with the yuca fries.

FOR 1 SERVING OF CUTLETS:
CALORIES: 320
PROTEIN: 10 GRAMS (0.5 BLOCK)
CARBOHYDRATES: 63 GRAMS (3 BLOCKS)
FAT: 4.5 GRAMS (0.5 BLOCK)

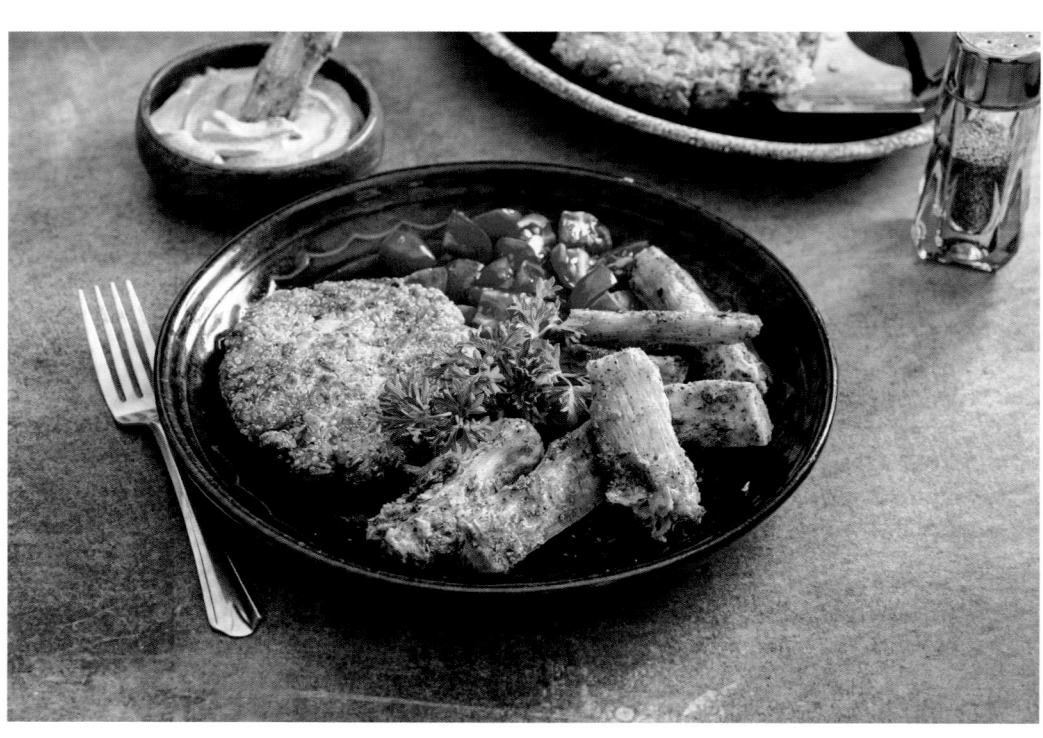

YUCA FRIES WITH CHIPOTLE CASHEW AIOLI

Yuca is a healthy, fat-free, gluten-free root vegetable that has a brown outer skin and white flesh. It's high in vitamins and iron and has even more fiber and potassium than potatoes. But all you need to know is that it's tasty as fuck.

SERVES 4

FOR THE YUCA FRIES

2 medium pieces fresh yuca

1 tablespoon sea salt, plus more for boiling

¼ cup extra-virgin olive oil

¼ cup safflower oil

1 tablespoon minced garlic

2 teaspoons paprika

2 teaspoons ground black pepper

½ teaspoon smoked paprika

FOR THE CHIPOTLE CASHEW AIOLI

1 cup Cashew Aioli (page 278)

2 teaspoons chipotle powder

1 MAKE THE FRIES: Trim both ends off the yuca roots and cut the yuca into 3- to 4-inch-thick rounds. Using a sharp knife, carefully cut a slit lengthwise in the skin of the yuca and peel.

2 Bring a large pot of well-salted water to a boil over medium-high heat. Add the yuca and cook until it is fork-tender, 20 to 25 minutes. Drain the yuca and let it cool completely.

3 Preheat the oven to 375°F. Cut the cooled yuca in half lengthwise and remove the inner root and any veins, then cut the yuca into 1-inch-thick "fingers."

4 In a medium bowl, whisk together the olive oil, safflower oil, garlic, paprika, the 1 tablespoon of salt, the pepper, and the smoked paprika. Toss the yuca fingers in the mixture and spread them in an even layer on a baking sheet. Bake until golden brown and crispy on all sides, about 25 minutes.

5 MAKE THE CHIPOTLE CASHEW AIOLI: In a small bowl, whisk the cashew aioli and chipotle powder until evenly incorporated.

6 Serve the yuca fries with the chipotle cashew aioli.

FOR 1 SERVING OF FRIES:
CALORIES: 610
PROTEIN: 4 GRAMS (0 BLOCKS)
CARBOHYDRATES: 75 GRAMS (4 BLOCKS)
FAT: 35 GRAMS (3.5 BLOCKS)

BB THE KING SEITAN

Just like the legendary jazz player, this dish has been a platinum staple in my dinner rotation since I first went vegan. **SERVES 4**

16 (1 × 4-inch) slices seitan

2 cups baby arugula

¼ cup Chimichurri (page 270)

¼ cup Horseradish Aioli (page 263)

1 Preheat a grill or grill pan over medium-high heat. Grill the seitan slices until browned and slightly crisp, 2 minutes per side.

2 Serve the seitan over the arugula and drizzle with the chimichurri and horseradish aioli.

FOR 1 SERVING:
CALORIES: 150
PROTEIN: 18 GRAMS (1 BLOCK)
CARBOHYDRATES: 5 GRAMS (0.5 BLOCK)
FAT: 7 GRAMS (0.5 BLOCK)

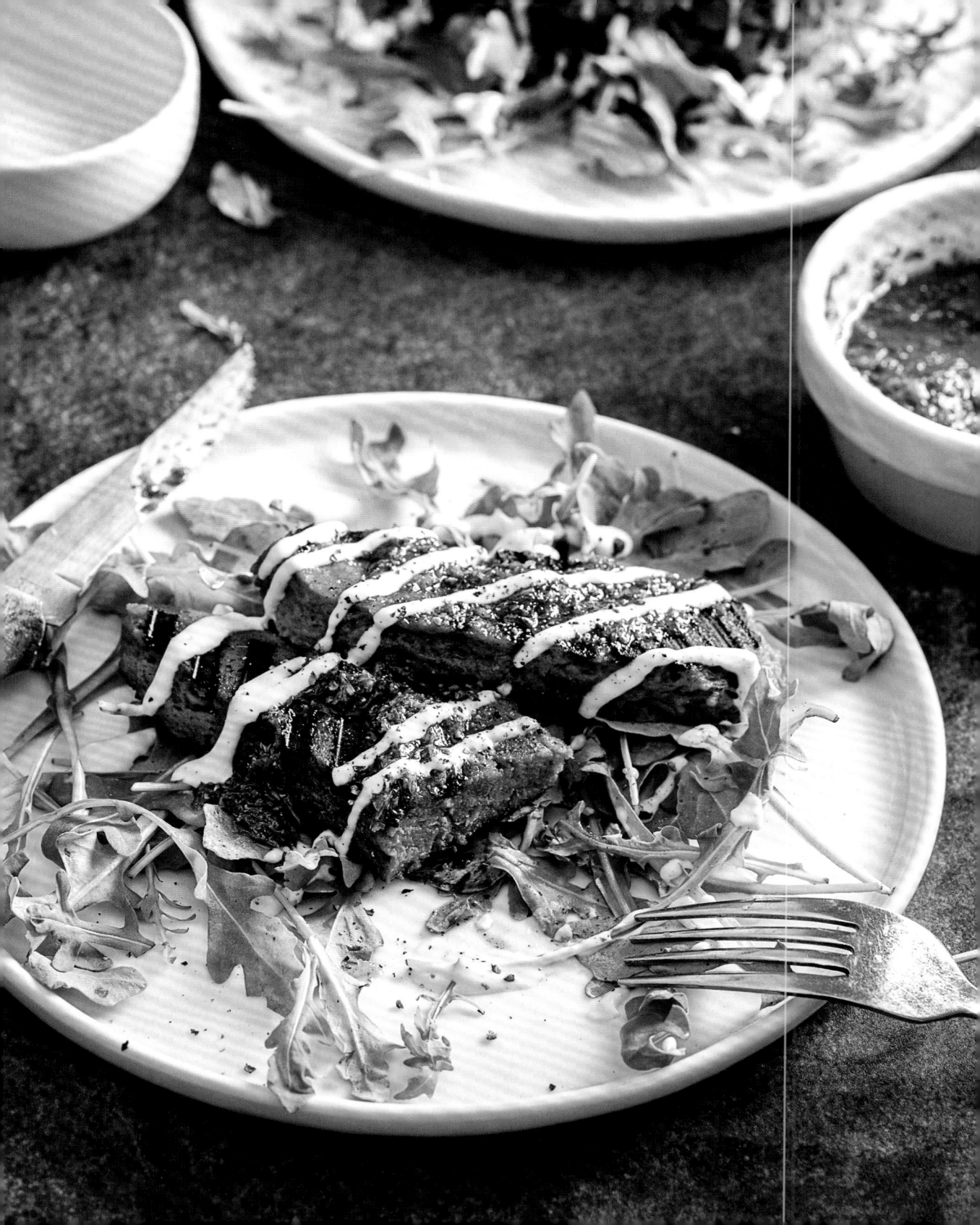

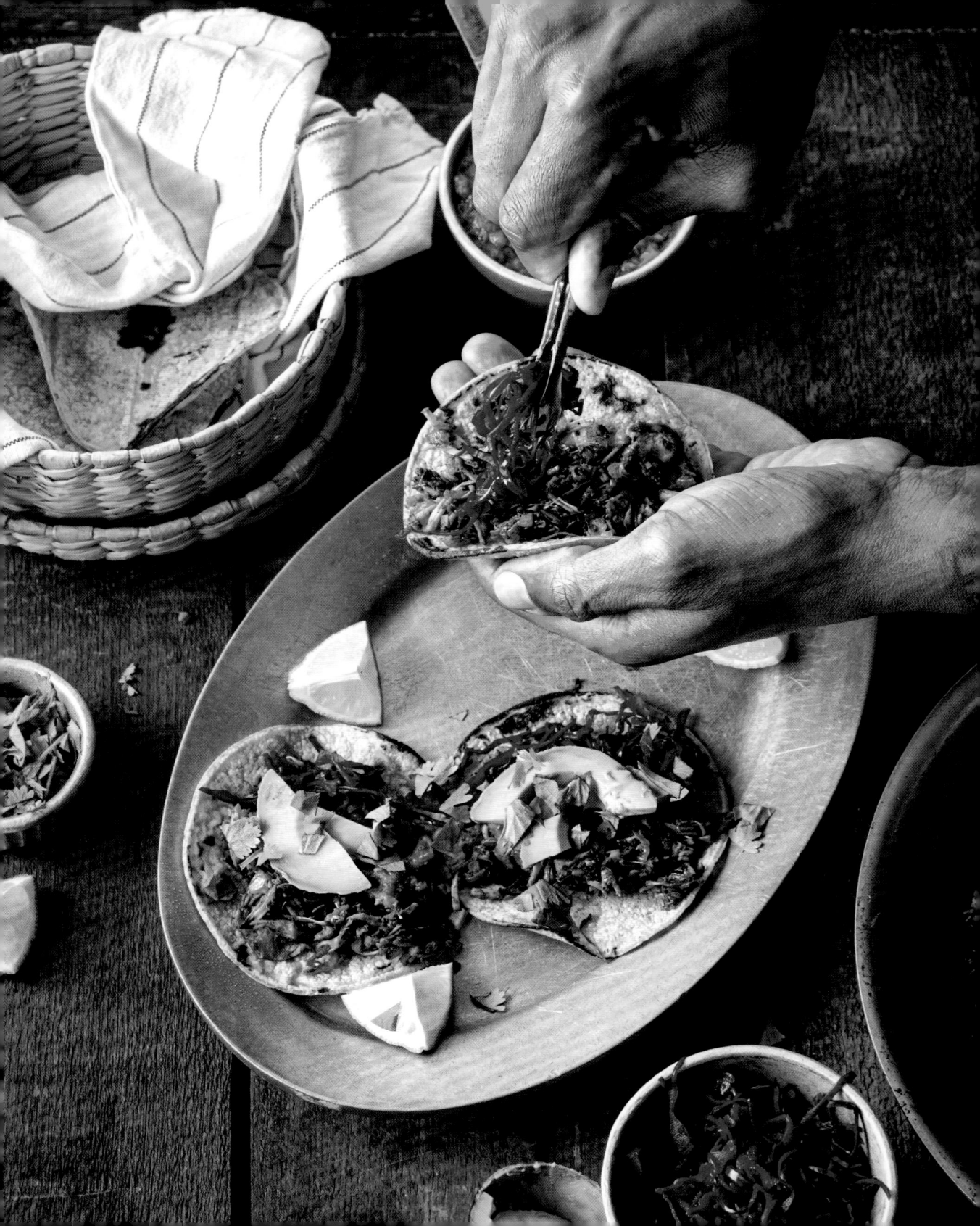

JACK U UP
STREET TACOS

I fell in love with street tacos during my monthly visits to Los Angeles, so I developed my own version using jackfruit as the base. Don't let jackfruit fool you—it can be sweet when it's ripe, but the unripened fruit has a really mild taste that takes on flavor well and gives you meat-like texture. **SERVES 4.**

FOR THE JACKFRUIT

¼ cup extra-virgin olive oil

1 cup diced yellow onion

2 tablespoons minced garlic

½ jalapeño, seeded and diced

1 tablespoon chili powder

1 tablespoon smoked paprika

2 teaspoons ground cumin

2 teaspoons ground coriander

2 teaspoons dried oregano

2 teaspoons sea salt

1 teaspoon ground black pepper

Pinch of cayenne pepper

1 (14-ounce) can or 2 (10.6-ounce) boxes young jackfruit (I like Native Forest and Upton's Naturals), drained and rinsed

¼ cup maple syrup

2 tablespoons fresh lime juice

FOR THE PICKLED PURPLE CABBAGE

3 cups thinly shredded purple cabbage

¼ cup apple cider vinegar

1 tablespoon agave nectar

1 teaspoon sea salt

FOR SERVING

About 4 corn tortillas

Roasted Tomato Salsa (page 273)

2 Hass avocados, peeled, pitted, and sliced

Chopped fresh cilantro

RECIPE CONTINUES >>

1 **MAKE THE JACKFRUIT:** Heat the olive oil in a large nonstick pan over medium-low heat. Add the onion, garlic, and jalapeño and cook until softened, 5 minutes. Reduce the heat to low and add the chili powder, smoked paprika, cumin, coriander, oregano, salt, black pepper, and cayenne and cook for another 5 minutes. Increase the heat to medium and add the jackfruit. Cook for 10 minutes, using the back of a wooden spoon to stir and break up the jackfruit as you cook. Add the maple syrup and lime juice and cook for another 10 minutes, or until it reaches the desired texture, continuing to stir and break up the mixture. Remove the pan from the heat and set aside.

2 **MAKE THE PICKLED CABBAGE:** In a large bowl, toss together the shredded cabbage, vinegar, agave, and salt. Use your hands to massage the cabbage so it begins to break down and soften. Set aside for at least 20 minutes to pickle. Drain any excess liquid from the cabbage before serving.

3 **SERVE:** Over a gas flame or on a grill pan over medium heat, grill the tortillas for barely 1 minute per side. (Alternatively, you can use a nonstick pan over low heat.) Top the tortillas with the jackfruit and pickled cabbage and finish with the roasted tomato salsa, sliced avocados, and chopped cilantro.

FOR 1 SERVING:
CALORIES: 580
PROTEIN: 9 GRAMS (0.5 BLOCK)
CARBOHYDRATES: 75 GRAMS (4 BLOCKS)
FAT: 31 GRAMS (3 BLOCKS)

CARIBBEAN
QUESA-RITOS

Before going vegan, I had a weakness for quesadillas and burritos. This recipe combines the best of both worlds and adds some Caribbean flava thanks to coconut lentils and plantains. You may have tried lentils before, but until you've had mine, you haven't lived. **SERVES 8**

FOR THE COCONUT LENTILS

2 tablespoons extra-virgin olive oil

½ cup diced yellow onion

1 tablespoon minced garlic

2 teaspoons ground coriander

2 teaspoons paprika

2 teaspoons ground ginger

2 teaspoons ground allspice

1 teaspoon chili powder

1 teaspoon sea salt, plus more to taste

½ teaspoon cinnamon

½ teaspoon ground black pepper

2 cups full-fat coconut milk

1 cup dried green lentils, sorted, rinsed, and any small stones discarded

½ cup filtered water

2 tablespoons fresh lime juice

FOR THE CARAMELIZED ONIONS

¼ cup extra-virgin olive oil

2 cups sliced yellow onions

1½ tablespoons maple syrup

½ teaspoon sea salt

FOR THE SEARED PLANTAINS

1 very ripe plantain, sliced ¼ inch thick on a diagonal

2 tablespoons extra-virgin olive oil

2 tablespoons agave nectar

1 teaspoon sea salt

½ teaspoon ground black pepper

FOR THE QUESA-RITOS

4 (12-inch) whole wheat tortillas

1 cup Jalapeño Cilantro Aioli (page 279), for serving

2 cups Mango Salsa (page 272), for serving

RECIPE CONTINUES >>

1 **MAKE THE COCONUT LENTILS:** In a large pot over medium heat, heat the oil and add the onion. Cook, stirring, until the onion is softened, about 8 minutes. Stir in the garlic, coriander, paprika, ginger, allspice, chili powder, salt, cinnamon, and pepper and cook until fragrant, 1 to 2 minutes. Add the coconut milk, lentils, and water and bring to a boil. Reduce the heat to low, cover, and simmer until the lentils are fully cooked, 35 to 40 minutes. Remove the pot from the heat.

2 Using a handheld immersion blender, blend the lentils in pulses until the mixture is slightly creamy but retains some texture, about 1 minute. You could also do this by transferring the lentils to a blender. Stir in the lime juice and adjust the salt to taste.

3 **MAKE THE CARAMELIZED ONIONS:** In a large pan over medium heat, heat the oil. Add the onions, maple syrup, and salt and cook, stirring occasionally, until the onions are very soft and sweet, about 20 minutes.

4 **MAKE THE PLANTAINS:** Heat a large pan over medium-high heat.

5 In a medium bowl, toss together the plantain, oil, agave, salt, and pepper. Sear the plantain slices until golden brown, about 2 minutes per side. Remove the pan from the heat, leaving the plantains in the pan to stay warm.

6 **ASSEMBLE THE QUESA-RITOS:** Over a gas flame or on a grill pan over medium heat, grill the tortillas for barely 1 minute per side. (Alternatively, you can use a nonstick pan over low heat.) Set aside under a kitchen towel to keep warm.

7 Fill each tortilla with 1 cup of the lentils and about ½ cup of the caramelized onions, then fold it up into a quesadilla shape. Top each quesa-rito with ¼ cup of the jalapeño aioli, ½ cup of the mango salsa, and ½ cup of the plantains.

FOR 1 QUESA-RITO (2 SERVINGS):
CALORIES: 590
PROTEIN: 12 GRAMS (0.5 BLOCK)
CARBOHYDRATES: 60 GRAMS (3 BLOCKS)
FAT: 37 GRAMS (3.5 BLOCKS)

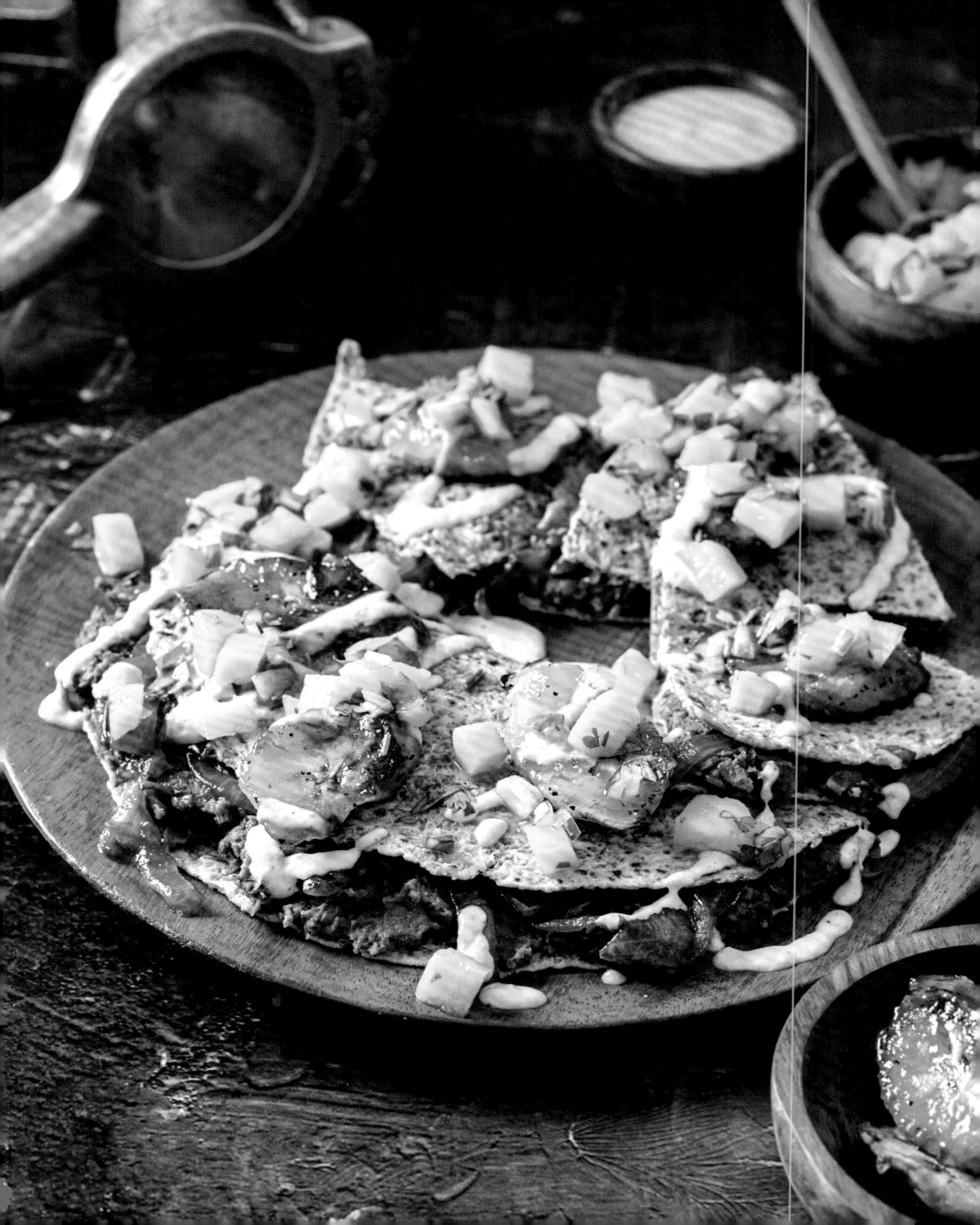

CHAPTER 20

EXTRA DRIP:
Sauces and Other Extras

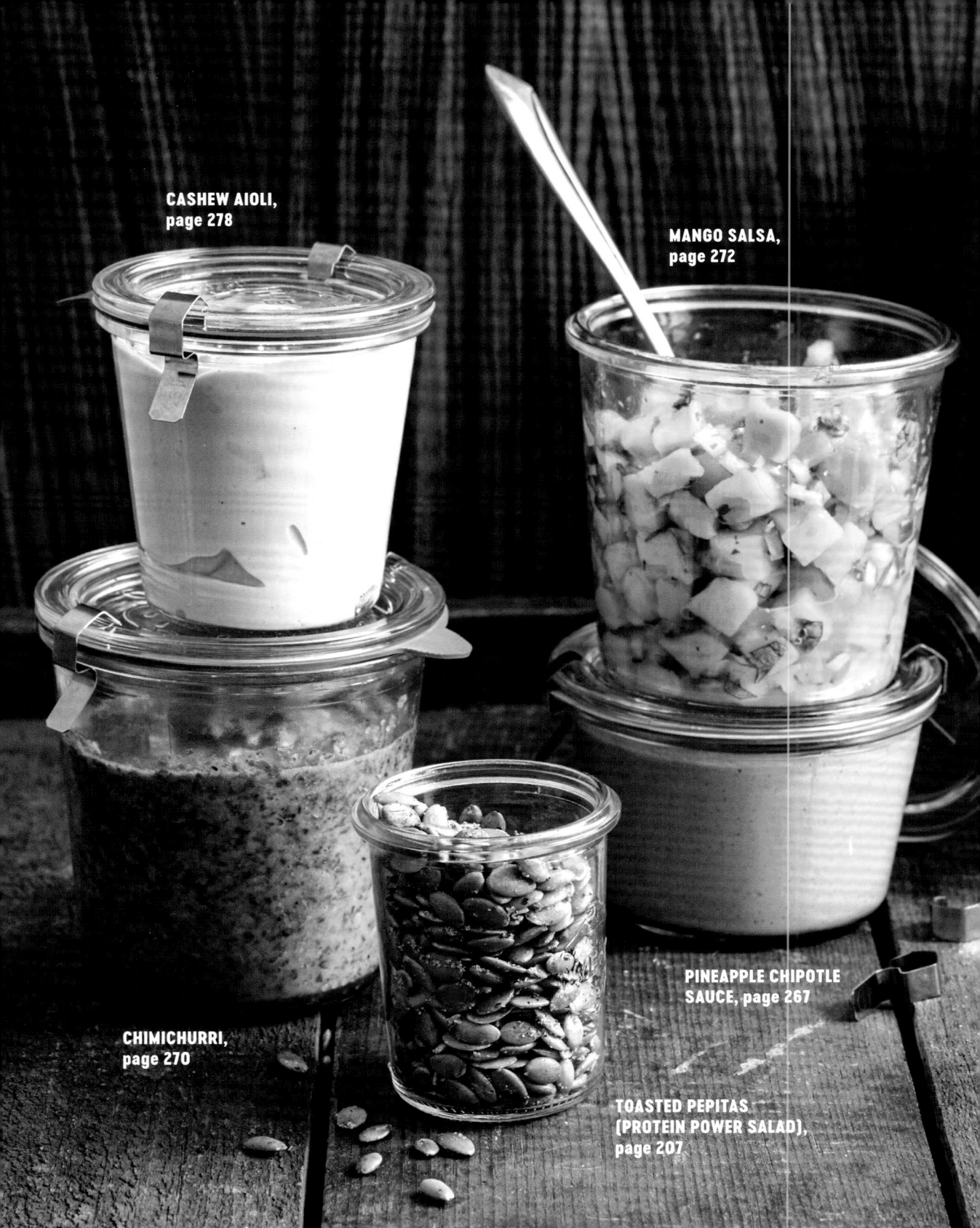

CASHEW AIOLI,
page 278

MANGO SALSA,
page 272

CHIMICHURRI,
page 270

PINEAPPLE CHIPOTLE
SAUCE, page 267

TOASTED PEPITAS
(PROTEIN POWER SALAD),
page 207

HOLY MOLY GUACAMOLE

I mean, that's pretty much what you're gonna say as soon as your taste buds experience this. Your avocados will thank you. **MAKES 2 TO 3 CUPS**

3 Hass avocados, peeled and pitted

½ cup chopped fresh cilantro

¼ cup finely diced red onion

¼ cup fresh lime juice

½ jalapeño, stemmed, seeded, and minced

1 garlic clove, minced

½ teaspoon sea salt, plus more to taste

In a medium bowl, add the avocados, cilantro, onion, lime juice, jalapeño, garlic, and salt. Use a fork to gently smash the avocados and incorporate the ingredients, leaving some chunks for texture. Taste and adjust the seasoning as desired.

FOR 1 TABLESPOON:
CALORIES: 150
PROTEIN: 3 GRAMS (0 BLOCKS)
CARBOHYDRATES: 6 GRAMS (0.5 BLOCK)
FAT: 15 GRAMS (1.5 BLOCKS)

HORSERADISH AIOLI

This sauce is made from plant-based ingredients, but you'd never guess it based on its luscious, creamy texture. With the big-time kick it gets from the horseradish, you'll want to slather this on just about anything. **MAKES 2 CUPS**

1 cup Cashew Aioli
(page 278)

2 tablespoons
freshly grated or
jarred prepared
horseradish

2 tablespoons
fresh lemon juice

2 tablespoons
agave nectar

1 teaspoon minced
garlic

In a high-speed blender or food processor, add the cashew aioli, horseradish, lemon juice, agave, and garlic, and blend until completely smooth. Store in an airtight container in the refrigerator for up to 1 week.

FOR 1 TABLESPOON:
CALORIES: 120
PROTEIN: 3 GRAMS (0 BLOCKS)
CARBOHYDRATES: 9 GRAMS (0.5 BLOCK)
FAT: 7.5 GRAMS (1 BLOCK)

EXTRA DRIP

PEANUT HOISIN SAUCE

A sweet, tangy homemade hoisin and rich, creamy peanuts team up to make a powerhouse sauce that packs a big flavor punch with a nice, light texture. I especially like using this for marinating tofu, seitan, and veggies. **MAKES ABOUT 2 CUPS**

½ cup sesame oil

¼ cup brown rice vinegar

¼ cup molasses

¼ cup unsweetened peanut butter

¼ cup tamari soy sauce

1 tablespoon chopped garlic

1 tablespoon chopped jalapeño, seeds removed for less heat

1 tablespoon chopped shallot

1 teaspoon ground black pepper

In a high-speed blender, add the sesame oil, vinegar, molasses, peanut butter, tamari, garlic, jalapeño, shallot, pepper, and ½ cup of water and blend until completely smooth. Store in an airtight container in the refrigerator for up to 5 days.

FOR ¼ CUP:
CALORIES: 110
PROTEIN: 2 GRAMS (0 BLOCKS)
CARBOHYDRATES: 5 GRAMS (0.5 BLOCK)
FAT: 10 GRAMS (1 BLOCK)

WALNUT VINAIGRETTE

Sometimes you feel like a nut, and sometimes you just feel like a tangy, mustard-based vinaigrette that harnesses the power of the walnut to make it just a little bit creamy.

MAKES ABOUT 1½ CUPS

¼ cup walnuts

¼ cup maple syrup

¼ cup apple cider vinegar

2 tablespoons minced shallot

2 teaspoons stone-ground mustard

1 teaspoon minced garlic

1 teaspoon sea salt, plus more to taste

¼ teaspoon ground black pepper, plus more to taste

½ cup extra-virgin olive oil

In a high-speed blender, add the walnuts, maple syrup, vinegar, shallot, mustard, garlic, salt, and pepper and blend on medium speed until smooth. With the blender on low speed, stream in the oil and blend until fully emulsified. Adjust the seasoning as needed. Store in an airtight container in the refrigerator for up to 5 days.

FOR 1 TABLESPOON:
CALORIES: 105
PROTEIN: 9 GRAMS (0.5 BLOCK)
CARBOHYDRATES: 15 GRAMS (1 BLOCK)
FAT: 6 GRAMS (0.5 BLOCK)

PEANUT JALAPEÑO
CRUMBLE

With just two ingredients you can make a crunchy, protein-packed kick that can be added to any dish.

MAKES ABOUT 2/3 CUP

2/3 cup roasted, salted peanuts

1 tablespoon chopped jalapeño

In a food processor, add the peanuts and jalapeño and pulse until the mixture resembles a rough crumble.

FOR 1 TABLESPOON:
CALORIES: 78
PROTEIN: 3.25 GRAMS (0 BLOCKS)
CARBOHYDRATES: 3.25 GRAMS (0 BLOCKS)
FAT: 6.5 GRAMS (0.5 BLOCK)

PINEAPPLE CHIPOTLE
SAUCE

If you don't like spicy and sweet with a kickass taste, then this isn't for you . . . What am I saying? You're gonna love this sauce no matter what. **MAKES 2 CUPS**

⅔ cup chopped or cubed fresh pineapple

¼ cup brown rice vinegar

¼ cup sesame oil

¼ cup coconut nectar

¼ cup sunflower seeds

2 tablespoons grated fresh ginger

1 tablespoon chopped garlic

1 tablespoon chopped shallot

1 teaspoon chipotle powder

In a high-speed blender, add the pineapple, vinegar, sesame oil, coconut nectar, sunflower seeds, ginger, garlic, shallot, and chipotle powder and blend until completely smooth. Store in an airtight container in the refrigerator for up to 5 days.

FOR ¼ CUP:
CALORIES: 280
PROTEIN: 3 GRAMS (0 BLOCKS)
CARBOHYDRATES: 20 GRAMS (1 BLOCK)
FAT: 22 GRAMS (2 BLOCKS)

RED WINE VINAIGRETTE

A dressing as classic as the UB40 jam. **MAKES 1½ CUPS**

½ cup red wine vinegar

2 large garlic cloves

2 teaspoons Dijon mustard

½ teaspoon sea salt

½ teaspoon ground black pepper

1 cup extra-virgin olive oil

In a high-speed blender, add the vinegar, garlic, mustard, salt, and pepper and blend until completely smooth. With the blender on low speed, stream in the oil and blend until fully emulsified. Store in an airtight container in the refrigerator for up to 1 week.

FOR 1 TABLESPOON:
CALORIES: 80
PROTEIN: 0 GRAMS (0 BLOCKS)
CARBOHYDRATES: 0 GRAMS (0 BLOCKS)
FAT: 9 GRAMS (1 BLOCK)

TAHINI GINGER
DRESSING

When you combine the sweet, hot kick of ginger with the savory, bitter, nutty creaminess of tahini, you get a show unlike any other your mouth has witnessed.

MAKES ABOUT 2 CUPS

¾ cup tahini

¼ cup tamari soy sauce

2 tablespoons fresh lemon juice

¼ cup grated fresh ginger

2 teaspoons chopped garlic

1 teaspoon ground black pepper

In a high-speed blender, add the tahini, tamari, lemon juice, ginger, garlic, pepper, and ½ cup of water and blend until completely smooth, about 1 minute. Store in an airtight container in the refrigerator for up to 5 days.

FOR 1 TABLESPOON:
CALORIES: 60
PROTEIN: 2 GRAMS (0 BLOCKS)
CARBOHYDRATES: 1.3 GRAMS (0 BLOCKS)
FAT: 5.3 GRAMS (0.5 BLOCK)

CHIMICHURRI

I'm all about the herb . . . in my sauce. This bright sauce combines parsley, cilantro, and oregano to make a versatile condiment that enhances the flavor of whatever you put it on.

MAKES ABOUT 2 CUPS

2 cups fresh parsley leaves

1 cup fresh cilantro leaves

½ cup extra-virgin olive oil

¼ cup fresh lime juice

1 small shallot, chopped

2 tablespoons fresh oregano leaves

2 tablespoons apple cider vinegar

1 tablespoon agave nectar

1 tablespoon minced garlic

½ teaspoon sea salt

½ teaspoon ground black pepper

¼ teaspoon crushed red pepper

In a high-speed blender, add the parsley, cilantro, olive oil, lime juice, shallot, oregano, vinegar, agave, garlic, salt, black pepper, and crushed red pepper. Pulse until the herbs have broken down but the mixture still retains some texture, about 1 minute. Store in an airtight container in the refrigerator for up to 5 days.

FOR 1 TABLESPOON:
CALORIES: 33.6
PROTEIN: 0 GRAMS (0 BLOCKS)
CARBOHYDRATES: 3 GRAMS (0 BLOCKS)
FAT: 2.5 GRAMS (0.5 BLOCK)

BADASS VEGAN

CASHEW CRUMBLE

Unlike most crumbles that you find on baked goods, this one is more of a savory garnish and has a light texture that's perfect for topping salads, bowls, and soups.

MAKES ABOUT 1 CUP

1 cup raw cashews

2 teaspoons sesame oil

1 teaspoon sea salt

In the bowl of a food processor, add the cashews, sesame oil, and salt. Pulse until the cashews are crumbled into tiny pieces, about 30 seconds. Be careful not to overprocess—we're not making cashew butter!

FOR 1 TABLESPOON:
CALORIES: 84
PROTEIN: 2.5 GRAMS (0 BLOCKS)
CARBOHYDRATES: 2.5 GRAMS (0 BLOCKS)
FAT: 7.5 (1 BLOCK)

MANGO SALSA

A Caribbean version of a traditional tomato-based salsa that makes some sweet love to your taste buds. **MAKES ABOUT 2 CUPS**

2 cups diced mango

¼ cup finely diced red onion

¼ cup finely chopped fresh cilantro

2 tablespoons fresh lime juice

½ teaspoon sea salt

In a medium bowl, add the mango, onion, cilantro, lime juice, and salt and mix gently to combine. Store in an airtight container in the refrigerator for up to 3 days.

FOR 2 TABLESPOONS:
CALORIES: 15
PROTEIN: 0 GRAMS (0 BLOCKS)
CARBOHYDRATES: 3 GRAMS (0 BLOCKS)
FAT: 0 GRAMS (0 BLOCKS)

ROASTED TOMATO SALSA

A classic in my house—I use it for everything from dip to salad dressing. Very versatile, low in calories, and—dammit—it just tastes good AF. **MAKES ABOUT 2 CUPS**

4 Roma tomatoes

½ teaspoon extra-virgin olive oil

1 teaspoon sea salt, plus more to taste

2 garlic cloves, peeled

1 jalapeño, left whole

¼ cup roughly chopped fresh cilantro

¼ cup roughly chopped yellow onion

1 Preheat the oven to 375°F.

2 In a medium bowl, gently toss the tomatoes with the olive oil and a pinch of salt. Transfer the tomatoes, garlic cloves, and jalapeño to a baking sheet. Roast the vegetables for 15 minutes and set aside to cool.

3 Carefully remove the stem and seeds from the jalapeño. Add half of the jalapeño (or the whole thing if you like it spicy!) to a high-speed blender, along with the roasted tomatoes, roasted garlic, cilantro, onion, and the 1 teaspoon of salt. Blend until well mixed but not completely smooth. Taste and adjust the salt as desired. Store in an airtight container in the refrigerator for up to 5 days.

FOR 2 TABLESPOONS:
CALORIES: 5
PROTEIN: 0 GRAMS (0 BLOCKS)
CARBOHYDRATES: 2 GRAMS (0 BLOCKS)
FAT: 0 GRAMS (0 BLOCKS)

CILANTRO LIME
DRESSING

This dressing will have your taste buds dancing whether you use it as a marinade or drizzle it over your favorite leafy greens. **MAKES ABOUT 2 CUPS**

¼ cup fresh lime juice

2 tablespoons apple cider vinegar

1 tablespoon agave nectar

2 tablespoons minced red onion

2 teaspoons stone-ground mustard

2 teaspoons ground cumin

2 teaspoons ground coriander

1 teaspoon sea salt

¼ teaspoon cayenne pepper

1 cup extra-virgin olive oil

½ cup fresh cilantro leaves

In a high-speed blender, add the lime juice, vinegar, agave, onion, mustard, cumin, coriander, salt, and cayenne and blend until smooth. With the blender on low speed, stream in the oil and blend until fully emulsified. Add the cilantro and blend until smooth. Store in an airtight container in the refrigerator for up to 5 days.

FOR 1 TABLESPOON:
CALORIES: 74
PROTEIN: 0.5 GRAM (0 BLOCKS)
CARBOHYDRATES: 2 GRAMS (0 BLOCKS)
FAT: 8 GRAMS (1 BLOCK)

SPICY CHILI LIME
DRESSING

A dressing or marinade with a dropkick hit of Thai chilies.

MAKES ABOUT 2 CUPS

½ cup fresh lime juice

¼ cup agave nectar

¼ cup tamari soy sauce

¼ cup sesame oil

¼ cup thinly sliced scallions

2 tablespoons finely chopped fresh Thai basil

2 tablespoons finely chopped fresh cilantro

2 teaspoons minced garlic

1 teaspoon thinly sliced Thai chili

¼ teaspoon sea salt, plus more to taste

In a medium bowl, whisk together the lime juice, agave, tamari, sesame oil, scallions, Thai basil, cilantro, garlic, chili, and salt. Taste and adjust the seasoning as needed. Store in an airtight container in the refrigerator for up to 5 days.

FOR 1 TABLESPOON:
CALORIES: 27.5
PROTEIN: 0.5 GRAM (0 BLOCKS)
CARBOHYDRATES: 2.5 GRAMS (0 BLOCKS)
FAT: 2 GRAMS (0 BLOCKS)

EXTRA DRIP

ALMOND GINGER
DRESSING

If you can have sweet and spicy at the same time . . . why would you choose anything else? **MAKES 3 CUPS**

¾ cup raw almonds, soaked overnight, drained, and rinsed

¼ cup plus 2 tablespoons tamari soy sauce

¼ cup plus 2 tablespoons fresh lime juice

2 tablespoons chopped shallot

2 tablespoons maple syrup

2 tablespoons chopped fresh ginger

1 teaspoon chopped garlic

1 teaspoon dulse flakes

¼ teaspoon cayenne pepper, plus more to taste

¼ cup extra-virgin olive oil

In a high-speed blender, add the almonds, tamari, lime juice, shallot, maple syrup, ginger, garlic, dulse, cayenne, and 2 tablespoons of water and blend on medium speed until completely smooth. With the blender on low speed, stream in the oil and blend until fully emulsified. Taste and adjust the seasoning as needed. Store in an airtight container in the refrigerator for up to 5 days.

FOR 1 TABLESPOON:
CALORIES: 39
PROTEIN: 0.5 GRAM (0 BLOCKS)
CARBOHYDRATES: 2.5 GRAMS (0 BLOCKS)
FAT: 3.5 GRAMS (0 BLOCKS)

CASHEW SOUR CREAM

This recipe turns simple ingredients into a rich, tangy sour cream that's better than the real thing. **MAKES ABOUT 3 CUPS**

2 cups raw cashews, soaked overnight, drained, and rinsed

1 cup filtered water

½ cup fresh lemon juice

1½ tablespoons apple cider vinegar

2 teaspoons nutritional yeast

½ teaspoon sea salt

In a high-speed blender, add the cashews, water, lemon juice, vinegar, nutritional yeast, and salt. Blend until completely smooth, stopping the blender to scrape down the sides as needed. Store in an airtight container in the refrigerator for up to 5 days.

FOR 1 TABLESPOON:
CALORIES: 51
PROTEIN: 2 GRAMS (0 BLOCKS)
CARBOHYDRATES: 2 GRAMS (0 BLOCKS)
FAT: 4.5 GRAMS (0.5 BLOCK)

CASHEW AIOLI

Aioli is just a fancy way of saying mayonnaise. Use this sauce anywhere and anytime you'd use mayo. **MAKES 2¹/₂ CUPS**

2 cups raw cashews, soaked overnight, drained, and rinsed

½ cup filtered water

2 teaspoons fresh lemon juice

2 teaspoons apple cider vinegar

1 teaspoon nutritional yeast

1 teaspoon sea salt

½ teaspoon Dijon mustard

½ cup extra-virgin olive oil

In a high-speed blender, add the cashews, water, lemon juice, vinegar, nutritional yeast, salt, and Dijon, and blend until smooth. With the blender on low speed, stream in the oil and blend until fully emulsified. Store in an airtight container in the refrigerator for up to 5 days.

FOR 1 TABLESPOON:
CALORIES: 87
PROTEIN: 2 GRAMS (0 BLOCKS)
CARBOHYDRATES: 2 GRAMS (0 BLOCKS)
FAT: 8.5 GRAMS (1 BLOCK)

JALAPEÑO CILANTRO
AIOLI

This creamy condiment uses the cashew aioli as a base and flavors it up with green heat and fresh cilantro.

MAKES ABOUT 3 CUPS

1 tablespoon extra-virgin olive oil

¼ cup diced yellow onion

3 large jalapeños, seeded and diced

1 garlic clove, minced

½ cup filtered water

½ teaspoon sea salt

2 cups Cashew Aioli (opposite)

¼ cup finely chopped fresh cilantro

Heat the olive oil in a small saucepan over medium heat. Add the onion, jalapeños, and garlic and cook until the onion is translucent, 5 minutes. Add the water and salt and bring to a simmer. Reduce the heat to low and cook until most of the water has evaporated, about 8 minutes. Remove the pan from the heat and allow the mixture to cool completely. Stir in the cashew aioli and cilantro. Store in an airtight container in the refrigerator for up to 5 days.

FOR 1 TABLESPOON:
CALORIES: 47
PROTEIN: 0.5 GRAM (0 BLOCKS)
CARBOHYDRATES: 0.5 GRAM (0 BLOCKS)
FAT: 4.5 GRAMS (0.5 BLOCK)

BALSAMIC VINAIGRETTE

A classic dressing that gets an assist from the tag team of Dijon and black pepper for an added kick. **MAKES ABOUT 1½ CUPS**

¾ cup high-quality balsamic vinegar

1 tablespoon Dijon mustard

2 teaspoons agave nectar

1 to 2 garlic cloves

½ teaspoon sea salt

½ teaspoon ground black pepper

¾ cup extra-virgin olive oil

In a high-speed blender, add the vinegar, mustard, agave, garlic, salt, and pepper and blend until completely smooth. With the blender on low speed, stream in the olive oil and blend until fully emulsified. Store in an airtight container in the refrigerator for up to 5 days.

FOR 1 TABLESPOON:
CALORIES: 65
PROTEIN: 0 GRAMS (0 BLOCKS)
CARBOHYDRATES: 0.5 GRAM (0 BLOCKS)
FAT: 7 GRAMS (0.5 BLOCK)

SWEET MISO
DIPPING SAUCE

Miso brings some sweet-salty umami that combines with agave to give you an addictive sauce to drizzle over all the things. **MAKES ABOUT 1 CUP**

½ cup agave nectar

¼ cup white miso

1 tablespoon tamari soy sauce

1 tablespoon fresh lemon juice

1 tablespoon minced fresh ginger

2 tablespoons sesame oil

In a high-speed blender, add the agave, miso, tamari, lemon juice, and ginger and blend until completely smooth. With the blender on low speed, slowly stream in the oil and blend until fully emulsified. Store in an airtight container in the refrigerator for up to 10 days.

FOR 1 TABLESPOON:
CALORIES: 40
PROTEIN: 0.5 GRAM (0 BLOCKS)
CARBOHYDRATES: 6.25 GRAMS (0.5 BLOCK)
FAT: 1.5 GRAMS (0 BLOCKS)

CHAPTER 21

DESSERTS

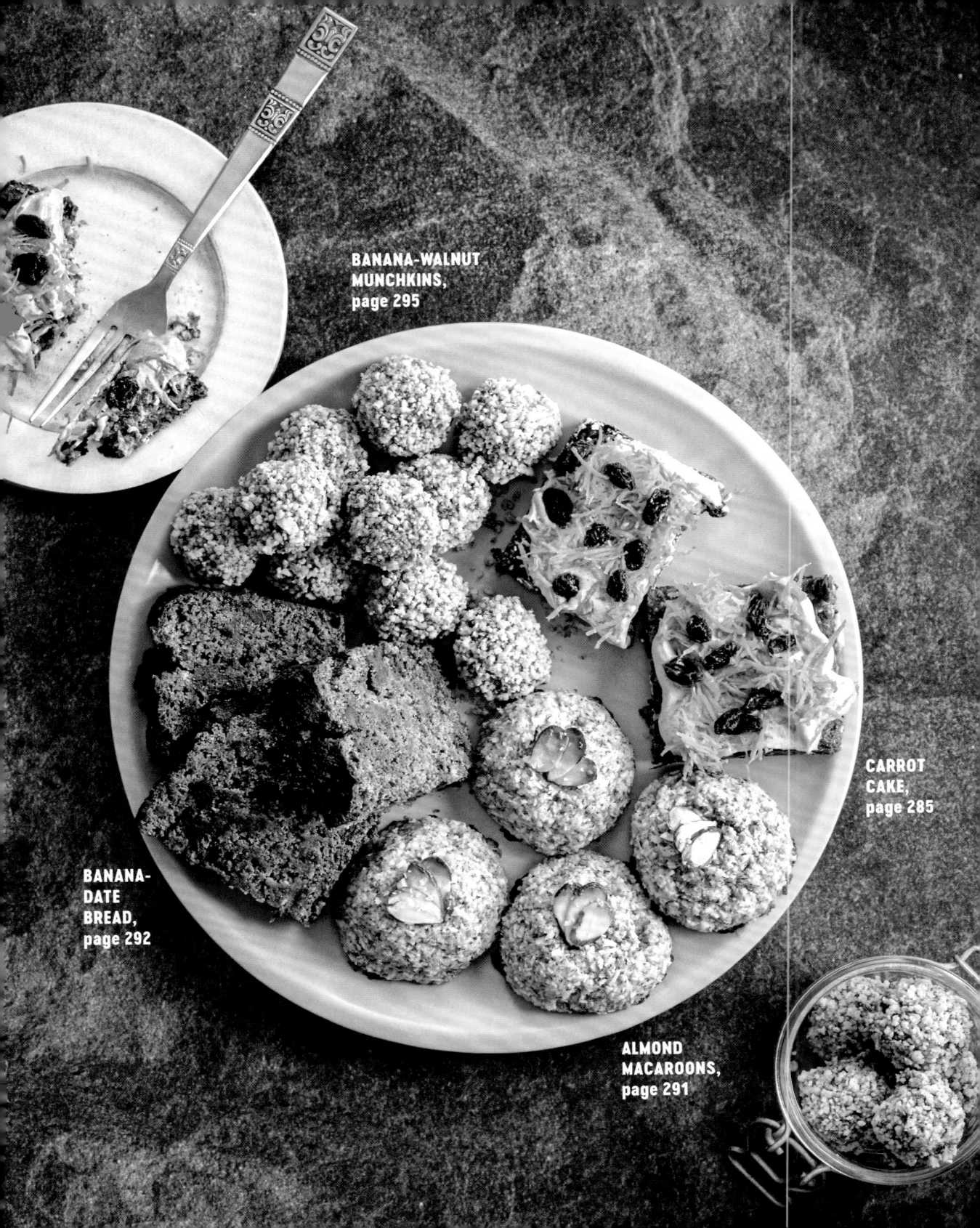

BANANA-WALNUT
MUNCHKINS,
page 295

CARROT
CAKE,
page 285

BANANA-
DATE
BREAD,
page 292

ALMOND
MACAROONS,
page 291

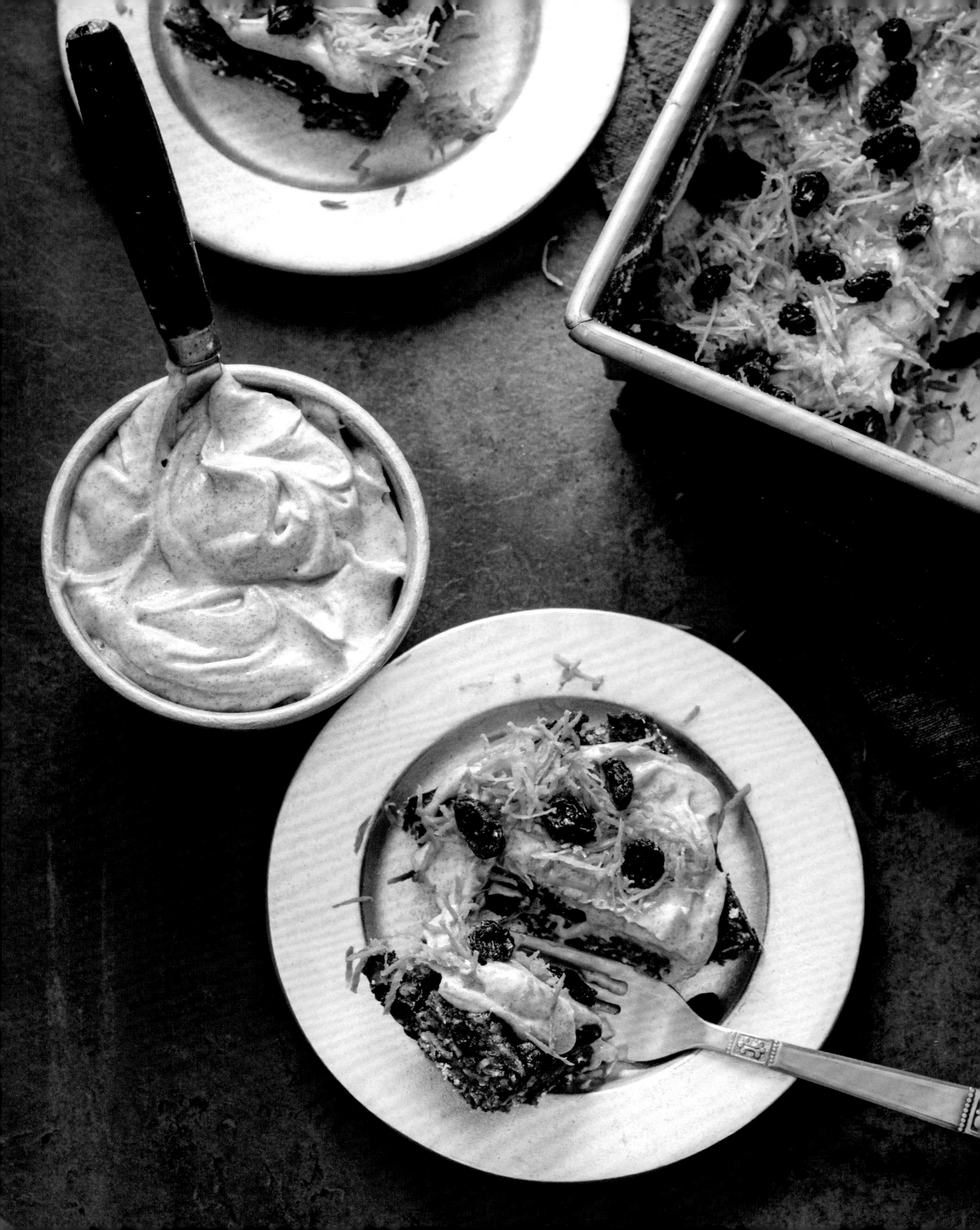

CARROT CAKE

With its dense, moist texture and sweet but not too sweet flavor, this cake-bar mash-up is enough to make even Bugs proud. **MAKES 1 (8-INCH) CAKE (16 SERVINGS)**

FOR THE CAKE

1 cup rolled oats

½ cup walnuts

½ cup raisins

1 teaspoon ground cinnamon

12 Medjool dates, pitted

2 bananas

½ cup Almond Milk (page 179) or store-bought

1 tablespoon flaxseeds

1½ teaspoons sunflower seeds

1 teaspoon vanilla paste or vanilla extract

FOR THE ICING

1 cup raw cashews, soaked for 6 hours, drained, and rinsed well

8 Medjool dates, pitted

½ cup Almond Milk (page 179) or store-bought

¼ cup fresh lemon juice

1 cup shredded carrots

½ cup raisins

1 MAKE THE CAKE: Preheat the oven to 350°F.

2 In a food processor, add about half the oats and process until they form a very fine flour. Measure out and reserve about 1 tablespoon of the oat flour for the baking pan. Transfer the remaining oat flour to a large bowl and add the remaining whole oats.

3 In the food processor, add the walnuts and pulse until the nuts are roughly chopped. Add the chopped walnuts, raisins, and cinnamon to the oat flour and stir to combine.

4 In the food processor, add the dates, bananas, milk, flaxseeds, sunflower seeds, and vanilla and blend until smooth. Transfer to the oat flour mixture and mix thoroughly to combine.

5 Sprinkle the reserved oat flour on the bottom of an 8 × 8-inch baking pan. Spread the cake batter in an even

RECIPE CONTINUES >>

layer in the pan. Bake until the cake is golden brown and the center is firm, about 30 minutes. Let cool for 20 to 30 minutes and transfer the cake to a serving plate.

6 **MAKE THE ICING:** In a high-speed blender, add the soaked cashews, dates, milk, lemon juice, and ½ cup of water and blend until smooth.

7 Spread the icing evenly over the cake. Decorate the top of the cake with the shredded carrots and raisins. Cover any leftovers and store at room temperature.

FOR 1 SERVING:
CALORIES: 220
PROTEIN: 4 GRAMS (0.5 BLOCK)
CARBOHYDRATES: 41 GRAMS (2 BLOCKS)
FAT: 7 GRAMS (0.5 BLOCK)

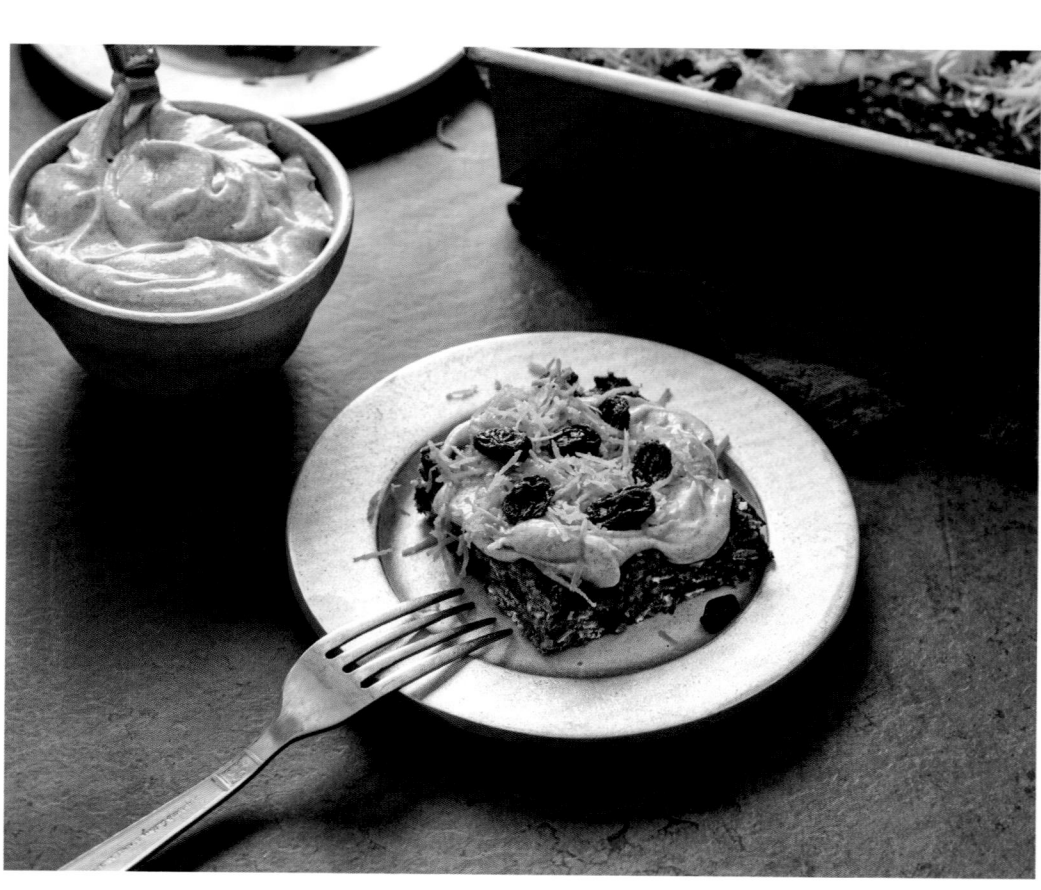

APPLE PIE

This ain't your mama's apple pie . . . but once you let her taste this recipe, she'll understand why you stopped eating hers. **SERVES 8**

FOR THE CRUST

Vegan butter (such as Earth Balance), for the pan

1½ cups gluten-free flour mix (such as Bob's Red Mill)

⅓ cup vegetable shortening

¼ cup cold water

2 tablespoons granulated sugar

2 teaspoons apple cider vinegar

½ teaspoon sea salt

¼ teaspoon baking powder

FOR THE FILLING

2 pounds apples (about 4), peeled, cored, and sliced ¼ inch thick

⅓ cup packed brown sugar

3 tablespoons granulated sugar

2 teaspoons vanilla extract

1 tablespoon molasses

2 teaspoons ground cinnamon

FOR THE CRUMBLE TOPPING

1 cup chopped pecans

⅔ cup gluten-free flour mix (such as Bob's Red Mill)

⅔ cup packed brown sugar

¼ cup vegan butter (such as Earth Balance)

Pinch of sea salt

1 **MAKE THE CRUST:** Preheat the oven to 350°F. Grease a 9-inch pie pan with vegan butter and set aside.

2 In a large bowl, combine the flour, shortening, water, sugar, vinegar, salt, and baking powder. Mix and knead by hand until the mixture is smooth. Use your hands to press the mixture into the prepared pie pan, forming a crust.

3 Bake until the crust is just starting to brown, 12 to 15 minutes. Set aside and leave the oven on.

4 **MAKE THE FILLING:** In a large bowl, toss together the sliced apples, brown sugar, granulated sugar, vanilla, molasses, and cinnamon. Transfer the apple mixture to the prebaked crust and set aside.

5 **MAKE THE CRUMBLE TOPPING:** In a medium bowl, add the pecans, flour, brown sugar, butter, and salt. Use a

RECIPE CONTINUES >>

fork or mix by hand until the mixture is well combined. Scatter the crumble mixture on top of the apple filling in an even layer.

6 Bake until the crumble topping is deeply browned, about 40 minutes. Let cool for 5 to 10 minutes before serving. Cover any leftovers and store at room temperature.

FOR 1 SERVING:
CALORIES: 520
PROTEIN: 5 GRAMS (0.5 BLOCK)
CARBOHYDRATES: 72 GRAMS (3.5 BLOCKS)
FAT: 26 GRAMS (2.5 BLOCKS)

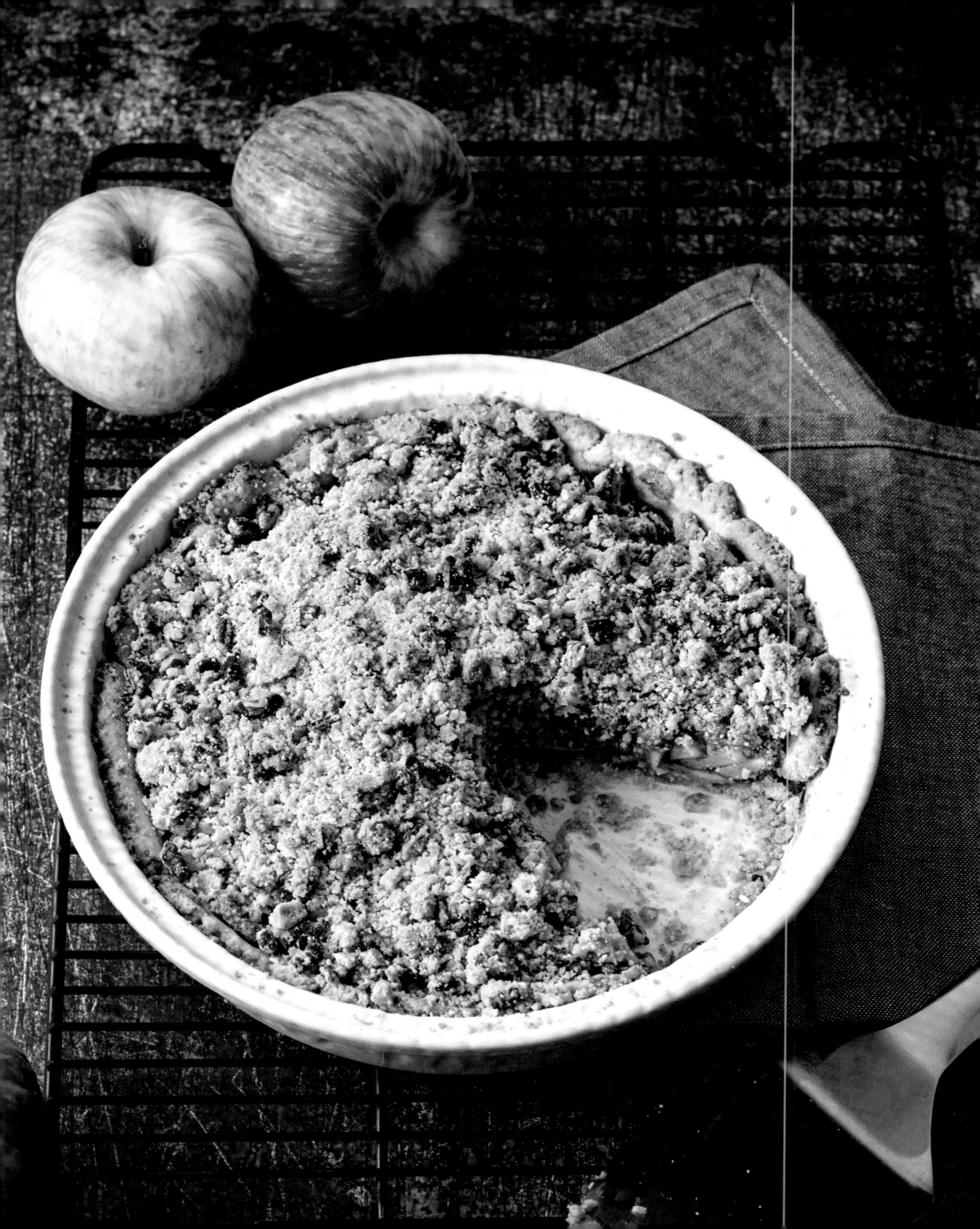

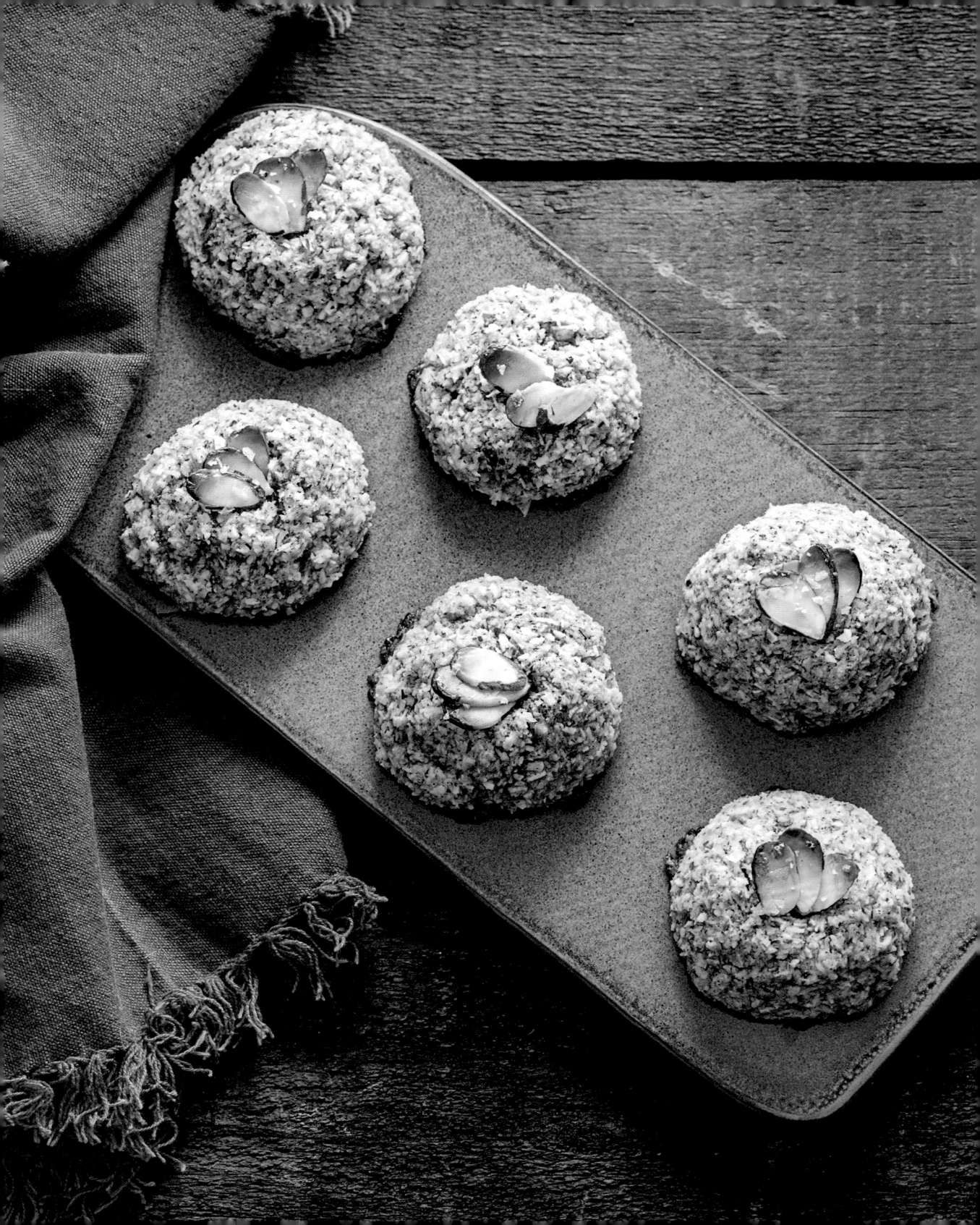

ALMOND MACAROONS

I dare you to make these sweet bites of joy and not pop the whole batch into your mouth before you can share 'em.

MAKES ABOUT 10

1½ cups unsweetened shredded coconut

½ cup plus 2 tablespoons almond flour

½ cup plus 2 tablespoons maple syrup

2 tablespoons plus 2 teaspoons vegan butter, softened

2 teaspoons vanilla paste

¼ teaspoon sea salt

¼ cup sliced almonds

1 teaspoon agave nectar

Pinch of flaky sea salt (such as Maldon)

1 Preheat the oven to 350°F. Line a baking sheet with parchment paper.

2 In a medium bowl, add the coconut, almond flour, maple syrup, butter, vanilla, and sea salt and mix well using your hands. Scoop the mixture into roughly ¼-cup portions and roll them into balls. Set the balls on the prepared baking sheet.

3 In a small bowl, toss together the sliced almonds, agave, and flaky salt. Arrange 3 almond slices on top of each portioned ball. Bake until golden brown, about 15 minutes. Store any leftover macaroons in an airtight container.

FOR 1 MACAROON:
CALORIES: 200
PROTEIN: 2 GRAMS (0 BLOCKS)
CARBOHYDRATES: 18 GRAMS (1 BLOCK)
FAT: 15 GRAMS (1.5 BLOCKS)

BANANA-DATE BREAD

I've always been a big fan of the banana-date duo, so now we're just leveling up to, you guessed it, banana-date bread. **MAKES 1 LOAF (10 SERVINGS)**

½ cup coconut oil, melted, plus more for greasing the pan

2 cups whole wheat flour

2 teaspoons baking soda

2 teaspoons potato starch

2 teaspoons ground cinnamon

2½ cups pitted Medjool dates

6 very ripe bananas

½ cup Almond Milk (page 179) or store-bought

½ cup vegan chocolate chips

1 Preheat the oven to 375°F. Grease a standard loaf pan with coconut oil and set aside.

2 In a large bowl, sift together the whole wheat flour, baking soda, potato starch, and cinnamon. Set aside.

3 In a food processor, add the dates and bananas and process until very smooth. Add the banana-date mixture to the dry ingredients and whisk to combine. Add the almond milk and coconut oil and whisk again until smooth. Fold in the chocolate chips.

4 Pour the mixture into the prepared loaf pan. Bake until a toothpick inserted in the center comes out clean and the top of the loaf is golden brown, about 1 hour. If the top of the loaf starts to get too dark before the center is done, cover the loaf with foil as it finishes baking. Once cool, cover any leftovers and store at room temperature.

FOR 1 SERVING:
CALORIES: 450
PROTEIN: 6 GRAMS (0.5 BLOCK)
CARBOHYDRATES: 84 GRAMS (4 BLOCKS)
FAT: 14 GRAMS (1.5 BLOCKS)

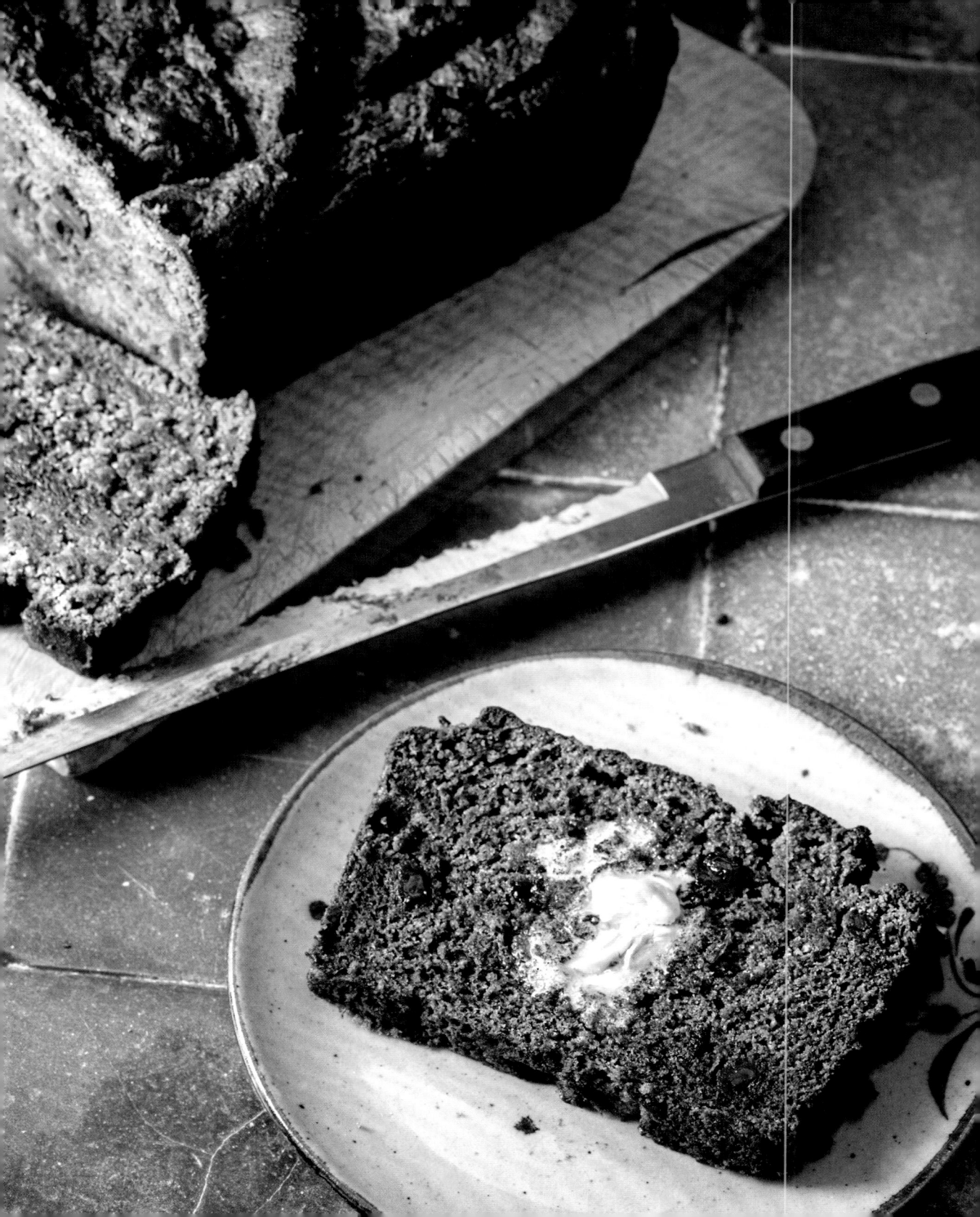

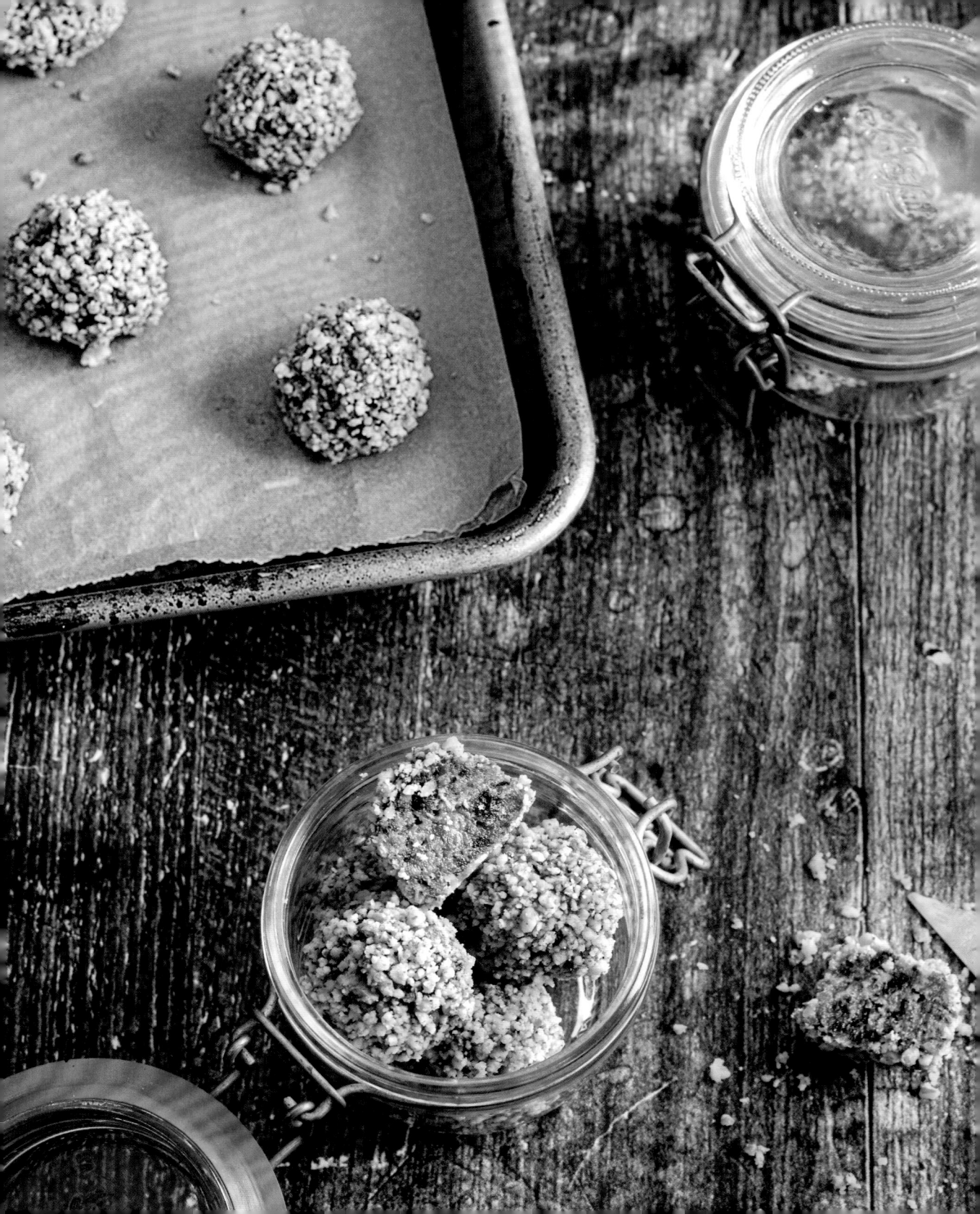

BANANA-WALNUT
MUNCHKINS

This recipe will have you breaking up with your regular doughnut holes and calling these munchkins your new boo.

MAKES ABOUT 25

3 cups walnuts

12 Medjool dates, pitted

1 large very ripe banana

¼ teaspoon ground cinnamon

Pinch of sea salt

1 Preheat the oven to 250°F. Line a baking sheet with parchment paper.

2 In a food processor, add 1 cup of the walnuts and process until fine crumbs form. Transfer the walnut crumbs to a wide, shallow bowl and set aside.

3 In the food processor, add the remaining 2 cups walnuts, the dates, banana, cinnamon, and salt and process until the mixture is uniform, about 2 minutes.

4 Using a tablespoon measure, portion and roll the mixture into small balls. Roll each ball in the walnut crumbs until thoroughly coated and set on the prepared baking sheet. Bake for 20 to 25 minutes, rotating the tray halfway through baking. Let the munchkins cool completely before serving. Store any leftover munchkins in an airtight container for up to 5 days.

FOR 3 MUNCHKINS:

CALORIES: 360
PROTEIN: 7 GRAMS (0.5 BLOCK)
CARBOHYDRATES: 36 GRAMS (2 BLOCKS)
FAT: 23 GRAMS (2.5 BLOCKS)

BANANAS ON A DATE

This is the deluxe version of what I shared on page 115. With spices like cinnamon and allspice, the dates know they're gonna seal the deal. **SERVES 4**

12 Medjool dates, pitted

½ teaspoon ground cinnamon

½ teaspoon ground allspice

4 bananas, sliced

½ cup unsweetened shredded coconut

¼ cup crushed pecans

1 In a high-speed blender, add the dates, cinnamon, allspice, and ½ cup of water and blend until completely smooth.

2 Divide the bananas among four bowls and top with the date mixture. Sprinkle the coconut and pecans on top and serve.

FOR 1 SERVING:
CALORIES: 425
PROTEIN: 4 GRAMS (0.5 BLOCK)
CARBOHYDRATES: 83 GRAMS (4 BLOCKS)
FAT: 12 GRAMS (1 BLOCK)

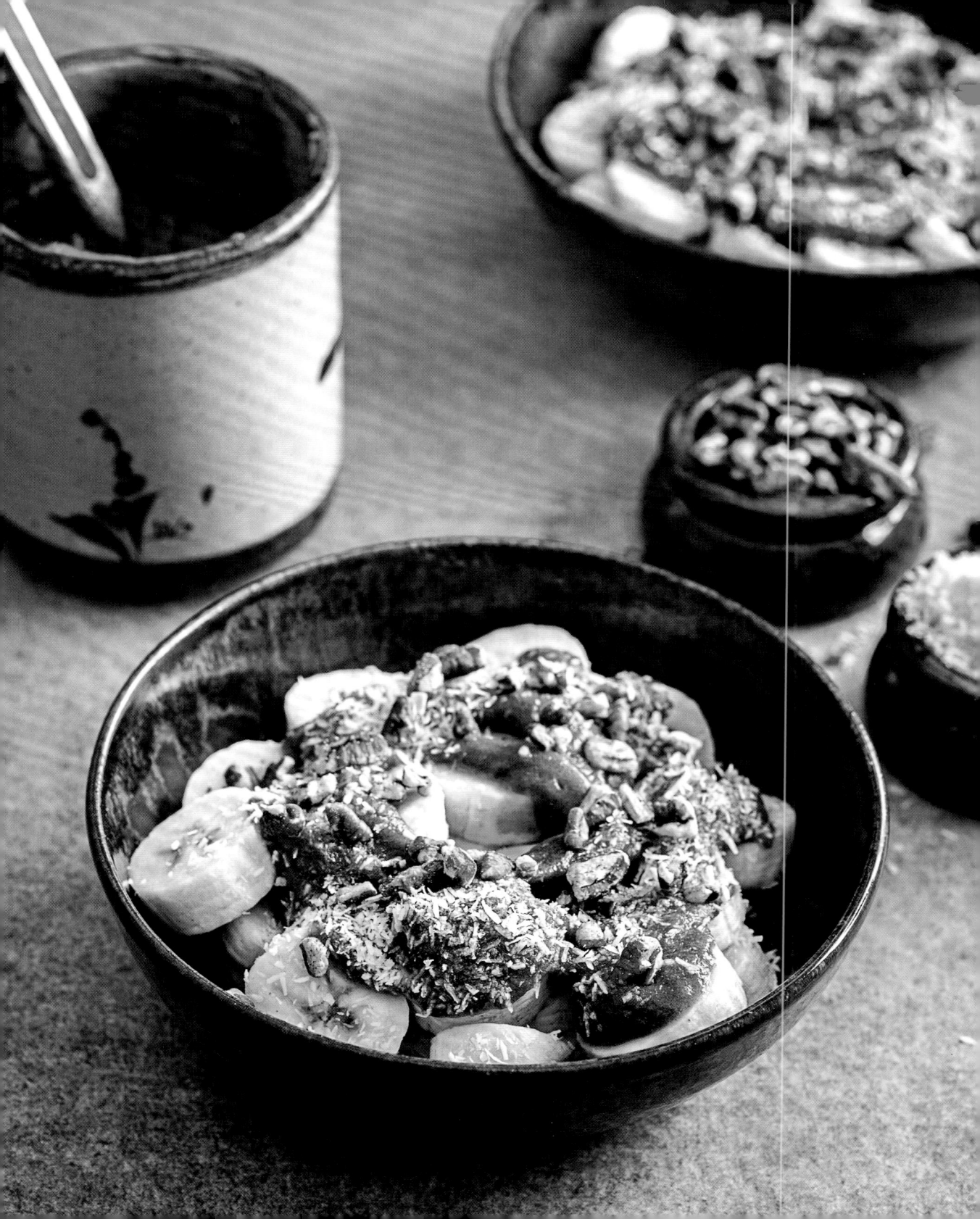

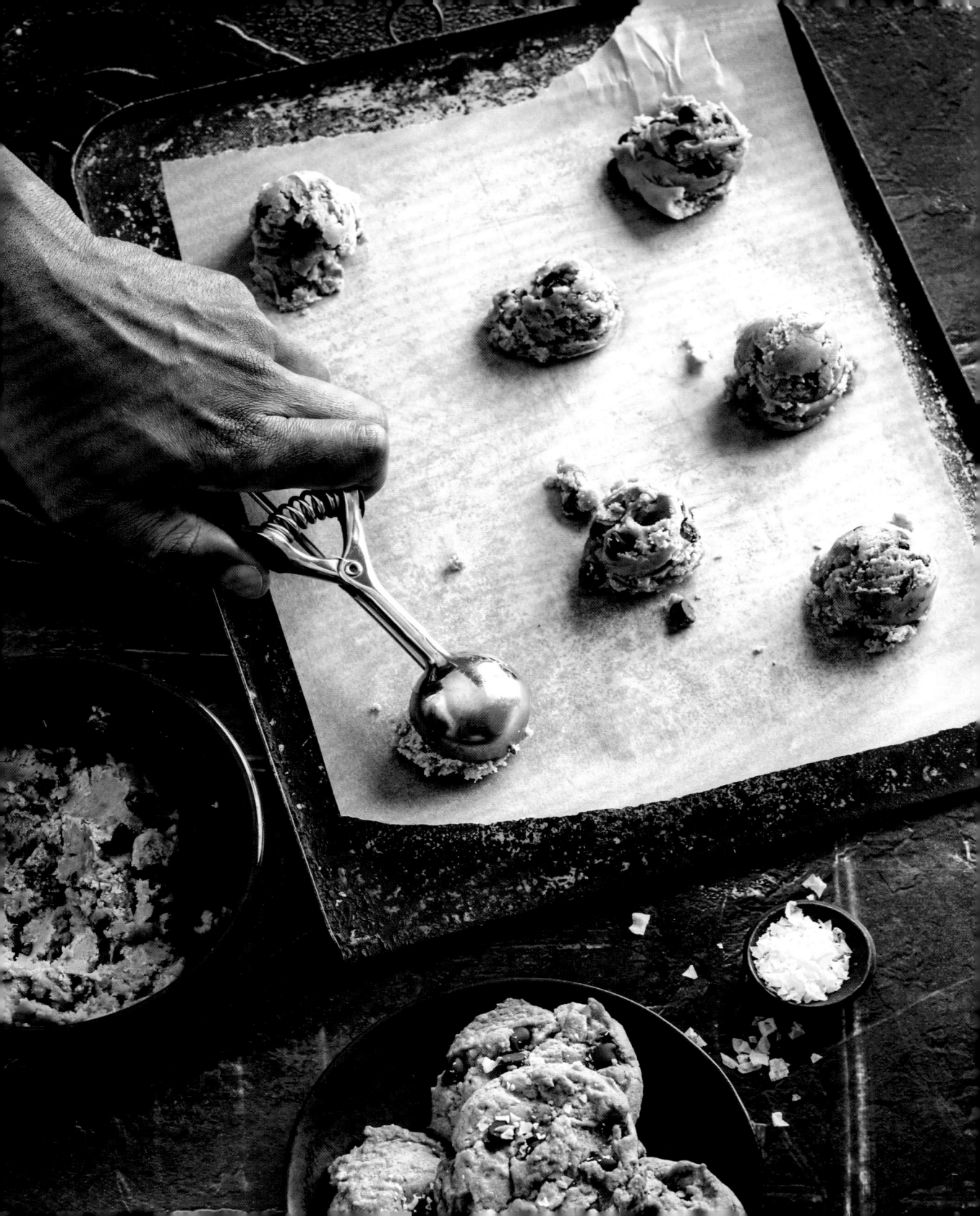

CHOCOLATE CHIP
COOKIES

If everyone ate my chocolate chip cookies, I think we could get a little closer to solving the world's problems.

MAKES 24 COOKIES

1¼ cups packed light brown sugar

½ cup coconut oil, slightly softened

2 teaspoons vanilla paste

¼ cup coconut milk

¼ cup unsweetened applesauce

2⅓ cups all-purpose flour

1 teaspoon baking soda

½ teaspoon sea salt

1 cup vegan chocolate chips

Flaky sea salt (such as Maldon)

1 Preheat the oven to 375°F. Line two large baking sheets with parchment paper.

2 In the bowl of a stand mixer fitted with the paddle attachment, add the brown sugar, coconut oil, and vanilla. Beat on medium speed until creamy, about 2 minutes. Add the coconut milk and applesauce and beat on low speed until combined, about 1 minute.

3 In a medium bowl, whisk together the flour, baking soda, and salt. Add the flour mixture to the brown sugar mixture and beat on low speed until combined, 1 to 2 minutes. The batter will be very thick. Fold in the chocolate chips.

4 Using a spoon, scoop mounds of dough about the size of golf balls (about 3 tablespoons) onto the

RECIPE CONTINUES >>

prepared baking sheets, leaving a few inches between cookies.

5 Bake until the edges are golden, 9 to 10 minutes. Sprinkle the cookies with flaky salt while they're still warm. Let the cookies cool on the baking sheets for 15 minutes. Store any leftover cookies in an airtight container for up to 7 days.

FOR 1 COOKIE:
CALORIES: 220
PROTEIN: 3 GRAMS (0 BLOCKS)
CARBOHYDRATES: 31 GRAMS (1.5 BLOCKS)
FAT: 11 GRAMS (1 BLOCK)

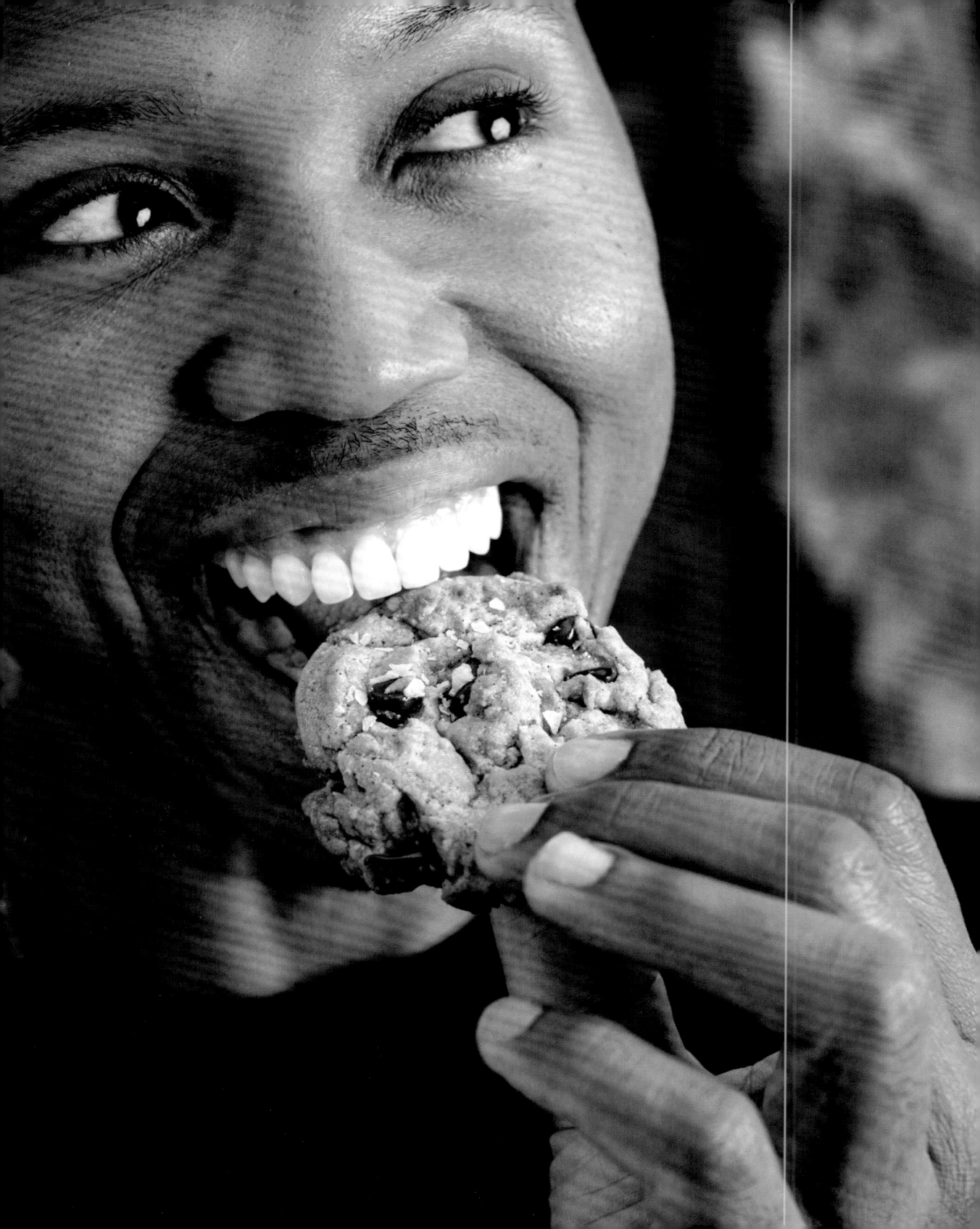

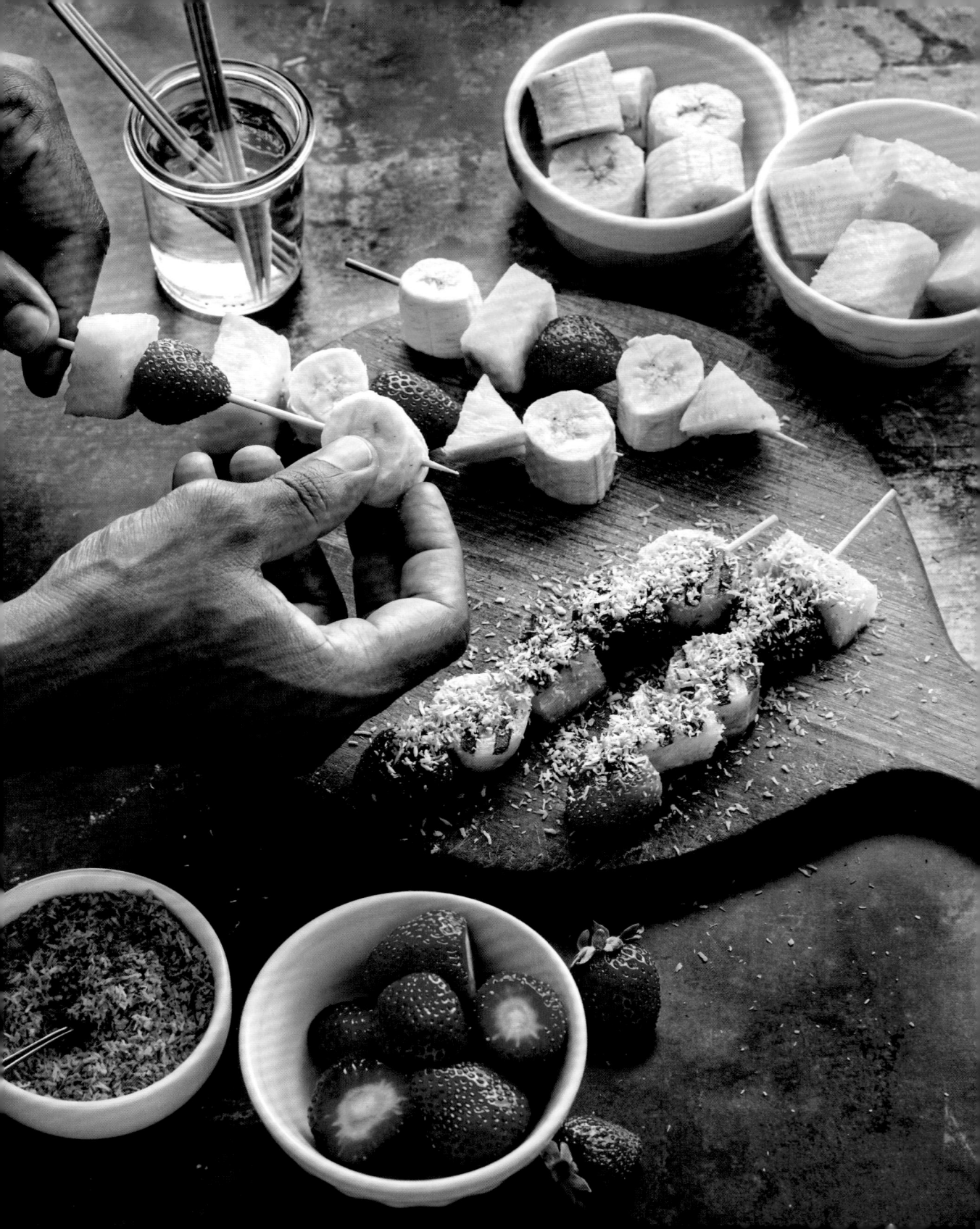

FRUIT KEBOB AND WEAVE

Yeah, you've had fresh banana, pineapple, and strawberries, but don't come at me until you've tried them grilled and topped with toasted coconut. **MAKES 6 (6-INCH) SKEWERS**

2 cups cubed fresh pineapple (about 1½-inch cubes)

2 bananas, sliced into 1½-inch rounds

12 strawberries, hulled

6 (6-inch) skewers, soaked in water if wooden

2 tablespoons melted coconut oil

½ cup toasted unsweetened shredded coconut

1 Heat a grill to medium.

2 Thread the pineapple, bananas, and whole strawberries onto the skewers and brush with the melted coconut oil. Grill the fruit skewers for about 2 minutes per side, uncovered.

3 Transfer the fruit skewers to a plate, sprinkle with the coconut, and serve.

FOR 1 KEBAB:
CALORIES: 140
PROTEIN: 1 GRAM (0 BLOCKS)
CARBOHYDRATES: 17 GRAMS (1 BLOCK)
FAT: 9 GRAMS (1 BLOCK)

SUMMER BERRY PIE

You know I love me a smoothie, so I figured why not bake one into a pie so tasty that everyone's gonna be asking for the recipe. Seriously, you'll win any cookout with this one.

MAKES 1 (8-INCH) PIE (16 SERVINGS)

FOR THE CRUST

8 ounces pitted Medjool dates (12 to 14 dates)

1 cup pecans

1 cup almonds

¼ teaspoon sea salt

FOR THE FILLING

1⅓ cups blueberries, plus more for serving

4 ounces pitted Medjool dates (6 dates)

2 bananas

2 tablespoons tapioca starch

⅔ cup sliced strawberries, plus more for serving

¼ cup halved raspberries, plus more for serving

1 tablespoon agave nectar

1 MAKE THE CRUST: In a food processor, add the dates, pecans, almonds, and salt and process until the mixture is nearly uniform and sticky. Press the date-nut mixture firmly into an 8-inch pie pan and set aside.

2 MAKE THE FILLING: Preheat the oven to 350°F.

3 In a food processor, add ⅔ cup of the blueberries, the dates, bananas, and tapioca starch and process until smooth.

4 Transfer the mixture to a large bowl and fold in the remaining ⅔ cup blueberries, the strawberries, and the raspberries. Pour into the crust.

5 Bake until the filling is bubbling and the crust is browned, 30 minutes. Let cool to room temperature before serving, or refrigerate and serve chilled. Garnish the top of the pie with the extra berries and drizzle with the agave. Cover any leftovers.

FOR 1 SERVING:
CALORIES: 170
PROTEIN: 3 GRAMS (0 BLOCKS)
CARBOHYDRATES: 23 GRAMS (1 BLOCK)
FAT: 9 GRAMS (1 BLOCK)

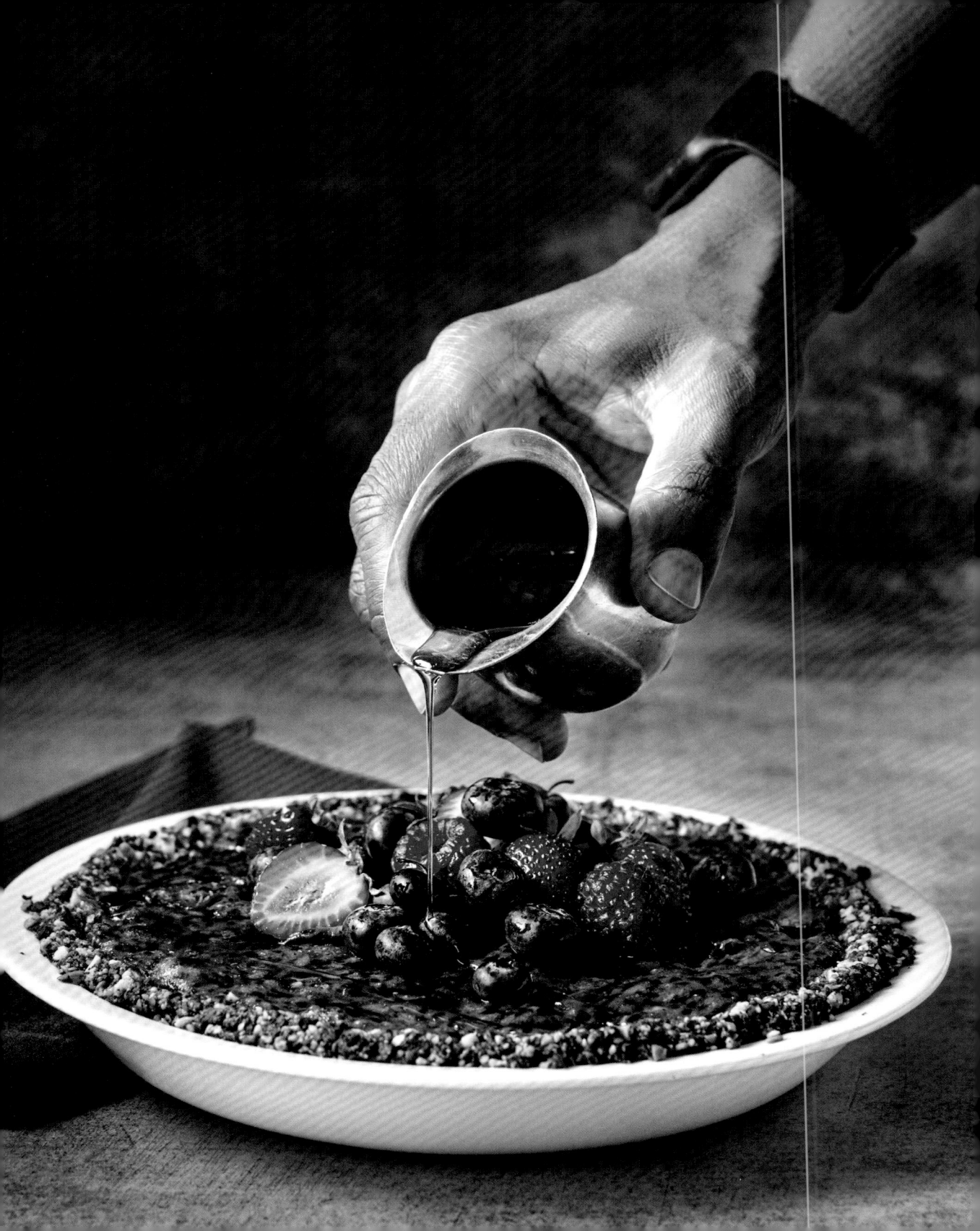

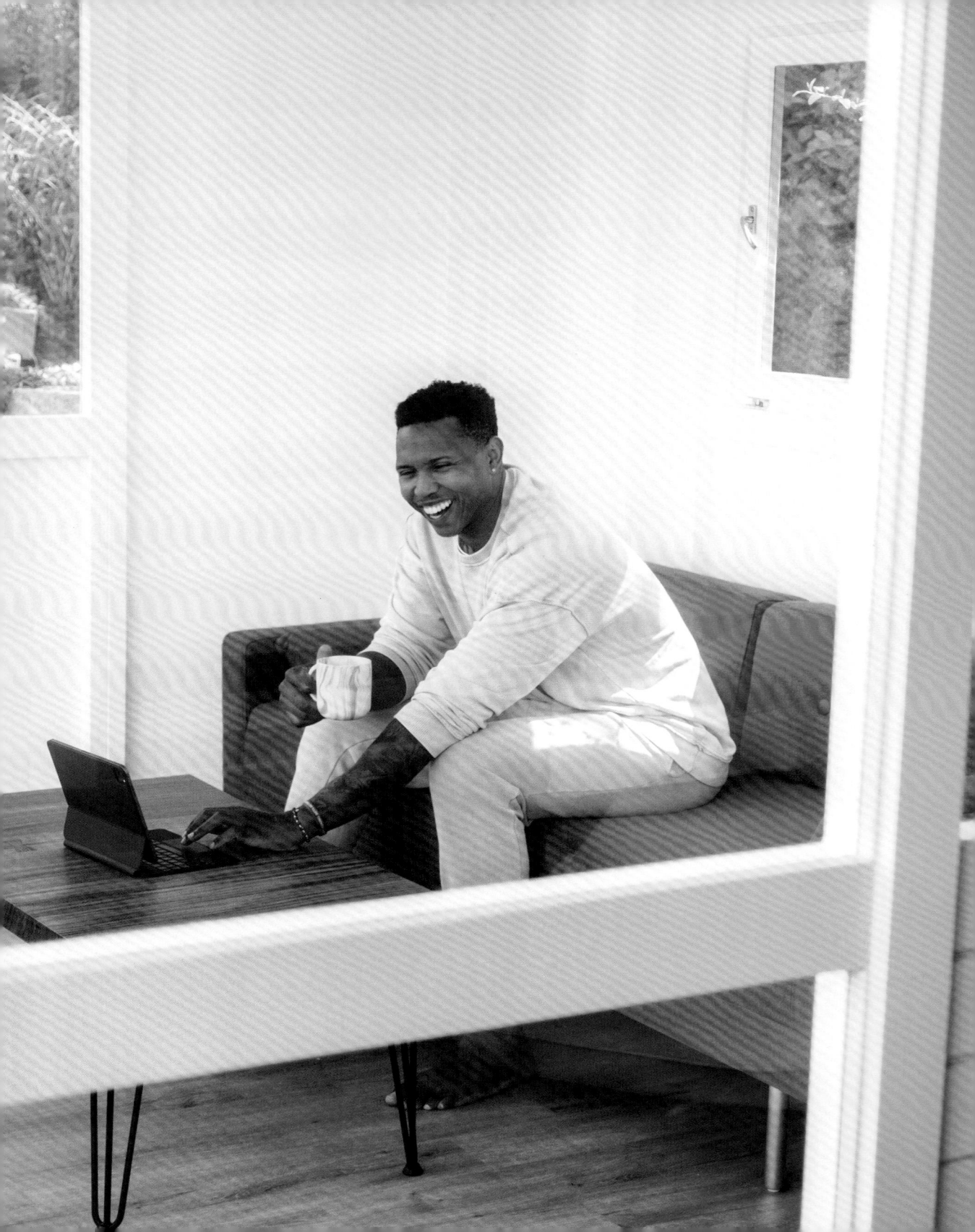

ACKNOWLEDGMENTS

My life has been a series of different chapters, and just like any book or novel, I have so many characters in my story. While this list may seem extensive at first glance, there are still so many characters I may have missed, not because I don't love them, but because they either showed up a little too early in the book or popped up in a later chapter. And so are the characters in my life. If you read this and know me personally, don't think that I didn't put you on the list out of malice or bad intentions . . . blame it on my head and not my heart.

FAMILY

Camellia Lewis, my mother, who adopted her grandson (who was born a crack baby) when she was already in her forties and could have just moved on with her life. I owe you everything.

Joey Lewis, my brother, who took me in like a father and made sure I always stayed on the right path (most of the time, lol).

David Lewis, my brother, who honestly is my closest friend on this earth, who took me under his wing even when he could have rejected the idea of me coming into the family.

Elizabeth Lewis, my niece. I love how we have just grown to where we are now, from you rolling your eyes at me as a baby to me being your favorite uncle, lol.

Ana Reyes Lewis, my wife, the love of my life, who has helped me become the best version of myself and also allows me to live out this crazy dream of healing the world. You don't even know how amazing you are.

Pax Reyes Lewis, my Peace, my first-born, the child I never knew I needed but couldn't see life without.

Marz Reyes Lewis, my fighter. I see signs of me every time you breathe. You, your sister, and your mother are my "Peace on Marz."

Sophia Hood, I didn't get to spend much time with you, but you were where my legacy began as far as I can remember.

I promise to keep our lineage going and to keep learning more about how we got here from the kings and queens that we are.

Brian Pickett Lewis, my brother. Wow, man, I'm choking up just typing this. I have had so much death around me, but none hit me like yours, man. There are so many times I want to text or call you when something amazing happens and then it hits me. I will never forget what you told me about how I am doing important work, and I can't stop because while it may have been too late for you, I am helping so many. I promise to never stop and to "Get it DONE."

Howard Love, my uncle, who never looked at me as an annoyance or as in the way. Who took me to the Vashon Center and Wohls as a little kid to hoop with my cousin even though we were little kids playing against grown men. That little lesson taught me to not fear anyone. I miss you, Unc. RIP.

Charles Humphrey, my uncle. Wow, you taught me so much about how to be there for my family. I still laugh about the time we all went to Tampa and we laughed so hard at Mom . . . :)

Francisco Reyes, Pop, we may not be blood, but you have taken me in and loved me as if I were yours. I have learned so much from you, and I love our talks and discussions.

Adela Reyes, Moms, you are the absolute best, and I am so thankful for you and your love and kindness.

Marva McKnight, my Granny I met later in life, but I feel as if you have been with me since day one.

Rebecca Williams, my auntie. How can it be that I didn't meet you till I was twenty-one, but we instantly became so close? I love you, Auntie, and I am so thankful that you are always there, no matter if it's a phone call or a road trip.

Monique King, my sister. We don't talk every day, but I still feel like no matter how much time passes without us having a conversation, we pick up like we never left.

FRIENDS

Anthony Love, my family, my friend. We literally went to nursery school, elementary school, middle school, and high school together. Out of forty-three years, I can say I only remember having one argument and we were like thirteen, lol. Love you, man.

Craig Coleman, my day one. I can't even talk about half the things we have done but you already know "what it is."

K. S. Kallous—Carlos Boldon, Terrance Gant, Ed Covington, Steven Harris, Robert Arbuthnot, Shaun Scott. My line brothers, not many will understand all we went through together, but it's not for them to understand. Love y'all, and I am honored to be your Ankor. YOYO.

Kappa Alpha Psi Fraternity Inc., I am so thankful for the bond and brotherhood. Major shoutout to all the Nupes out there.

Philip Lay, my fraternity brother who encouraged me to move to Florida to go to grad school. I will never forget you telling me that you may not have had any money to help me, but that anything that you could do to help me with the move, you had my back.

Star Amun, I had always claimed that I wanted to be vegan but was always a hypocrite, and you would call me out on it to the point where I always had your voice in my ear telling me how great the transition would be.

Rafael Ogando, you don't even know it, but you opened my eyes to a whole new world. I always tell the story of us being roommates in Fort Lauderdale and going grocery shopping only for you to school me on the difference between a plantain and a banana . . .

Gary Jouett, my boy who taught me what Seventh-day Adventist even was and also told me more about the vegetarian lifestyle (before I went vegan) and always had my back.

Ben Tario—RAT!!! Man, you don't even know how you changed my life, bro. While in grad school at Nova Southeastern, I was dead broke, and having you as my boss for work-study in the athletic department was perfect, and we formed a bond forever. I'll never forget the time we were driving to the football tournament we were playing in, and we stopped in the most racist truck stop I think either one of us could have imagined and even you as a blond-haired, blue-eyed brother were nervous as hell too. On the way back, we made sure not to stop there even though we needed gas, lol.

Brion Ross—TOO $HORT, my brother for real. There weren't many Black students in the grad programs while we were there, and not only did we have football, but we had a Midwest connection. You know you got a brother for life.

William Barnes—Big Nupe. Man, you have always had my back no matter what the situation, and you were the one that took me to my first casting call even though I was nervous as hell . . . you helped to build that confidence I needed.

Jimmy Thoppil, my Indian brother who not only opened my life to the Indian community but opened your home to me when I was basically living in my car and took me in. I love you, bro.

Jose Gonzalez—Silar, man, it's been a long time, but you and I had a bond early in all those basketball tourneys and I am thankful for you opening your doors to me too, bro.

Jim Morris, my mentor who opened my eyes not only to the world of fasting but also to mental strength. People often ask me how I got you to become my mentor and I always say, I just simply asked. To me you will always be the original Badass Vegan.

Torre Washington, my brother at arms, the bond has been strong since day one, fam. You don't know how grateful I am for your brotherhood. I still remember our conversation about ten years ago when we were laughing at the fact that I only had twelve dollars in my bank account, but we knew that it would get better if we stayed focused and kept grinding . . . IRON SHARPENS IRON.

Dominick Thompson, my brother from another. So funny how alike we are, from being from the Midwest, to our upbringings, to our paths, to veganism. We may bump heads from time to time, but it's always all love and we know that the next day we will be laughing and talking about what vegan spot we are hitting up.

Robert Cheeke, my twin. Many don't know it, but we have the same birthday. I appreciate everything you have done for the vegan movement and how you and I bonded from day one. Over a decade later, and you are still helping me out (this book being the latest helping hand).

John Salley, my mentor, my brother who is always there when I need him no matter if he is in L.A. or London.

Rich Roll, my bro, I tell you from time to time . . . but I truly mean it when I say that you are just an inspiration to me, bro. I'll just keep following in your footsteps.

Greg Alzone, I almost don't have any words for how dope of a human you are, brother. You do so much to help people that many never even see or know about, and you don't even look for any publicity or mention. You are just a dope human. Thank you so much for your friendship.

Chris Paul, I appreciate you believing in my dream to help heal our people. Everything you do for the community is so genuine and from a place of love that anyone who is graced to have witnessed your work also feels empowered to do the same.

Rachel Holtzman, you are a damn magician. I know for a fact that I wouldn't have made this book turn out the way it did without your patience and skill. I am so glad to have had you be a part of my first book.

Jackie Sobon, thanks so much for taking the time to make these dishes pop the way they did. You are amazing behind the camera, but the way you turn a dish into art is crazy.

Cassie Fuertez, Adam Codeus, and Davy Greenberg, you three are just so damn dope behind the lens. Thank you so much for having the patience to help me create this timepiece.

Tara Punzone, you aren't just a chef, you are so much more than that; you are a goddess in the kitchen with the dishes you create. Without you teaching me and sharing your knowledge, this book wouldn't have the amazing dishes that it has.

Keegan Kuhn, man, we have been through more in the last six years than anyone will ever know. Beyond making *They're Trying to Kill Us* together, we have created something even greater . . . a brotherhood. Love you, bro.

Cedric the Entertainer, my frat brother,

who always represented our frat and our city and put us on the map. I appreciate you and everything you have done for me, YOYO.

Lucia Watson and the whole Avery team, thank you so much for believing in my vision and bringing it to life. You made this experience so seamless. I can't wait to do it again—what do you say?

Kareem Cook, Nupe, thank you so much for not just being my business partner, my frat brother, and my friend, but thank you for believing in the mission of healing the community. Keep changing the world—you know I will be right there by your side.

Style P, my bro, I'm so thankful for all you have done not only for me but for the community. Love is Love.

Janis Donnaud, my agent . . . I can't thank you enough for all your help during this process. You are definitely the master at this, and now I understand why you sit on the Game of Thrones.

Alicia Acklin, my childhood friend, who always had my back and would always buy my lunch for me all through high school because you knew how bad all the other kids talked about the obese kid with the glasses bringing out his brown bag lunch.

Damon Dash, bro, you are one of the realest out there. Always looking to uplift and always there when I need you. Many aren't ready for the truth you give out but it's the truth we need.

Terry Talley, Uncle Terry, I miss you. You did so much for me, but nothing stands out like the time you took me to see *The Last Dragon* and changed my life. I learned that day that I could be my own superhero and help the world.

Murphy Lee and Kyjuan, YO brothers, y'all definitely showed me what it was to love the Lou but still think globally.

To my Hood Family, I know we don't talk every day but you know how much I love you all.

ACKNOWLEDGMENTS

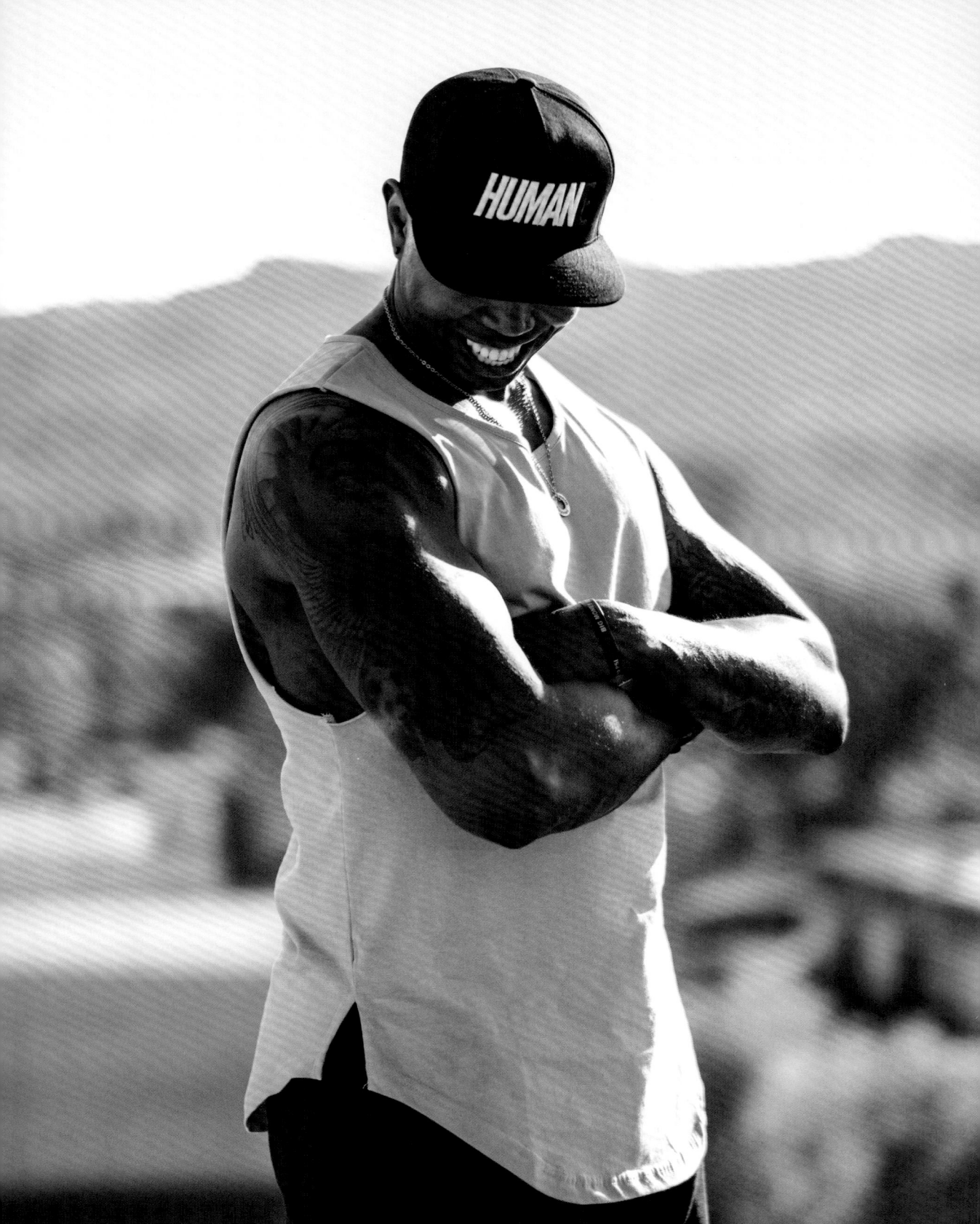

INDEX

Note: Page numbers in *italics* indicate photos, and page numbers in parentheses indicate intermittent references.

BADASS VEGAN

INDEX

BADASS VEGAN

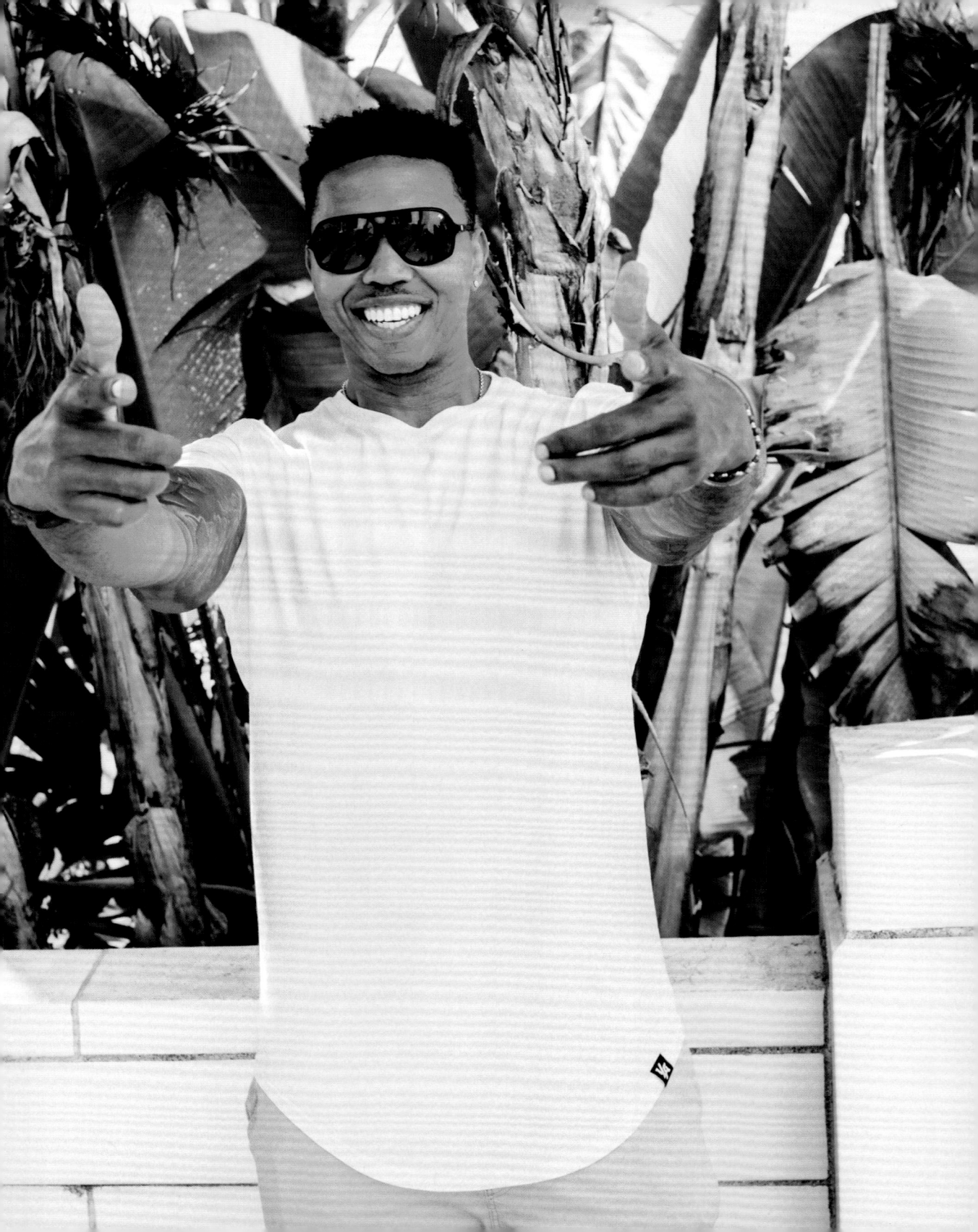